T0264081

Cardiovascular Magnetic Resonance in Heart Failure

Guest Editors

RAYMOND J. KIM, MD
DUDLEY J. PENNELL, MD, FRCP, FACC

HEART FAILURE CLINICS

www.heartfailure.theclinics.com

Consulting Editors
RAGAVENDRA R. BALIGA, MD, MBA
JAMES B. YOUNG, MD

Founding Editor
JAGAT NARULA, MD, PhD

July 2009 • Volume 5 • Number 3

SAUNDERS an imprint of ELSEVIER, Inc.

W.B. SAUNDERS COMPANY
A Division of Elsevier Inc.

1600 John F. Kennedy Boulevard • Suite 1800 • Philadelphia, Pennsylvania 19103-2899

http://www.theclinics.com

HEART FAILURE CLINICS Volume 5, Number 3
July 2009 ISSN 1551-7136, ISBN-13: 978-1-4377-1225-4, ISBN-10: 1-4377-1225-8

Editor: Barbara Cohen-Kligerman

Heart Failure Clinics (ISSN 1551-7136) is published quarterly by Elsevier Inc., 360 Park Avenue South, New York, NY 10010-1710. Months of publication are January, April, July, and October. Business and editorial offices: 1600 John F. Kennedy Boulevard, Suite 1800, Phliadelphia, PA 19103-2899. Customer service office: 11830 Westline Industrial Drive, St. Louis, MO 63146. Periodicals postage paid at New York, NY, and additional mailing offices. Subscription prices are USD 193.00 per year for US individuals, USD 320.00 per year for US institutions, USD 67.00 per year for US students and residents, USD 232.00 per year for Canadian individuals, USD 367.00 per year for Canadian institutions, USD 247.00 per year for international individuals, USD 367.00 per year for international institutions, and USD 85.00 per year for Canadian and foreign students/residents. To receive student and resident rate, orders must be accompanied by name of affiliated institution, date of term, and the *signature* of program/residency coordinator on institution letterhead. Orders will be billed at individual rate until proof of status is received. Foreign air speed delivery is included in all *Clinics* subscription prices. All prices are subject to change without notice. **POSTMASTER:** Send address changes to *Heart Failure Clinics*, Elsevier Journals Customer Service, 11830 Westline Industrial Drive, St. Louis, MO 63146. **Customer Service: 1-800-654-2452 (US and Canada). From outside of the US and Canada, call 314-453-7041. Fax: 314-453-5170. For print support, e-mail: JournalsCustomerService-usa@elsevier.com. For online support, e-mail: JournalsOnlineSupport-usa@elsevier.com.**

Reprints. For copies of 100 or more of articles in this publication, please contact the Commercial Reprints Department, Elsevier Inc., 360 Park Avenue South, New York, NY 10010-1710. Tel.: 212-633-3812; Fax: 212-462-1935; E-mail: reprints@elsevier.com.

Heart Failure Clinics is covered in *MEDLINE/PubMed (Index Medicus)*.

Printed and bound by CPI Group (UK) Ltd, Croydon, CR0 4YY

Transferred to Digital Print 2011

Cover artwork courtesy of Umberto M. Jezek.

Contributors

CONSULTING EDITORS

RAGAVENDRA R. BALIGA, MD, MBA
Assistant Chief, Division of Cardiovascular
Medicine, and Professor of Internal Medicine,
The Ohio State University, Columbus, Ohio

JAMES B. YOUNG, MD
Chairman and Professor, Department
of Medicine, Lerner College of Medicine; and
George and Linda Kaufman Chair, Cleveland
Clinic Foundation, Case Western Reserve
University, Cleveland, Ohio

GUEST EDITORS

RAYMOND J. KIM, MD
Director, Duke Cardiovascular Magnetic
Resonance Center, Duke University Medical
Center, Durham, North Carolina

DUDLEY J. PENNELL, MD, FRCP, FACC
Director, CMR Unit, Royal Brompton Hospital;
and Professor, Department of Cardiology,
Imperial College London, London, United
Kingdom

AUTHORS

ROBERT W.W. BIEDERMAN, MD, FACC
Director of Cardiovascular MRI, Associate
Professor of Medicine, Drexel University
College of Medicine; and Division of
Cardiology, Allegheny General Hospital,
Pittsburgh, Pennsylvania

RUEDIGER BRAUN-DULLAEUS, MD
Professor of Medicine, Director of the
Department of Cardiology, Otto-von-Guericke-
University, Magdeburg, Germany

OTAVIO R. COELHO-FILHO, MD
Cardiovascular Division, Department of
Medicine, Brigham and Women's Hospital,
Boston, Massachusetts

SCOTT D. FLAMM, MD
Cardiovascular Medicine, Heart and Vascular
Institute; and Head, Cardiovascular Imaging
Laboratory, Imaging Institute, Cleveland Clinic,
Cleveland, Ohio

JOHN D. GRIZZARD, MD
Assistant Professor, Department of Radiology,
Virginia Commonwealth University Medical
Center, Richmond, Virginia

FRANK GROTHUES, MD
Associate Professor of Medicine, Department
of Cardiology, Otto-von-Guericke-University,
Magdeburg, Germany

ANNE S. KANDERIAN, MD
Cardiovascular Medicine, Heart and Vascular
Institute; and Cardiovascular Imaging
Laboratory, Imaging Institute, Cleveland Clinic,
Cleveland, Ohio

HAN W. KIM, MD
Assistant Professor, Department of Medicine,
Duke Cardiovascular Magnetic Resonance
Center, Duke University Medical Center,
Durham, North Carolina

RAYMOND J. KIM, MD
Director, Duke Cardiovascular Magnetic
Resonance Center, Duke University Medical
Center, Durham, North Carolina

RAYMOND Y. KWONG, MD, MPH, FACC
Cardiovascular Division, Department of
Medicine, Brigham and Women's Hospital,
Boston, Massachusetts

MAULIK D. MAJMUDAR, MD
Fellow, Department of Medicine, Duke
Cardiovascular Magnetic Resonance Center,
Duke University Medical Center, Durham,
North Carolina

SAUL G. MYERSON, MD, MRCP
Clinical Fellow and Consultant Cardiologist,
Department of Cardiovascular Medicine,
University of Oxford, John Radcliffe Hospital,
Headley Way, Oxford, United Kingdom

LEELAKRISHNA NALLAMSHETTY, MD
Department of Radiology, Brigham and
Women's Hospital, Boston,
Massachusetts

RORY O'HANLON, MRCPI
CMR Fellow, CMR Unit, Royal Brompton
Hospital, London, United Kingdom

DUDLEY J. PENNELL, MD, FRCP, FACC
Director, CMR Unit, Royal Brompton
Hospital; and Professor, Department of
Cardiology, Imperial College London, London,
United Kingdom

SUBHA V. RAMAN, MD, MSEE
Associate Professor of Internal Medicine,
Division of Cardiovascular Medicine, The Ohio
State University, Columbus, Ohio

VIKAS K. RATHI, MD, FACC
Associate Director of Cardiovascular MRI;
Assistant Professor of Medicine, Drexel
University College of Medicine; and Division
of Cardiology, Allegheny General Hospital,
Pittsburgh, Pennsylvania

RAHUL RENAPURKAR, MD
Cardiovascular Imaging Laboratory, Imaging
Institute, Cleveland Clinic, Cleveland, Ohio

ANNAMALAI SENTHILKUMAR, MD
Fellow, Department of Medicine, Duke
Cardiovascular Magnetic Resonance Center,
Duke University Medical Center, Durham,
North Carolina

DIPAN J. SHAH, MD, FACC
Assistant Professor of Medicine, Weill Cornell
Medical College; Director, Cardiac Magnetic
Resonance Imaging, The Methodist DeBakey
Heart & Vascular Center, Houston, Texas

CHETAN SHENOY, MBBS
Fellow, Department of Medicine, Duke
Cardiovascular Magnetic Resonance Center,
Duke University Medical Center, Durham,
North Carolina

ORLANDO P. SIMONETTI, PhD
Associate Professor of Internal Medicine
and Radiology, Division of Cardiovascular
Medicine, The Ohio State University,
Columbus, Ohio

Contents

> This article presents a rationale for incorporating cardiovascular MR in the evaluation of patients who have heart failure and is organized in four parts. Part I defines the context of cardiovascular MR within standard clinical evaluation and among the many other modalities available for cardiovascular assessment in patients who have heart failure. Part II describes the techniques most useful in treating heart failure. Part III provides recommended approaches for the standard heart failure cardiovascular MR examination. Part IV concludes with perspectives on the appropriate use and incorporation of cardiovascular MR in the evaluation and management of patients who have heart failure.

> Cardiovascular magnetic resonance (CMR) is an accurate, reproducible and well-validated imaging technique for the measurement of left ventricular and right ventricular volumes, function, and mass. In patients who have heart failure, CMR is ideally suited both for the initial assessment of fundamental parameters of cardiac function and longitudinal follow-up. Because of its accuracy, the decision to implement therapeutic measures based on cutoff values for ventricular ejection fraction can be made with confidence. Because the above-mentioned parameters correlate with morbidity and mortality, CMR can be used to estimate the prognosis of an individual patient and to obtain surrogate parameters in clinical trials. The process of ventricular remodeling after cardiac injury and reverse remodeling using medical and interventional therapy can be assessed using relatively small sample sizes, which puts CMR in the forefront of imaging techniques in remodeling research.

> Approximately two thirds of patients with heart failure have underlying coronary artery disease. In the setting of ischemic heart disease, cardiovascular magnetic resonance has demonstrated usefulness in two ways: for the detection of coronary artery disease and for the assessment of myocardial viability in consideration for revascularization. This article discusses the use of cardiovascular magnetic resonance for the detection of coronary artery disease. The purpose of this article is to provide readers with a brief overview of each of the cardiovascular magnetic resonance techniques, their relative strengths, and their relative weaknesses. Because adenosine stress cardiovascular magnetic resonance is currently the most widely used clinically, it is the primary focus of this article.

Contents

Cardiovascular MRI can assess multiple markers of myocardial viability in a single examination. Its accuracy is at least equivalent to, if not superior to, that of other currently available noninvasive imaging techniques, including positron emission tomography. The greater spatial resolution afforded by cardiovascular MRI, especially with the delayed-enhancement MRI (DE-MRI) technique, combined with the breadth and depth of correlative pathologic data, makes cardiovascular MRI a particularly powerful tool for detecting viable and irreversibly damaged myocardium. A wealth of clinical data exist, including data from multicenter efforts, to establish DE-MRI as a new gold standard in myocardial viability assessment. As the high accuracy and broad scope of DE-MRI are recognized, the technique will gain wider clinical use for analysis of dysfunctional myocardium and be integrated into the diagnostic and therapeutic algorithm.

In patients who have heart failure, treatment and survival are directly related to the cause. Clinically, as a practical first step, patients are classified as having either ischemic or non-ischemic cardiomyopathy, a delineation usually based on the presence or absence of epicardial coronary artery disease. However, this approach does not account for patients with non-ischemic cardiomyopathy who also have coronary artery disease, which may be either incidental or partly contributing to myocardial dysfunction (mixed cardiomyopathy). By allowing direct assessment of the myocardium, delayed-enhancement cardiovascular magnetic resonance (DE-CMR) may aid in addressing these conundrums. This article explores the use of DE-CMR in identifying ischemic and non-ischemic myopathic processes and details a systematic approach to determine the cause of cardiomyopathy.

There is often considerable phenotypic overlap in hypertrophic and infiltrative cardiomyopathies. This overlap creates difficulties, when using routine imaging modalities, in arriving at a conclusive diagnosis. Cardiovascular magnetic resonance (CMR) can make diagnosis easier and more certain. Used with gadolinium contrast agent for tissue characterization, CMR offers a superior field of view and temporal resolution, enabling clinicians to make more confident assessments of etiology. CMR may also be a useful modality for stratifying risk and monitoring treatment responses over time in patients with hypertrophic or infiltrative cardiomyopathies. This article highlights the role of CMR in the assessment and, if relevant, the risk stratification of hypertrophic and infiltrative cardiomyopathies.

Cardiovascular magnetic resonance is able to provide a comprehensive assessment of valvular and hemodynamic function, including quantification of valve regurgitation and other flows, and accurate cardiac volumes and mass for assessing the effect on both ventricles. Combined with the ability to image all areas of the heart (including difficult areas, such as the right ventricle and pulmonary veins), it is an ideal technique for investigating patients who have heart failure in whom these areas need to be examined.

Magnetic resonance is known to be a superior modality for the evaluation of pericardial disease and intracardiac masses because of its unmatched capacity for tissue characterization and high spatial resolution. New real-time sequences complement the standard morphologic imaging of the pericardium with dynamic image acquisitions that also can provide hemodynamic information indicative of constriction. Magnetic resonance also is becoming increasingly recognized as a superior modality for the detection and characterization of intracardiac thrombus. This article reviews the use of magnetic resonance imaging for the evaluation of pericardial disease and the detection of intracardiac thrombus, with particular emphasis on the newer pulse sequences currently available for cardiac imaging.

This article focuses on the role of cardiovascular magnetic resonance (CMR) in understanding the physiology of diastolic function and on the future applications of CMR as they relate to diastolic function evaluation. CMR has a demonstrated potential to define diastolic function and quantify its properties, in terms of active and passive stages, and its relaxation and compliance characteristics. CMR is also useful for assessing inflow and myocardial velocities, and untwisting properties of the chamber and myocardium, thus providing insights not fully available in other invasive and noninvasive strategies. CMR, which offers the necessary capabilities to evaluate the complex structure of the right ventricle, can serve in the future as the standard for evaluating diastolic function as it currently does for systolic function.

In coronary artery disease (CAD), cardiac magnetic resonance (CMR) imaging can integrate several types of pulse-sequence examinations (eg, myocardial perfusion, cine wall motion, T2-weighted imaging for myocardial edema, late gadolinium enhancement, and CMR angiography) that can provide anatomic, functional, and physiologic information about the heart in a single imaging session. Because of this ability to interrogate myocardial physiology using different pulse sequence techniques within a single CMR session, this technique has been recognized increasingly in many centers as the test of choice for assessing patients who present with cardiomyopathy of undetermined cause. This article first reviews the current evidence supporting the prognosticating role of CMR in assessing CAD and then discusses CMR applications and prognostication in many non-coronary cardiac conditions.

Heart Failure Clinics

VISIT THE CLINICS ONLINE!

Access your subscription at:
www.theclinics.com

Editorial
Using a Magnet to Strike Gold

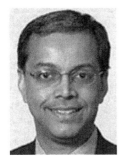
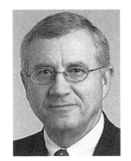

Ragavendra R. Baliga, MD, MBA   James B. Young, MD
Consulting Editors

Cardiac magnetic resonance (CMR) imaging is rapidly emerging as the procedure of first choice in the management of patients who have heart failure (HF). It has been argued that all patients with newly diagnosed HF should undergo CMR to detect structural and functional abnormalities that are usually not detected by conventional imaging techniques. In HF patients, a typical approach includes the assessment of morphology and function, characterization of the nature of the cardiomyopathy, and risk stratification.

CMR now should be considered the gold standard for the assessment of cardiac morphology. The ability of CMR to image in any plane without the need for optimal transthoracic imaging windows allows for substantial flexibility in the interrogation of abnormal heart structures. This characteristic can be used to determine specific structural or functional abnormalities that may not be best "captured" in conventional imaging planes. The CMR images can accurately and reproducibly assess both left and right ventricular chamber sizes, wall thickness, and mass. Moreover, the ability of CMR to characterize the composition of abnormal tissue allows the detection of constrictive pericarditis, which causes HF or infiltrative cardiomyopathies such as amyloidosis. It is, therefore, extraordinarily helpful in separating those patients who have significant pericardial constriction and might benefit after pericardiectomy from those whose primary abnormality is driven more by myocardial restriction.

CMR is not only useful for determining morphology but also for functional assessment. Advances in cine assessment (resulting in faster image acquisition) and high spacial resolution (making planimetry of interface between the left ventricular cavity and the myocardium accurate) have resulted in easy and reproducible assessment of left ventricular and right ventricular function in normal and HF patients. Regional myocardial function can also be determined using the myocardial tagging technique. Tagging is also useful in assessing rotation, contraction, and strain in the subendocardial, midwall, and subepicardial layers of the left ventricular wall. CMR can also be used to determine myocardial perfusion, including contractile reserve and perfusion reserve. Dobutamine stress cine CMR is used to detect ischemia-induced wall motion abnormalities, whereas adenosine stress perfusion imaging allows early detection of subendocardial perfusion defects that are not detected by conventional methods.

Delayed-enhancement CMR is particularly useful in evaluating patients who have HF. The high spacial resolution provided by this technique, along with its ability to detect nonviable myocardium, makes it useful for differentiating ischemic from nonischemic myocardial disorders and detecting myocardial scarring. In patients who have ischemic disease, the epicardium typically is involved because coronary artery disease progresses as a wavefront from the epicardium to the endocardium. Isolated midwall or epicardial hyperenhancement strongly suggests a nonischemic etiology. The ability of delayed-enhancement technique to detect scarring makes it uniquely positioned in the early noninvasive detection of sudden death among a variety of cardiac

Heart Failure Clin 5 (2009) ix–x
doi:10.1016/j.hfc.2009.03.001
1551-7136/09/$ – see front matter © 2009 Published by Elsevier Inc.

heartfailure.theclinics.com

disorders. Furthermore, with the development of pacemakers and defibrillators that are CMR compatible, CMR could likely be used in all HF patients. It is a radical proposition to suggest moving from the traditional imaging modalities or echocardiography and cineradiography but one that is now supported by a tremendous wealth of data and experience. Never before has the cardiologist been rewarded with a diagnostic image that truly allows one to "get what you see."

In this issue, Drs. Pennel and Kim have assembled authors who are international experts in the exciting and rapidly evolving field of CMR. In these articles, it is clear that CMR is not only the gold standard for assessing morphology and function, but also is emerging as the gold standard in the assessment of myocardial perfusion and ischemia, making the magnet a useful tool for striking gold!

Ragavendra R. Baliga, MD, MBA
The Ohio State University
Columbus, OH, USA

James B. Young, MD
Division of Medicine
Lerner College of Medicine
Cleveland Clinic
Cleveland, OH, USA

E-mail addresses:
Ragavendra.Baliga@osumc.edu (R.R. Baliga)
YOUNGJ@ccf.org (J.B. Young)

Preface

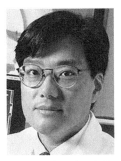
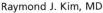
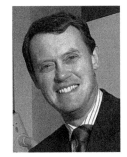

Raymond J. Kim, MD   Dudley J. Pennell, MD, FRCP, FACC
Guest Editors

Although heart failure is a common disorder, it is complex and there are a myriad of important clinical questions that must be answered to optimize patient management. What is the etiology? Is there left ventricular systolic dysfunction? Is there diastolic dysfunction? Is the heart remodeling, and, if so, is the remodeling process responding to therapy? How about secondary processes such as ventricular thrombus formation and changing hemodynamics with worsening valvular competency? Who should get revascularization? An implantable cardioverter defibrillator?

It is rare when a clinical tool can even begin to approach the exhaustive demands of clinical practice. In this regard, we are delighted, as guest editors for this issue of *Heart Failure Clinics*, to present a state-of-the-art review of cardiovascular magnetic resonance (CMR) in heart failure. In the articles that follow, an important distinguishing attribute of CMR—its versatility—will become abundantly clear. From a single 45–60 minute examination, CMR allows a comprehensive assessment of structure and function, viability and perfusion, and valvular function and hemodynamics, among others. For many of these, CMR is considered the "gold standard" approach.

The contributors, all international experts with vast expertise in clinical CMR, have performed admirably in providing a succinct yet thorough review of the topics. The articles range from an introduction of the CMR techniques that are commonly used in a heart failure examination to a discussion of the value of CMR for the purposes of risk stratification and prognostication. We hope that readers will find this issue to be not only stimulating but also of practical value for the routine management of their heart failure patients.

Raymond J. Kim, MD
Duke Cardiovascular Magnetic Resonance Center
Duke University Medical Center
Durham, NC, USA

Dudley J. Pennell, MD, FRCP, FACC
Royal Brompton Hospital
Imperial College London
London, UK

E-mail addresses:
rjkim@duke.edu (R.J. Kim)
DJ.Pennell@rbht.nhs.uk (D.J. Pennell)

doi:10.1016/j.hfc.2009.03.002

heartfailure.theclinics.com

The CMR Examination in Heart Failure

Subha V. Raman, MD, MSEE*, Orlando P. Simonetti, PhD

KEYWORDS

- Heart failure • Magnetic resonance imaging • Prognosis
- Etiology • Cardiomyopathy • Ischemic heart disease
- Viability • Biopsy

Heart failure (HF) is a leading cause of hospitalization, death, and disability in most developed countries, forming a significant social and economic burden for patients, families, and health care systems.[1,2] The prevalence of HF remains undeterred in the modern era, thanks at least in part to advances in rescuing patients with previously deadly conditions, such as acute ST-segment elevation myocardial infarction who survive to face sequelae such as HF many years after the initial event. Reducing morbidity and mortality caused by HF requires correct diagnosis, risk stratification, and institution of appropriate treatment.[3] Although clinical assessment forms the cornerstone in the initial evaluation of the patient with HF,[4,5] selection of appropriate therapies relies on a thorough understanding of cardiovascular structure and function typically beyond that which can be gleaned from bedside examination and routine tests, such as electrocardiography (ECG) and serologic evaluation. Such an understanding may be efficiently provided by cardiovascular MR (CMR) using an array of techniques ranging from segmental wall motion assessment to molecular myocardial characterization. This article presents a rationale for incorporating CMR in the evaluation of patients who have HF and is organized as follows. Part I defines the context of CMR within standard clinical evaluation and among the many other modalities available for cardiovascular assessment in patients who have HF. Part II describes the techniques most useful in imaging HF. Part III provides recommended approaches for the standard HF CMR examination. Part IV

concludes with perspectives on the appropriate use and incorporation of CMR in the evaluation and management of patients who have HF.

The clinician's first step in determining if and what type of diagnostic test to use in evaluating a patient who has HF is to enumerate the clinical questions to be answered. Typically, imaging helps answer questions related to (1) etiology, (2) cardiac function, and (3) cardiac structure. Etiologic questions start with ruling out the most common causes of left ventricular (LV) dysfunction, such as atherosclerotic heart disease. This historically has relied heavily on catheter-based coronary angiography, although the advent of CMR has afforded more widespread acknowledgment that coronary angiography misclassifies HF cause in 13% of patients.[6] Many other common causes that benefit from imaging, particularly CMR, include hypertensive heart disease (extent of hypertrophy and fibrosis), myocardial infiltrative disorders, inflammatory conditions, congenital heart disease (complex anatomy and physiology), and arrhythmic disorders' myocardial substrate.

Questions related to cardiac performance seek quantification of LV systolic function, LV diastolic function, and stress function; right ventricular (RV) function may be particularly relevant in patients with congenital heart disease, pulmonary hypertension, and valvular heart disease. Although not necessarily indicative of functional status, global measures of cardiac function, such as ejection fraction, are widely used in the initial classification and risk stratification of patients who have HF. RV function has relevance not only as a primary

The Ohio State University, Columbus, OH, USA
* Corresponding author. Internal Medicine, Division of Cardiovascular Medicine, The Ohio State University, 200 DHLRI, 473 West 12th Avenue, Columbus, OH 43210.
E-mail address: raman.1@osu.edu (S.V. Raman).

Heart Failure Clin 5 (2009) 283–300
doi:10.1016/j.hfc.2009.02.002
1551-7136/09/$ – see front matter © 2009 Elsevier Inc. All rights reserved.

endpoint in right heart conditions but also in the evaluation of patients with left HF being considered for procedures such as shunt closure or valve repair. Additional structural questions that require definitive assessment include presence and severity of valvular heart disease, intracardiac shunts, and pericardial disease. Bedside evaluation should guide this set of queries, although occasionally patient habitus, eccentricity of valvular jets, or equilibration of right and left heart pressures may obscure detection of valvular heart disease or shunts on physical examination. Clues such as signs of right HF with or without pulmonary venous congestion must be recognized to help direct the imaging evaluation appropriately.

The breadth of questions to be answered in the initial evaluation of a patient who has HF coupled with increasing pressures to deliver cost-effective care mandate efficient use of diagnostic modalities to answer these questions. Inaccurate or indeterminate diagnoses may prevent implementation of optimal therapies most likely to improve the underlying conditions and inappropriately increase downstream costs. Presumptively treating hypertensive heart disease in a patient with undiagnosed chronic ischemic heart disease, for instance, misses the opportunity to treat atherosclerosis at the macro- and microvascular levels and positively impact myocardial performance and outcomes. Conversely, recognizing instances in which severity of LV dysfunction exceeds that expected based on extent of obstructive coronary artery disease should prompt further myocardial characterization, because revascularization alone in this population is unlikely to be sufficient for complete recovery of viable myocardium. Suspecting secondary causes of HF in the appropriate clinical setting can direct the imaging examination toward the most likely among the differential diagnoses (**Box 1**).

Typical tests used in the initial evaluation of patients who have HF include 12-lead surface ECG, chest roentgenography, and echocardiography. Virtually all patients undergo ECG upon initial assessment because of its ease and simplicity. Although it rarely provides sufficient information to determine cause, prognosis, and treatment strategy in HF, abnormalities in the setting of other studies that are inconclusive should prompt consideration of myocardial disease (**Fig. 1**). This is especially true for genetic cardiomyopathies in which the ECG provides distinct information compared with the predominantly morphologic and functional data yielded by cardiac imaging tests. QRS duration has been heavily relied on to select patients for device therapie,s such as cardiac resynchronization, although it has poor predictive value in determining which

| **Box 1** |
| **Secondary causes of heart failure** |

Ischemic heart disease

Hypertension

Valvular disease

Intracardiac shunts

Pericardial disease

Metabolic disorders (eg, thyroid disease, diabetes, acromegaly, catecholamine excess)

Infiltrative diseases

    Sarcoidosis

    Amyloidosis

    Glycogen storage diseases

Toxins (eg, alcohol, cocaine)

Pregnancy

Sustained tachyarrhythmias

patients are likely to respond to cardiac resynchronization.[7] Chest roentgenography is frequently a first test performed in the acute HF setting, particularly when cardiac versus pulmonary causes remain in the differential diagnosis. Simple findings from upright, well-penetrated posteroanterior roentgenography, such as increased cardiothoracic ratio and pulmonary vascular congestion, have value that is unfortunately diminished in mosts chest roentgenographs obtained in the often dyspneic, nonsupine patient who has acute HF with anteroposterior projection.[8] Serologic testing, such as brain natriuretic peptide levels, has shown the limitation of distinguishing cardiac from pulmonary cause of dyspnea by physical examination and chest roentgenography alone.[9]

It is uncommon in current clinical settings to encounter a patient sent to the CMR laboratory for HF evaluation who has not already undergone echocardiography. Echocardiography provides an assessment of LV systolic and diastolic function and a survey of structural abnormalities such as valvular, pericardial, and shunt conditions. All of this is delivered at the bedside, if necessary, given the portable nature of the modality. It is less clear what echocardiography provides in terms of definitive diagnosis in cases other than significant valvular disease, intracardiac shunt, or gross pericardial abnormality. Surface echocardiography alone performs poorly in distinguishing ischemic from nonischemic cardiomyopathy and viable from nonviable thinned myocardium given its limited spatial resolution and contrast mechanisms for tissue characterization. Although its prognostic

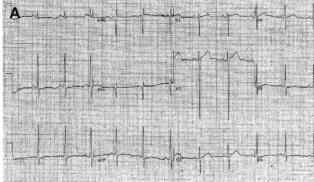
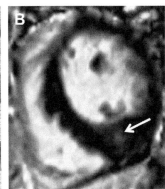

Fig. 1. Recognition of cardiomyopathy was afforded by ECG in this 15-year-old athlete with syncope. (*A*) ECG shows increased QRS voltage although potentially within the range of normal based on age and repolarization abnormality. Echocardiography was unremarkable; however, CMR was pursued based on the ECG findings. (*B*) Cine imaging showed asymmetric hypertrophy of the inferior LV myocardium and focal hyperenhancement on late postgadolinium imaging. Subsequent genotyping revealed a novel mutation in the myosin heavy chain gene consistent with hypertrophic cardiomyopathy.

value in HF is particularly good with Doppler evaluation as a surrogate for filling pressures, recognition of myocardial fibrosis or infiltrative disease remains challenging based on acoustic properties alone. Many patients also have poor acoustic windows, the *sine qua non* for adequate echocardiography, as a result of obese body habitus, lung hyperinflation, or chest wall edema; contrast echocardiography partially— but not consistently—overcomes these limitations.[10]

Other modalities used in the initial evaluation of patients who have HF include nuclear imaging, particularly rest-redistribution thallium and positron emission tomography for myocardial viability.[11] Extensive literature confirms limited spatial resolution resulting in difficulty distinguishing nontransmural from transmural scar with nuclear imaging. The exposure of patients to significant doses of ionizing radiation should reserve use of these modalities to patients for whom CMR cannot be offered because of contraindications.[12,13] Endomyocardial biopsy of the native heart is subject to sampling error, increased risk of perforation, and other complications associated with invasive cardiac catheterization and is infrequently required in the contemporary evaluation of new-onset HF.[14] Clinical suspicion of conditions such as giant cell myocarditis do warrant tissue diagnosis, given the implications regarding treatment selection and prognosis.[15] Invasive hemodynamics, although not routinely recommended, may be useful for confirmation of pulmonary hypertension, shunt physiology, and demonstration of response to vasodilator therapy and may be performed in conjunction with imaging and other tests.[16] Serologic testing, such as brain natriuretic peptides provides global assessment to complement local information on myocardial disease afforded by high-quality imaging.

Histopathologic studies have identified specific substrate for adverse outcomes in HF, including myocardial fibrosis, ischemia/vasculopathy, and edema.[17–21] Fibrosis or scar itself may influence cardiac structure and function over time and render a segment of myocardium abnormal with respect to systolic and diastolic function. Scar intermingled with viable myocytes may form substrate for re-entrant ventricular arrhythmias. Ischemia may result from epicardial coronary disease and microvascular disease; over time it leads to myocyte swelling and necrosis. Remodeling from dilatation alters annular size, which, in turn, impairs function of the mitral and tricuspid valve complexes. Recently, increased recognition of the role played by intracardiac vortex flow further underscored the ill effects of ventricular remodeling. Finally, intra- and interventricular dyssynchrony remain ill-defined substrates for adverse outcomes in patients who have HF. For imaging to improve outcomes in HF, it should identify and quantify myocardial fibrosis, ischemia, remodeling, and other characteristics that, if better characterized, may be better targeted for interventions to reduce morbidity and mortality. The next section illustrates how CMR uniquely provides such comprehensive information.

PRINCIPLES OF CARDIOVASCULAR MAGNETIC RESONANCE TECHNIQUES IN HEART FAILURE

The combinations of radiofrequency pulses, magnetic field gradient pulses, data sampling strategies, and image reconstruction methods that make up MRI pulse sequence programs are virtually unlimited. These pulse sequence variations are used in CMR to generate an enormous range of image characteristics based on sensitivity to the MR relaxation parameters T1, T2, and T2* and motion, flow, diffusion, and other physiologic processes. Sequence parameters that control spatial resolution, temporal resolution, and scan time can be traded off to achieve diagnostic image quality in almost any patient, provided the patient has no contraindications to MRI (eg, claustrophobia, implanted pacemakers or defibrillators). This tremendous flexibility has resulted in a wide range of methods to evaluate cardiac structure and function and characterize many of the changes in myocardial tissue associated with HF. This section provides a brief description of some of the more important CMR techniques currently in use.

Cine Imaging

Cine imaging of cardiac function, valve function, and blood flow is a key component of any CMR examination of patients with known or suspected HF. Bright-blood cine imaging sequences have been shown to provide highly accurate and reproducible measurements of LV and RV volumes and LV mass.[22–24] Image planes can be precisely and reproducibly prescribed in any arbitrary orientation, permitting volume and mass measurement by three-dimensional integration without the need for geometric assumptions. This factor is especially important given the chamber dilatation and remodeling that often accompany HF.

The most commonly applied method for cardiac cine imaging uses a segmented, balanced steady-state free precession (SSFP) acquisition with retrospective ECG gating[25] and parallel data acquisition.[26,27] SSFP rapidly generates bright-blood images with high signal and high spatial and temporal resolution. Spoiled gradient echo is also used for some types of cine imaging, but bright-blood signal depends on flow through the image plane with this technique. SSFP image contrast depends primarily on the ratio of relaxation parameters T2/T1, which gives rise to a roughly 3:1 contrast ratio between blood and myocardium that is relatively independent of blood flow. This last point is especially important in imaging the failing heart in which function may be severely impaired and intracardiac flow velocities reduced. SSFP is sensitive to magnetic field homogeneity, which has limited its application at 3 T and higher field strengths.

Some typical cine imaging parameters are listed in **Table 1**. Generally, each slice plane is acquired in a short breath-hold of eight to ten heartbeats,

which results in a cine loop depicting a single, composite cardiac cycle. Using this "segmented" approach to data acquisition, a fraction of the data is acquired every heartbeat for each of multiple images or frames across the cardiac cycle. Segmented acquisition relies on reproducible cardiac motion and positioning of the heart from one beat to the next and requires regular cardiac rhythm and the patient's ability to breath-hold. "Real-time" images, on the other hand, are acquired as a series of complete images in rapid succession, without physiologic synchronization, directly analogous to echocardiography.[28] This rapid acquisition mode has been made possible by recent advances in MRI hardware and data acquisition methods, although spatial and temporal resolution are sacrificed somewhat relative to segmented acquisition as shown by the typical parameters listed in **Table 1** and images shown in **Fig. 2**. The primary advantage of real-time acquisition is its insensitivity to breathing motion or arrhythmia, which makes it a robust method that can be used to obtain diagnostic cine images in virtually any patient. Cine imaging may be performed under resting conditions and during graded infusion of dobutamine, with the latter being especially helpful in demonstrating inotropic reserve or ischemia in appropriate clinical scenarios.

Velocity-Encoded Cine

It is possible to encode information into the magnitude and the phase of the complex MRI signal. Although in most CMR methods only the magnitude image is reconstructed, phase-velocity imaging encodes the instantaneous velocity into the phase of each image pixel.[29,30] Motion or flow of tissue or blood causes a phase shift relative to stationary tissue. The sensitivity to motion and ratio of signal phase to velocity can be precisely controlled. There are other causes of phase shift in the MRI signal, such as local field inhomogeneity and tissue fat content. Accurate velocity mapping requires additional data in the form of a phase reference image, which typically requires the interleaved acquisition of a second complete image data set using a pulse sequence designed to have no sensitivity to velocity. Assuming all other extraneous sources of phase remain constant between the two acquisitions, calculating a phase-difference results in accurate estimation of velocity (**Fig. 3**). In the reconstructed "phase images," pixel intensity is directly proportional to velocity, and the sign (positive or negative) indicates direction. The accuracy of the method has been well validated and shown to be valuable in

Table 1
Breath-hold cine and real-time cine magnetic resonance

	Breath-Hold Cine	Real-Time Cine
TR	2.7	2.4
TE	1.2	1.0
Flip angle (typical)	80	70
Slice thickness	8 mm	8 mm
Field of view (typical)	290 mm×360 mm	270 mm×360 mm
Matrix (typical)	154×256	80×192
Pixel dimensions (typical)	1.9 mm×1.4 mm	3.4 mm×1.9 mm
Lines per segment	14	—
Temporal resolution	38 ms	65 ms
Cardiac synchronization	Yes, retrospective gating	No
Parallel acceleration	2x	3x
Scan time (per slice)	7 heartbeats	3 sec

Typical pulse sequence parameters.

the evaluation of valve flow, intracardiac flow, and myocardial tissue velocity.[31–35]

MRI phase-velocity imaging is a variation on the cine techniques already described, although generally it uses a gradient echo rather than a SSFP type sequence. Segmented acquisition methods are typically used to generate a two-dimensional map of blood and tissue velocity in one direction at multiple cardiac phases during a short breath-hold. The requirement of phase reference data and the use of the slower spoiled gradient echo techniques mean that velocity maps are generally of somewhat lower spatial and/or temporal resolution than conventional cine. These limitations have been overcome recently through the use of parallel acquisition methods that reduce data requirements and accelerate scans through the use of multiple parallel receiver coils.[36] Parallel acquisition techniques have become standard for most cardiac imaging methods on all vendors' systems.

Valve flow, intracardiac flow, and myocardial tissue motion may require measurement of velocities in all three directions (x, y, z) to be fully characterized. Phase-velocity can be extended to multiple directions and to three-dimensional volume rather than single-slice acquisition, but at the expense of scan time and/or temporal resolution.

Myocardial Strain Mapping

Although cine imaging provides structural and functional information regarding wall motion, wall thickening, and valve function, CMR techniques also have been developed to measure

intramyocardial motion and estimate myocardial strain, or local tissue deformation, which may be a more sensitive indicator of regional dysfunction. Intramyocardial motion imaging has not yet reached clinical practice, but three basic methods have been developed to acquire this information: phase-velocity mapping, tissue tagging, and DENSE (displacement encoding with stimulated echoes).[37–39] Strain can be estimated from phase-velocity data, but tracking of tissue displacement from velocity data can be complicated. Tagging provides tissue displacement information directly, but with low spatial resolution. DENSE directly encodes tissue displacement into the phase of the MR signal, providing a pixel-by-pixel map of tissue displacement at multiple cardiac phases (**Fig. 4**). Circumferential (E_{cc}) and radial (E_{rr}) strains are easily calculated from the displacement maps.[40] Clinical applications for this method are still under evaluation.

Myocardial Tissue Characterization

One of the primary advantages of CMR over other cardiac imaging modalities is its flexibility and sensitivity to a variety of tissue parameters. This can be especially relevant in the diagnosis of several causes of HF. Imaging techniques that are sensitive to MR relaxation time constants T1, T2, and T2* all play a role in CMR of HF. T1-weighted imaging is typically used in combination with gadolinium-based MRI contrast agents designed to shorten T1 relaxation, causing signal enhancement in T1-weighted images. T2- and T2*-weighted imaging methods, on the other hand, are generally used without contrast agent

Segmented, breath-hold   Real-time

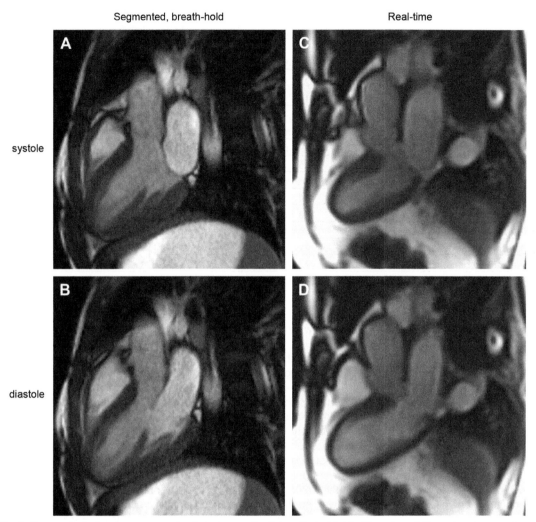

Fig. 2. Segmented cine images acquired during patient breath-hold (*A, B*) and real-time cine images from a different patient acquired during free-breathing (*C, D*). Higher spatial and temporal resolution of segmented cine provides clearer depiction of valve structures, but this method requires breath-hold and regular cardiac rhythm, whereas real-time cine does not.

injection to assess native changes that reflect tissue pathologies.

Perfusion imaging

Myocardial perfusion can be assessed by rapid acquisition of T1-weighted images during intravenous bolus injection of gadolinium contrast agent.[41] CMR perfusion imaging is a "first-pass" technique; dynamic enhancement of the myocardium reflects the delivery of contrast agent to the tissue via the coronary circulation. Pharmacologic vasodilatation using either adenosine or dipyridimole is typically used to accentuate regional myocardial flow differences, although perfusion CMR recently was demonstrated immediately after treadmill exercise.[42] Myocardium supplied by a stenotic vessel or diseased microvasculature

demonstrates slower enhancement, a lower peak signal, and a longer time to reach peak signal than normally perfused tissue (**Fig. 5**). Images (ideally covering the entire heart) of multiple slice planes must be acquired repeatedly and in rapid succession to monitor the first-pass of contrast agent through the myocardium. Modern pulse sequences permit acquisition of four or five slices in a single cardiac cycle with adequate spatial resolution, temporal resolution, and image quality to reliably detect subendocardial perfusion deficits.

Late gadolinium enhancement

Late gadolinium enhancement (LGE) imaging of the heart has gained wide acceptance as the preferred method for detection of focal myocardial

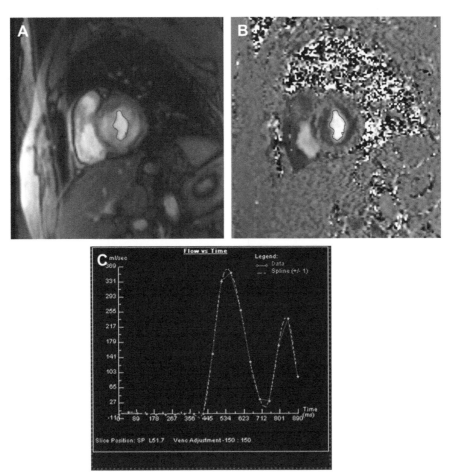

Fig. 3. CMR phase velocity mapping of transmitral valve flow. Magnitude (*A*) and phase-velocity (*B*) images are shown from a single diastolic frame. Pixel intensity in phase map (*B*) is proportional to velocity. The graph of volume flow versus time (*C*) illustrates E and A waves of flow through a manually drawn region defining the mitral valve orifice.

necrosis or fibrosis. Specific patterns of enhancement have been associated with some causes of LV HF.[43,44] Any of the commercially available gadolinium-based MRI contrast agents can be used effectively for LGE, although none currently has a US Food and Drug Administration indication for imaging the heart. All of these agents rapidly diffuse across the capillary membranes after injection and distribute in the interstitial space without penetrating intact cell membranes; all cause shortening of tissue T1 relaxation proportional to concentration. Within approximately 10 minutes after injection, the contrast agent reaches a quasi-equilibrium state, although slow continual washout takes place as it is excreted by the kidneys. It has been shown that the equilibrium volume of distribution of gadolinium is higher in necrotic or fibrotic myocardium than in viable myocardium.[45] The relative concentration of gadolinium per gram of tissue is higher, causing greater

T1 shortening in dead or scarred tissue than in viable tissue (**Fig. 6**).[46] The native T1 of viable myocardium is approximately 977 msec; 15 minutes after injection of 0.15 mmol/kg gadolinium, the T1 of viable myocardium drops to approximately 500 msec, whereas the T1 of infarcted myocardium reaches values typically less than 400 msec.[47] This T1 difference is the basic mechanism exploited by the LGE technique to differentiate nonviable from viable myocardial tissue.

Although several variants exist, the underlying method common to all LGE sequences has remained consistent for the past decade. Inversion-recovery magnetization preparation with the inversion time (TI) set to null viable tissue is used to create high contrast between viable and nonviable myocardial tissue. The most frequently applied method uses a segmented gradient echo acquisition, typically collecting one image over

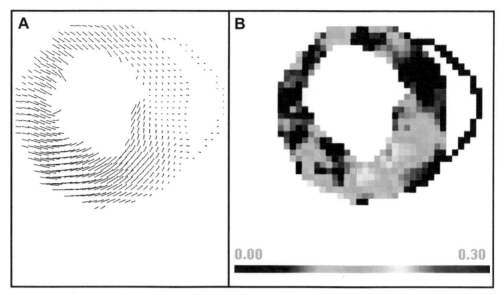

Fig. 4. Example of short-axis displacement encoded imaging (DENSE) in an animal model of segmental myocardial dysfunction. End-systolic displacement map (*A*) shows minimal displacement of tissue in the anterior-apical septum. Circumferential strain map (*B*) shows corresponding region of low strain.

a short breath-hold of 10 to 16 heart beats.[48] Common variations include segmented three-dimensional, single-shot two-dimensional,[49] navigator respiratory gating, parallel imaging, SSFP, and phase-sensitive reconstruction.[50] Single-shot methods that acquire the entire image in less than one heartbeat are insensitive to cardiac arrhythmias and breathing motion. Similar to real-time cine imaging, some compromise is made in spatial and temporal resolution, but the tradeoff for diagnostic image quality in patients with severe arrhythmias or inability to breath-hold is often worthwhile. Delayed enhancement also has been demonstrated successfully at 3 T, with improved SNR compared with 1.5 T.[51] Although the underlying mechanism is common to all techniques, these variations have made LGE a robust method with demonstrated diagnostic use in a range of diseases that cause necrosis, fibrosis, and inflammation of the myocardium.

Although LGE has been successful in detection of focal myocardial pathologies, it is expected that diffuse fibrosis, inflammation, or infiltration can cause global changes in the T1 relaxation of myocardium after gadolinium injection.[52] It may be difficult to detect such changes using standard methods, because LGE relies on the relative signal differences between viable and nonviable tissues. T1 mapping methods, although not yet in widespread use, can be used to quantitatively measure global changes in myocardial T1 that may be caused by diffuse pathologic changes. A promising and practical method for myocardial T1

measurement recently was described[47] and used to show global T1 shortening not evident with conventional LGE in patients with chronic aortic regurgitation.[52] The basic strategy for T1 mapping is to acquire multiple images at different inversion-recovery delay times (TI) and then to fit a T1-recovery curve to these images on a pixel-by-pixel basis. For this method to be broadly effective, normal myocardial T1 values must be established and the timing and dose of gadolinium standardized, because they affect the measured T1 post-contrast.

T2 and T2* imaging

The transverse relaxation parameters, T2 and T2*, are known to reflect pathologic changes in tissue. T2 is closely associated with tissue water content, and T2-weighted imaging methods can be used to detect inflammation and edema associated with acute myocardial infarction and myocarditis. T2-weighted CMR is generally performed using a spin-echo based acquisition with a long echo time (TE) for T2 sensitivity, in combination with a "black-blood" preparation pulse to suppress signal from blood.[53] An additional inversion-recovery pulse with a short inversion time (STIR) is often applied to suppress signal from epicardial fat and further accentuate the contrast between edematous and normal tissue.[53] The result is an image in which edematous tissue with high water content appears significantly brighter than normal tissue (**Fig. 7**). The most commonly used technique uses a segmented acquisition method

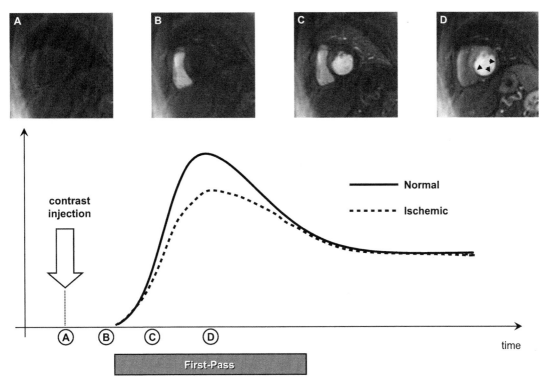

Fig. 5. Time course of myocardial signal enhancement during first-pass perfusion. Each image (*A–D*) corresponds to the labeled time points after bolus intravenous injection of gadolinium contrast agent. Contrast agent passes through the right-ventricle (*B*) and left-ventricle (*C*) blood pools before enhancing the myocardium (*D*). Ischemic territory (*arrowheads*) in inferior wall is seen as a region of low signal intensity (*D*).

(turbo- or fast-spin-echo) to acquire a single image over a short breath-hold, although single-shot methods that acquire an entire image in a single heartbeat are also applied. These methods are known to suffer from motion and flow artifacts that can lead to myocardial signal dropout and enhanced signal from static blood on the endocardial surface of the ventricle[54] but have proved valuable in the characterization of acute myocardial inflammation.[55–57] T2-weighted CMR is an ongoing focus of research, and several new methods recently were proposed to address the known limitations of current techniques.[58,59]

The relaxation parameter T2* has been correlated with tissue iron, and T2*-weighted CMR methods can be used in the evaluation of HF caused by iron overload.[60] T2*-weighted images show abnormal signal loss in iron-overloaded myocardium. Because iron overload often affects the myocardium globally, however, focal changes in signal intensity may not be evident on T2*-weighted images. T2* sensitivity depends on TE in a gradient-echo pulse sequence, and acquisition of a series of images over a range of TE enables quantitative estimation of T2*. T2* quantification allows evaluation of global changes in myocardial T2*, and a threshold has been established (T2*

< 20 msec) to indicate significant iron overload. A direct estimate of iron content in milligrams per gram of tissue can be computed using the formula: $[Fe]_{R2}^* = .0254 \times R2^* + 0.202$, which has been shown to correlate well with direct mass spectroscopy measurements of explanted tissue.[61]

Spectroscopy

Beyond indirect and qualitative evaluation of pathologic changes in myocardial tissue based on MRI relaxation parameters with and without contrast agent injection, MR spectroscopy offers the potential to directly measure the biochemistry and energy use of myocardial tissue.[31] P spectroscopy provides for the examination of phosphocreatine, ATP, and inorganic phosphate levels.[62–64] Although ^{31}P spectroscopy of the human heart was first demonstrated in the 1980s, the acquisition of in vivo cardiac spectra has proved to present technical challenges that have prevented robust clinical applications of this technology to date, and its use remains relegated to one of a research tool. Hydrogen (^{1}H) spectroscopy recently showed promise as a means to measure myocardial triglyceride levels in vivo.[65–67] This technique may help elucidate links among

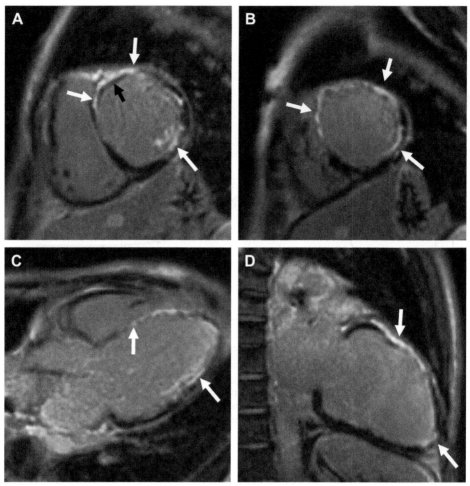

Fig. 6. LGE shows extensive myocardial scarring in this patient as high signal intensity (*white arrows*) in short-axis (*A, B*) and long-axis (*C, D*) views. Signal from viable myocardium is "nulled" by appropriate setting of inversion recovery time. Regions of "no-reflow" also may appear dark (*black arrow, A*) but typically are surrounded by hyperenhanced nonviable tissue.

adiposity, deposition of triglycerides in the myocardium, and HF.

Magnetic Resonance Angiography

Several methods exist for MR angiography (MRA) that may be useful in select HF CMR examinations, particularly in patients with suspected vascular anomalies or extracardiac shunts. Contrast-enhanced MRA is the most commonly applied method for angiography of large thoracic vessels. In this method, a three-dimensional image volume covering the area of interest is rapidly acquired in a short breath-hold during bolus injection of gadolinium contrast media. Data acquisition is timed to the passage of contrast agent through the vessels of interest (eg, aorta, pulmonary veins, pulmonary arteries). The high concentration of contrast agent in the blood results in a dramatic shortening of T1

and high signal intensity relative to background tissues. The signal difference between blood and background can be enhanced by subtraction of a precontrast dataset or "mask." With or without subtraction, the resulting three-dimensional angiography data can be displayed and interrogated using maximum intensity projection, volume rendering, or multi-planar reconstruction techniques. Other methods of MRA are available for patients with contraindications to contrast agents or who are unable to breath-hold.

THE STANDARD HEART FAILURE CARDIOVASCULAR MAGNETIC RESONANCE EXAMINATION

The standard HF CMR examination should include multiplanar cine imaging (horizontal long axis, vertical long axis, three-chamber, and contiguous

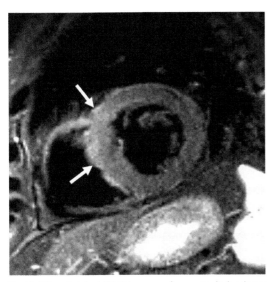

Fig. 7. T2-weighted STIR image of myocardial edema caused by acute myocardial infarction. Increase in tissue water leads to lengthening of T1 and T2 relaxation parameters, which causes increased signal intensity on T2-weighted STIR images. Additional radiofrequency pulses are used to suppress blood and fat signals and enhance contrast between edematous and normal myocardial tissue.

short axis covering the heart) and LGE acquisitions in similar planes, with additional elements based on the individual patient's history. Given the prevalence of ischemic heart disease, it may be beneficial to include stress with either adenosine perfusion imaging or dobutamine cine imaging to demonstrate (1) presence and extent of reversible ischemia and (2) inotropic reserve in patients being considered for revascularization to improve LV contractile function. Knowing the patient has obstructive coronary artery disease by prior angiography may preclude the need for stress imaging; however, defining the relative contribution of ischemia versus nonischemic processes, particularly in cases of severe LV dysfunction, may be useful to predict degree of improvement to be expected with coronary revascularization. In patients with LV dysfunction caused by recent myocardial infarction, recognizing microvascular obstruction can be done with either with first-pass perfusion[68] or LGE imaging,[69] does not require stress, and portends increased likelihood of major adverse cardiovascular events after myocardial infarction. Abnormal myocardial perfusion reserve in the absence of epicardial coronary artery disease indicates microvascular disease;[70] CMR may be the optimal modality to translate these findings to better understand entities such as the ill-defined "diabetic cardiomyopathy" that likely affects more patients than currently recognized because of lack of definitive diagnostic criteria.

Cine imaging is typically done using SSFP techniques. Note that patients who have HF may have significant orthopnea or other sources of dyspnea (eg, large pleural effusions and parenchymal lung disease), reducing image quality with breath-hold acquisitions. In such instances, or for patients with frequent ectopy or intermittent arrhythmias, real-time-cine imaging is a robust technique to provide regional wall motion assessment. The somewhat lower spatial and temporal resolution and lower image contrast do not preclude adequate segmental LV function interpretation, especially when considering such patients' typical acoustic windows. Quantification of LV volumes, mass, and ejection fraction are routinely reported as part of the HF CMR examination at our institution when using breath-hold, segmented cine data. Not infrequently, quantification of RV volumes and ejection fraction is also provided, given CMR's unique ability to reliable quantify the RV.[22] Recognizing its influence on left heart output and prognosis in a variety of cardiomyopathies underscores the need for accurate RV appraisal. Postprocessing should be done by experienced personnel facile with this aspect of data analysis to ensure consistency in technique and reproducibility of results. Quantification does impact prognosis[71] and selection of surgical therapies such as surgical ventricular restoration, which requires a certain preoperative volume to allow adequate cardiac performance postoperatively.[72] CMR does not rely on "segmental" versus "nonsegmental" regional wall motion abnormality to classify ischemic versus nonischemic cardiomyopathy, given much more definitive data provided by direct demonstration of infarct versus noninfarct scar with LGE imaging.

LGE is arguably the most important element of the CMR examination in HF. Midwall fibrosis on LGE indicates a nonischemic process and has been identified in idiopathic, hypertrophic,[73] and other genetic cardiomyopathies, such as those caused by mutations in lamin A/C,[74] the last being suspected in any cardiomyopathy patient with conduction system disease. Hypertrophic cardiomyopathy has, to date, been found to result from more than 200 different mutations both familiar and spontaneous; genotype alone performs poorly in predicting where an individual lies on the spectrum of prognosis from benign to lethal.[75] Even conventional criteria to stratify risk of sudden cardiac death in hypertrophic cardiomyopathy occasionally fail to identify high-risk patients.[76] In conjunction with CMR, however, the value of genotype-phenotype correlation becomes apparent. In a small group of families with hypertrophic cardiomyopathy caused by mutations in the troponin-I gene, Moon and colleagues[77] demonstrated distinct patterns of fibrosis from mild to severe that distinguished families with late-onset, mild disease from families with early onset, malignant phenotypes. Other studies have confirmed the predictive value of myocardial fibrosis by LGE in patients who have hypertrophic cardiomyopathy with complex ventricular arrhythmias.[78,79]

Beyond distinguishing the subendocardial infarct scar of ischemic heart disease from midwall fibrosis of nonischemic cardiomyopathy,[6] LGE has helped to define distinct patterns of hyperenhancement that occur more commonly in specific conditions. Myocarditis, for example, typically produces epicardial hyperenhancement (**Fig. 8**) and commonly involves the lateral LV myocardium,[80] a site not routinely sampled by endomyocardial biopsy unless directed by CMR. Sarcoidosis often results in mass-like LGE within the basal interventricular septum, corresponding to the noncaseating granulomas seen at histopathologic examination.[81,82] Amyloidosis produces a pattern of subendocardial enhancement with LGE and may be accompanied by a distinct appearance of the blood pool on LGE because of circulating amyloid protein (**Fig. 9**).[83] Beyond the qualitative appearance of myocardial amyloidosis, Maceira and colleagues[83] demonstrated the potential for T1 mapping to quantify changes caused by amyloid protein.

LGE corresponding to other myocardial infiltrates such as those seen in glycogen storage disorders,[84] infection-related cardiomyopathies such as Chagas disease,[85] and muscular dystrophy-associated cardiomyopathies have each been described and remain active areas of investigation.[86]

We routinely perform the following tests in addition to cine and LGE as part of our undiagnosed cardiomyopathy CMR protocol, often used by the referring physician who has made the diagnosis of cardiomyopathy but has not ascribed a specific cause: T2* imaging for iron cardiomyopathy, aortic valve through-plane velocity-encoded cine, and arteriovenous valve through-plan velocity-encoded cine. The two velocity-encoded cines allow one to rapidly assess for valvular insufficiency or stenosis, with more detailed acquisitions dictated based on results of this survey. Hemochromatosis is the most common autosomal dominant condition in the Western world, and patients with secondary iron overload (such as that caused by chronic transfusions in diseases such as thalassemia) may develop cardiomyopathy independently of liver disease. In primary and secondary iron overload, serologic measures of iron homeostasis perform poorly compared with CMR[60] in identifying cardiac involvement. The acquisition and analysis are simple and can be done with a single breath-hold scan each in the coronal and mid-short axis planes, the former for hepatic iron quantification and the latter for myocardial iron quantification. T2* shortening leads to signal dropout at longer TE (**Fig. 10**). The resulting multi-echo data can be used to calculate T2* on a pixel-by-pixel basis and generate a T2* map. Iron cardiomyopathy should be considered if T2* is less than 20 msec at 1.5 T; normative

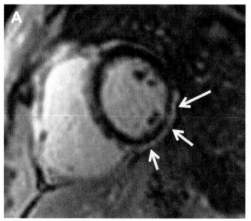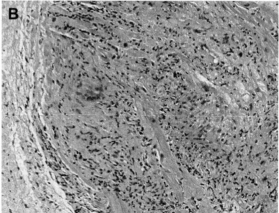

Fig. 8. Myocarditis in a 45-year-old man who presented with malaise, congestion, and ventricular tachycardia at 200 beats/min. There is hyperenhancement of the inferior and inferolateral walls (*arrows*) on late postgadolinium imaging (*A*). Subsequent endomyocardial biopsy showed extensive inflammatory infiltrates on hematoxylin and eosin staining (*B*).

A

B

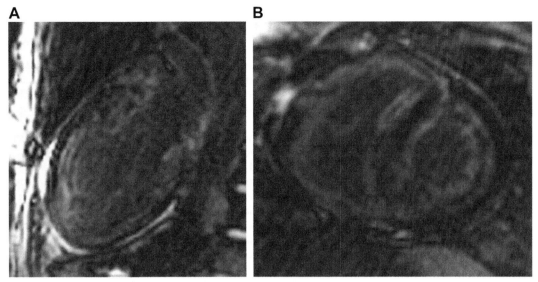

Fig. 9. Typical late postgadolinium enhancement imaging findings in a patient with cardiac amyloidosis. Note the subendocardial stripe of enhancement along with the dark signal intensity of the blood pool. These abnormalities are visible on vertical long-axis (A) and midventricular short-axis (B) views of the heart.

values have yet to be established at higher field strengths.

Much-maligned is CMR's role in diagnosing arrhythmogenic RV cardiomyopathy, a condition often suspected but rarely found in patients with ventricular arrhythmias. The tendency toward false-positive results with CMR results from variability in acquisition technique, undefined imaging findings at various points in the natural history of the disease, inappropriate use, and uncertainty in interpreting borderline imaging results. Most false-positive results arise from assigning pathologic fatty replacement based solely on noncontrast dark blood imaging of the myocardium with and without fat suppression. Studies incorporating LGE techniques to make the diagnosis[87] and

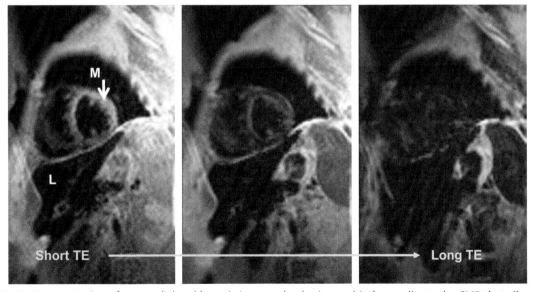

Fig. 10. Demonstration of myocardial and hepatic iron overload using multiecho gradient echo CMR that allows T2* quantification in tissues. Note that the liver (L) is dark even at the shortest TE and becomes even darker at longer TEs, whereas the myocardium (M) rapidly loses signal intensity at longer TEs as well. This patient presented with heart failure and a 15-year history of frequent blood transfusions for myelodysplasia.

review of histopathology[88] remind us that arrhythmogenic RV cardiomyopathy is really a disorder of fibro-fatty replacement and, to some extent, inflammation. Reliance exclusively on LGE without dark blood imaging may miss milder forms of the disease, underscoring the need for natural history studies using CMR and genetic or other confirmation. If compelled to do dark blood imaging with and without fat saturation in the CMR examination of the patient with ventricular arrhythmias or an arrhythmogenic RV cardiomyopathy family history, one is advised to carefully assess cine imaging for segmental RV abnormalities and LGE imaging for RV fibrosis before making the diagnosis.

With emergence of more robust T2-weighted imaging techniques,[59] demonstration of myocardial edema with CMR may hold significant appeal for patients with acute HF caused by myocarditis, offering insight into mechanisms of disease.[55] Not yet systematically explored is the potential for T2 imaging (and CMR in general) of posttransplant patients,[89] particularly where renal insufficiency caused by nephrotoxic immunosuppressive and other medications limit the use of gadolinium-based contrast agents. Also ripe for investigation is the assessment of LGE extent in patients referred for heart transplant consideration compared with commonly used endpoints, such as peak oxygen consumption; one may infer that extent of LGE, well established as inversely related to recovery of contractile function, might also have predictive value in determining survival without transplantation in end-stage patients.

Measurement of diastolic function with CMR in the HF examination currently depends on what technique is most frequently used and accurately quantified at a given center. Some sites favor mitral inflow and tissue velocity measurements using velocity-encoded cine acquisitions, with increasing evidence that quantification may be suitable for classification.[90] Others have incorporated routine performance of strain mapping, either with myocardial tagging[91] or displacement-encoded sensitivity imaging.[37]

MRA should be included in the evaluation of patients with cardiomyopathy caused by congenital heart disease and need not require contrast given excellent visualization of complex anatomy with whole-heart navigator-triggered techniques.[92] Other HF examinations that may incorporate MRA acquisitions include those for patients with bypass grafts being evaluated for suitability of internal mammary arteries for repeat revascularization procedures, because MRA performs well in visualizing these vessels and delineating existing conduit anatomy.[93]

THE ROLE OF CARDIOVASCULAR MAGNETIC RESONANCE IN HEART FAILURE EVALUATION AND MANAGEMENT

This article has presented extensive data to support the validity and unique ability of CMR to demonstrate cardiovascular structure and function and provide all of this information in such a way that it helps answer questions specific to the care of patients who have HF. These data would seem sufficient to support the use of CMR at least in the initial evaluation of patients with new-onset HF. As imaging comes under increasing scrutiny by payors, however, data on diagnostic value, prognostic validity, and accuracy in guiding treatment selection must be accompanied by data proving cost-effectiveness. Although considered an essential test in most centers where high-quality, dedicated teams perform CMR routinely for cardiomyopathy evaluation, cost-effectiveness analyses to date have not been performed at such centers of expertise. A prospective, randomized study in which patients who have new-onset HF are randomized to one of several initial diagnostic modalities has yet to be done. Until such a study is performed, one may consider existing data on reproducibility of CMR versus other modalities in patients who have HF.[23] Using quantitative measures such as LV volumes and ejection fraction that are routinely used in HF management, Grothues and colleagues showed considerably higher reproducibility for these endpoints. Considered from the perspective of clinical trial design, greater reproducibility in endpoints would afford sample size reductions of up to 95% by using CMR instead of echocardiography.

For individual patient analysis, consider the cost of uncertainty in serial assessment in, for instance, patients with severe aortic insufficiency in whom accurate, serial measurement of LV size is required to determine timing of valve replacement. Failure to detect a significant increase in LV end-systolic volume may delay appropriate valve surgery and increase patient care costs with continuing potentially ineffective medical therapies or worse, acute HF hospitalizations that might have been avoided with timely intervention. Such logic requires confirmation with rigorous cost-effectiveness analyses.

Consider the management of patients with Stages B through D HF,[3] which encompasses patients with structural heart disease with or without HF symptoms. First, to establish the presence of structural heart disease in Stage B patients requires accurate detection and quantification techniques. The clinician suspicious of structural heart disease typically starts with echocardiography, but CMR may be considered an alternative first-line choice to answer more specific myocardial questions, such as presence and extent of infiltrate or scar. If echo is used to determine need for CMR, inspecting the echocardiographic data helps gauge the need for CMR, particularly when poor acoustic window leaves essential questions regarding diagnosis and prognosis unanswered. Selecting appropriate patients for device therapy is especially important in Stage C HF.

Bleeker and colleagues[94] showed that simple presence or absence of posterolateral transmural scar by LGE performs well in distinguishing nonresponders from responders to cardiac resynchronization. Similar studies in selecting patients at risk for malignant arrhythmias could help refine patient selection for implantable cardiac defibrillators. Although well-established in determining likelihood of response to revascularization in ischemic heart disease,[95] CMR with LGE also performs well in predicting response to medical therapies such as beta-blockade in newly-diagnosed HF.[96] Before relegating Stage D patients to transplant evaluation or hospice, consider CMR with LGE for viability assessment. It may prove more cost-effective in the long-term, especially in the terminal stages of HF compared with prolonged, costly interventions that are unlikely to yield improvement in cardiac function. CMR also may yield insights as to underlying causes of disease that may have gone previously undetected.

The clinician understands that inaccurate or uncertain diagnosis of cause in HF may lead to prolonged courses of therapy that may be ineffective or even harmful. Conversely, precise initial diagnosis with CMR, particularly before deploying device therapies that may preclude examination with MR, can offer better selection of patients most likely to respond to interventions from medical to surgical to device therapies. Ultimately, incorporating CMR to reduce uncertainty in diagnosis and guide selection of beneficial therapies should help improve outcomes for patients who have HF.

REFERENCES

1. American Heart Association. Heart disease and stroke statistics: 2008 update. Dallas (TX): American Heart Association; 2008.
2. Redfield MM, Jacobsen SJ, Burnett JC, et al. Burden of systolic and diastolic ventricular dysfunction in the community: appreciating the scope of the heart failure epidemic. JAMA 2003;289(2):194–202.
3. Hunt SA, Abraham WT, Chin MH, et al. ACC/AHA 2005 guideline update for the diagnosis and management of chronic heart failure in the adult: a report of the American College of Cardiology/American Heart Association Task Force on Practice Guidelines (Writing Committee to Update the 2001 Guidelines for the Evaluation and Management of Heart Failure). Circulation 2005;112(12):e154–235.
4. Leier CV, Chatterjee K. The physical examination in heart failure. Part II. Congest Heart Fail 2007;13(2): 99–104.
5. Leier CV, Chatterjee K. The physical examination in heart failure. Part I. Congest Heart Fail 2007;13(1): 41–7.
6. McCrohon JA, Moon JCC, Prasad SK, et al. Differentiation of heart failure related to dilated cardiomyopathy and coronary artery disease using gadolinium-enhanced cardiovascular magnetic resonance. Circulation 2003;108(1):54–9.
7. Kass DA. Predicting cardiac resynchronization response by QRS duration: the long and short of it. J Am Coll Cardiol 2003;42(12):2125–7.
8. Collins SP, Lindsell CJ, Storrow AB, et al. Prevalence of negative chest radiography results in the emergency department patient with decompensated heart failure. Ann Emerg Med 2006;47(1):13–8.
9. Maisel AS, Krishnaswamy P, Nowak RM, et al. Rapid measurement of B-type natriuretic peptide in the emergency diagnosis of heart failure. N Engl J Med 2002;347(3):161–7.
10. Nemes A, Geleijnse ML, Krenning BJ, et al. Usefulness of ultrasound contrast agent to improve image quality during real-time three-dimensional stress echocardiography. Am J Cardiol 2007;99(2):275–8.
11. Di Carli MF, Maddahi J, Rokhsar S, et al. Long-term survival of patients with coronary artery disease and left ventricular dysfunction: implications for the role of myocardial viability assessment in management decisions. J Thorac Cardiovasc Surg 1998;116(6): 997–1004.
12. Schinkel AF, Poldermans D, Elhendy A, et al. Assessment of myocardial viability in patients with heart failure. J Nucl Med 2007;48(7):1135–46.
13. Gutberlet M, Frohlich M, Mehl S, et al. Myocardial viability assessment in patients with highly impaired left ventricular function: comparison of delayed enhancement, dobutamine stress MRI, end-diastolic wall thickness, and Tl201-SPECT with functional recovery after revascularization. Eur Radiol 2005; 15(5):872–80.
14. Cooper LT, Baughman KL, Feldman AM, et al. The role of endomyocardial biopsy in the management of cardiovascular disease: a scientific statement from the American Heart Association, the American College of Cardiology, and the European Society of Cardiology. Circulation 2007;116(19):2216–33.
15. Shields RC, Tazelaar HD, Berry GJ, et al. The role of right ventricular endomyocardial biopsy for idiopathic giant cell myocarditis. J Card Fail 2002;8(2): 74–8.

16. Binanay C, Califf RM, Hasselblad V, et al. Evaluation study of congestive heart failure and pulmonary artery catheterization effectiveness: the ESCAPE trial. JAMA 2005;294(13):1625–33.

17. Boyle A, Maurer MS, Sobotka PA. Myocellular and interstitial edema and circulating volume expansion as a cause of morbidity and mortality in heart failure. J Card Fail 2007;13(2):133–6.

18. Varnava AM, Elliott PM, Mahon N, et al. Relation between myocyte disarray and outcome in hypertrophic cardiomyopathy. Am J Cardiol 2001;88(3):275–9.

19. Delcayre C, Swynghedauw B. Molecular mechanisms of myocardial remodeling: the role of aldosterone. J Mol Cell Cardiol 2002;34(12):1577–84.

20. Struthers AD. Aldosterone-induced vasculopathy. Mol Cell Endocrinol 2004;217(1–2):239–41.

21. Frohlich ED. Fibrosis and ischemia: the real risks in hypertensive heart disease. Am J Hypertens 2001;14(6 Pt 2):194S–9S.

22. Grothues F, Moon JC, Bellenger NG, et al. Interstudy reproducibility of right ventricular volumes, function, and mass with cardiovascular magnetic resonance. Am Heart J 2004;147(2):218–23.

23. Grothues F, Smith G, Moon J, et al. Comparison of interstudy reproducibility of cardiovascular magnetic resonance with two-dimensional echocardiography in normal subjects and in patients with heart failure or left ventricular hypertrophy. Am J Cardiol 2002;90(1):29–34.

24. Pennell D. Ventricular volume and mass by CMR. J Cardiovasc Magn Reson 2002;4(4):507–13.

25. Carr JC, Simonetti O, Bundy J, et al. Cine MR angiography of the heart with segmented true fast imaging with steady-state precession. Radiology 2001;219(3):828–34.

26. Kellman P, Epstein FH, McVeigh ER. Adaptive sensitivity encoding incorporating temporal filtering (TSENSE). Magn Reson Med 2001;45(5):846–52.

27. Pruessmann KP, Weiger M, Boesiger P. Sensitivity encoded cardiac MRI. J Cardiovasc Magn Reson 2001;3(1):1–9.

28. Lee VS, Resnick D, Bundy JM, et al. Cardiac function: MR evaluation in one breath hold with real-time true fast imaging with steady-state precession. Radiology 2002;222(3):835–42.

29. Firmin DN, Nayler GL, Kilner PJ, et al. The application of phase shifts in NMR for flow measurement. Magn Reson Med 1990;14(2):230–41.

30. O'Donnell M. NMR blood flow imaging using multiecho, phase contrast sequences. Med Phys 1985;12(1):59–64.

31. Kondo C, Caputo GR, Semelka R, et al. Right and left ventricular stroke volume measurements with velocity-encoded cine MR imaging: in vitro and in vivo validation. AJR Am J Roentgenol 1991;157(1):9–16.

32. Firmin DN, Nayler GL, Klipstein RH, et al. In vivo validation of MR velocity imaging. J Comput Assist Tomogr 1987;11(5):751–6.

33. Hoeper MM, Tongers J, Leppert A, et al. Evaluation of right ventricular performance with a right ventricular ejection fraction thermodilution catheter and MRI in patients with pulmonary hypertension. Chest 2001;120(2):502–7.

34. Lee VS, Spritzer CE, Carroll BA, et al. Flow quantification using fast cine phase-contrast MR imaging, conventional cine phase-contrast MR imaging, and Doppler sonography: in vitro and in vivo validation. AJR Am J Roentgenol 1997;169(4):1125–31.

35. Jung B, Foll D, Bottler P, et al. Detailed analysis of myocardial motion in volunteers and patients using high-temporal-resolution MR tissue phase mapping. J Magn Reson Imaging 2006;24(5):1033–9.

36. Beerbaum P, Korperich H, Gieseke J, et al. Blood flow quantification in adults by phase-contrast MRI combined with SENSE: a validation study. J Cardiovasc Magn Reson 2005;7(2):361–9.

37. Aletras AH, Balaban RS, Wen H. High-resolution strain analysis of the human heart with fast-DENSE. J Magn Reson 1999;140(1):41–57.

38. Aletras AH, Ding S, Balaban RS, et al. DENSE: displacement encoding with stimulated echoes in cardiac functional MRI. J Magn Reson 1999;137(1):247–52.

39. Kim D, Gilson WD, Kramer CM, et al. Myocardial tissue tracking with two-dimensional cine displacement-encoded MR imaging: development and initial evaluation. Radiology 2004;230(3):862–71.

40. Wen H, Marsolo KA, Bennett E, et al. Adaptive postprocessing techniques for myocardial tissue tracking with displacement-encoded MRI. Radiology 2008;246(1):229–40.

41. Manning WJ, Atkinson DJ, Grossman W, et al. First-pass nuclear magnetic resonance imaging studies using gadolinium-DTPA in patients with coronary artery disease. J Am Coll Cardiol 1991;18(4):959–65.

42. Jekic M, Foster EL, Ballinger MR, et al. Cardiac function and myocardial perfusion immediately following maximal treadmill exercise inside the MRI room. J Cardiovasc Magn Reson 2008;10(1):3.

43. Bohl S, Wassmuth R, Abdel-Aty H, et al. Delayed enhancement cardiac magnetic resonance imaging reveals typical patterns of myocardial injury in patients with various forms of non-ischemic heart disease. Int J Cardiovasc Imaging 2008;24(6):597–607.

44. Mahrholdt H, Wagner A, Judd RM, et al. Delayed enhancement cardiovascular magnetic resonance assessment of non-ischaemic cardiomyopathies. Eur Heart J 2005;26(15):1461–74.

45. Rehwald WG, Fieno DS, Chen E-L, et al. Myocardial magnetic resonance imaging contrast agent

concentrations after reversible and irreversible ischemic injury. Circulation 2002;105(2):224–9.

46. Flacke SJ, Fischer SE, Lorenz CH. Measurement of the gadopentetate dimeglumine partition coefficient in human myocardium in vivo: normal distribution and elevation in acute and chronic infarction. Radiology 2001;218(3):703–10.

47. Daniel R, Messroghli DR, Walters K, et al. Myocardial T1 mapping: application to patients with acute and chronic myocardial infarction. Magn Reson Med 2007;58(1):34–40.

48. Simonetti OP, Kim RJ, Fieno DS, et al. An improved MR imaging technique for the visualization of myocardial infarction. Radiology 2001;218(1):215–23.

49. Chung YC, Simonetti OP, Kim RJ, et al. Infarct imaging in a single heart-beat. J Cardiovasc Magn Reson 2002;4(1):12–3.

50. Kellman P, Arai AE, McVeigh ER, et al. Phase-sensitive inversion recovery for detecting myocardial infarction using gadolinium-delayed hyperenhancement. Magn Reson Med 2002;47(2):372–83.

51. Bauner KUM, Muehling OM, Wintersperger BJM, et al. Inversion recovery single-shot TurboFLASH for assessment of myocardial infarction at 3 Tesla. Invest Radiol 2007;42(6):361–71.

52. Sparrow P, Messroghli DR, Reid S, et al. Myocardial T1 mapping for detection of left ventricular myocardial fibrosis in chronic aortic regurgitation: pilot study. AJR Am J Roentgenol 2006;187(6):W630–5.

53. Simonetti OP, Finn JP, White RD, et al. Black blood: T2-weighted inversion-recovery MR imaging of the heart. Radiology 1996;199(1):49–57.

54. Abdel-Aty H, Simonetti O, Friedrich MG. T2-weighted cardiovascular magnetic resonance imaging. J Magn Reson Imaging 2007;26(3):452–9.

55. Zagrosek A, Wassmuth R, Abdel-Aty H, et al. Relation between myocardial edema and myocardial mass during the acute and convalescent phase of myocarditis: a CMR study. J Cardiovasc Magn Reson 2008;10(1):19.

56. Schulz-Menger J, Wassmuth R, Abdel-Aty H, et al. Patterns of myocardial inflammation and scarring in sarcoidosis as assessed by cardiovascular magnetic resonance. Heart 2006;92(3):399–400.

57. Abdel-Aty H, Zagrosek A, Schulz-Menger J, et al. Delayed enhancement and T2-weighted cardiovascular magnetic resonance imaging differentiate acute from chronic myocardial infarction. Circulation 2004;109(20):2411–6.

58. Aletras AH, Kellman P, Derbyshire JA, et al. ACUT2E TSE-SSFP: a hybrid method for T2-weighted imaging of edema in the heart. Magn Reson Med 2008;59(2):229–35.

59. Kellman P, Aletras AH, Mancini C, et al. T2-prepared SSFP improves diagnostic confidence in edema imaging in acute myocardial infarction compared to turbo spin echo. Magn Reson Med 2007;57(5):891–7.

60. Anderson LJ, Holden S, Davis B, et al. Cardiovascular T2-star (T2*) magnetic resonance for the early diagnosis of myocardial iron overload. Eur Heart J 2001;22(23):2171–9.

61. Wood JC, Enriquez C, Ghugre N, et al. MRI R2 and R2* mapping accurately estimates hepatic iron concentration in transfusion-dependent thalassemia and sickle cell disease patients. Blood 2005;106(4):1460–5.

62. Neubauer S. The failing heart: an engine out of fuel. N Engl J Med 2007;356(11):1140–51.

63. Ten Hove M, Neubauer S. MR spectroscopy in heart failure: clinical and experimental findings. Heart Fail Rev 2007;12(1):48–57.

64. Ten Hove M, Neubauer S. The application of NMR spectroscopy for the study of heart failure. Curr Pharm Des 2008;14(18):1787–97.

65. Reingold JS, McGavock JM, Kaka S, et al. Determination of triglyceride in the human myocardium by magnetic resonance spectroscopy: reproducibility and sensitivity of the method. Am J Physiol Endocrinol Metab 2005;289(5):E935–9.

66. Szczepaniak LS, Dobbins RL, Metzger GJ, et al. Myocardial triglycerides and systolic function in humans: in vivo evaluation by localized proton spectroscopy and cardiac imaging. Magn Reson Med 2003;49(3):417–23.

67. Szczepaniak LS, Victor RG, Orci L, et al. Forgotten but not gone: the rediscovery of fatty heart, the most common unrecognized disease in America. Circ Res 2007;101(8):759–67.

68. Wu KC, Zerhouni EA, Judd RM, et al. Prognostic significance of microvascular obstruction by magnetic resonance imaging in patients with acute myocardial infarction. Circulation 1998;97(8):765–72.

69. Albert TS, Kim RJ, Judd RM. Assessment of no-reflow regions using cardiac MRI. Basic Res Cardiol 2006;101(5):383–90.

70. Panting JR, Gatehouse PD, Yang GZ, et al. Abnormal subendocardial perfusion in cardiac syndrome X detected by cardiovascular magnetic resonance imaging. N Engl J Med 2002;346(25):1948–53.

71. Marantz PR, Tobin JN, Wassertheil-Smoller S, et al. Prognosis in ischemic heart disease: can you tell as much at the bedside as in the nuclear laboratory? Arch Intern Med 1992;152(12):2433–7.

72. Lloyd SG, Buckberg GD. Use of cardiac magnetic resonance imaging in surgical ventricular restoration. Eur J Cardiothorac Surg 2006;29(Suppl 1):S216–24.

73. Moon JC, Reed E, Sheppard MN, et al. The histologic basis of late gadolinium enhancement cardiovascular magnetic resonance in hypertrophic cardiomyopathy. J Am Coll Cardiol 2004;43(12):2260–4.

74. Raman S, Sparks EA, Neff M, et al. Mid-myocardial fibrosis by cardiac magnetic resonance in patients with lamin A/C cardiomyopathy: possible substrate for diastolic dysfunction. J Cardiovasc Magn Reson 2007;9(6):907–13.

75. Keren A, Syrris P, McKenna WJ. Hypertrophic cardiomyopathy: the genetic determinants of clinical disease expression. Nat Clin Pract Cardiovasc Med 2008;5(3):158–68.

76. Maron BJ, Maron MS, Lesser JR, et al. Sudden cardiac arrest in hypertrophic cardiomyopathy in the absence of conventional criteria for high risk status. Am J Cardiol 2008;101(4):544–7.

77. Moon JC, Mogensen J, Elliott PM, et al. Myocardial late gadolinium enhancement cardiovascular magnetic resonance in hypertrophic cardiomyopathy caused by mutations in troponin I. Heart 2005;91(8):1036–40.

78. Dhoble A, Punnam SR, Abela GS. Likelihood of ventricular arrhythmias due to myocardial fibrosis in hypertrophic cardiomyopathy as detected by cardiac magnetic resonance imaging. J Am Coll Cardiol 2008;52(11):969.

79. Adabag AS, Maron BJ, Appelbaum E, et al. Occurrence and frequency of arrhythmias in hypertrophic cardiomyopathy in relation to delayed enhancement on cardiovascular magnetic resonance. J Am Coll Cardiol 2008;51(14):1369–74.

80. Mahrholdt H, Goedecke C, Wagner A, et al. Cardiovascular magnetic resonance assessment of human myocarditis: a comparison to histology and molecular pathology. Circulation 2004;109(10):1250–8.

81. Serra J, Monte G, Mello E, et al. Cardiac sarcoidosis evaluated by delayed-enhanced magnetic resonance imaging. Circulation 2003;107:e188–9.

82. Shimada T, Shimada K, Sakane T, et al. Diagnosis of cardiac sarcoidosis and evaluation of the effects of steroid therapy by gadolinium-DTPA-enhanced magnetic resonance imaging. Am J Med 2001; 110(7):520–7.

83. Maceira AM, Joshi J, Prasad SK, et al. Cardiovascular magnetic resonance in cardiac amyloidosis. Circulation 2005;111(2):186–93.

84. Moon JC, Sheppard M, Reed E, et al. The histological basis of late gadolinium enhancement cardiovascular magnetic resonance in a patient with Anderson-Fabry disease. J Cardiovasc Magn Reson 2006;8(3):479–82.

85. Rochitte CE, Oliveira PF, Andrade JM, et al. Myocardial delayed enhancement by magnetic resonance imaging in patients with Chagas' disease: a marker of disease severity. J Am Coll Cardiol 2005;46(8):1553–8.

86. Silva MC, Meira ZM, Gurgel Giannetti J, et al. Myocardial delayed enhancement by magnetic resonance imaging in patients with muscular dystrophy. J Am Coll Cardiol 2007;49(18):1874–9.

87. Tandri H, Saranathan M, Rodriguez ER, et al. Noninvasive detection of myocardial fibrosis in arrhythmogenic right ventricular cardiomyopathy using delayed-enhancement magnetic resonance imaging. J Am Coll Cardiol 2005;45(1):98–103.

88. Corrado D, Basso C, Thiene G, et al. Spectrum of clinicopathologic manifestations of arrhythmogenic right ventricular cardiomyopathy/dysplasia: a multicenter study. J Am Coll Cardiol 1997;30(6):1512–20.

89. Kim YJ, Kang SM, Hur J, et al. Images in cardiovascular medicine: chronic cardiac transplant rejection. Evaluation with magnetic resonance imaging. Circulation 2008;118(8):885–6.

90. Rathi VK, Doyle M, Yamrozik J, et al. Routine evaluation of left ventricular diastolic function by cardiovascular magnetic resonance: a practical approach. J Cardiovasc Magn Reson 2008;10(1):36.

91. Gotte MJ, Germans T, Russel IK, et al. Myocardial strain and torsion quantified by cardiovascular magnetic resonance tissue tagging: studies in normal and impaired left ventricular function. J Am Coll Cardiol 2006;48(10):2002–11.

92. Sorensen TS, Korperich H, Greil GF, et al. Operator-independent isotropic three-dimensional magnetic resonance imaging for morphology in congenital heart disease: a validation study. Circulation 2004; 110(2):163–9.

93. Stauder NI, Klumpp B, Stauder H, et al. Assessment of coronary artery bypass grafts by magnetic resonance imaging. Br J Radiol 2007;80(960):975–83.

94. Bleeker GB, Kaandorp TA, Lamb HJ, et al. Effect of posterolateral scar tissue on clinical and echocardiographic improvement after cardiac resynchronization therapy. Circulation 2006;113(7):969–76.

95. Kim RJ, Wu E, Rafael A, et al. The use of contrast-enhanced magnetic resonance imaging to identify reversible myocardial dysfunction. N Engl J Med 2000;343(20):1445–53.

96. Bello D, Shah DJ, Farah GM, et al. Gadolinium cardiovascular magnetic resonance predicts reversible myocardial dysfunction and remodeling in patients with heart failure undergoing beta-blocker therapy. Circulation 2003;108(16):1945–53.

Serial Assessment of Ventricular Morphology and Function

Frank Grothues, MD*, Ruediger Braun-Dullaeus, MD

KEYWORDS

- Magnetic resonance • Ventricular function
- Reproducibility • Ventricular remodeling • Heart failure

Cardiovascular magnetic resonance (CMR), with its versatility and ability to characterize soft tissue in conjunction with a lack of ionizing radiation, has evolved as a first line imaging tool for use in cases of several cardiac pathologies over the past decade.[1] One of the earliest applications of CMR was the assessment of cardiac morphology and cardiac function. The accurate and reproducible quantification of cardiac volumes, function, and mass constitute an elementary goal of any imaging modality. Although a single measurement of cardiac function can provide meaningful diagnostic and prognostic information, serial studies are essential to follow the course of the patient and the response to therapy. For assessing therapies in clinical trials, a highly reproducible technique is desirable. This review covers the current role of CMR in assessing morphologic and functional parameters in the context of heart failure, in the clinical and experimental settings.

THE IMPORTANCE OF MEASURING MORPHOLOGIC AND FUNCTIONAL PARAMETERS

Heart failure is the common final pathway of various heart diseases and is associated with a high rate of morbidity and a reduced quality of life. The incidence and prevalence in industrialized countries show a continuous rise as the result of higher life expectancy in an increasing proportion of the elderly population.[2] Primary or secondary cardiomyopathies, arterial hypertension, and coronary artery disease are the most common etiologies.[3]

A precise assessment of cardiac morphology and function allows an estimation of patients' rates of morbidity and mortality.[3-7] A reduced left ventricular (LV) ejection fraction has long been recognized as an independent predictor of adverse prognosis.[8,9] Furthermore, an increased LV mass is also associated with a higher mortality risk,[10-13] as are increased LV volumes.[8,9] In one postinfarction study, an enlarged end-systolic volume had an even greater predictive value for survival than a diminished ejection fraction.[8] Besides its use in estimating prognoses, LV function parameters are additionally used for therapeutic planning. For example, the main criteria for cardiac resynchronization therapy (CRT) using biventricular pacing[14,15] or the prevention of sudden cardiac death using implantable cardioverter defibrillators (ICD)[16-18] are largely based on the LV ejection fraction.

Another relevant aspect in patients who have heart failure is the ability to reliably detect deterioration of ventricular function over time, which enables timely planning of measures such as implantation of ventricular assist devices and heart transplantation. For this purpose, reproducible, noninvasive assessment of ventricular function is of pivotal importance.

Over the past decade, greater attention has also been paid to the contribution of right ventricular (RV) failure to morbidity and mortality associated with left-heart failure and pulmonary hypertension.[19,20] RV ejection fraction itself is an independent prognostic factor and provides additional clinical information.[21-23] Interestingly, even RV size alone seems to have a prognostic significance

Otto-von-Guericke-University, Magdeburg, Germany
* Corresponding author. Department of Cardiology, Otto-von-Guericke-University, Leipziger Strasse 44, D-39120 Magdeburg, Germany.
E-mail address: frank.grothues@med.ovgu.de (F. Grothues).

Heart Failure Clin 5 (2009) 301–314
doi:10.1016/j.hfc.2009.02.007

because patients with heart failure and similar degrees of LV and RV dilatation show worse clinical outcomes than do patients with disproportionate dilatation of the left ventricle (LV > RV).[24–26] Assessment of RV volume and function using conventional two-dimensional imaging techniques has long been hindered by the complex shape of the right ventricle, which made application of geometric models for quantification almost impossible. In contrast, tomographic imaging techniques such as CMR or CT do not suffer from this limitation and are, therefore, ideally suited.[27]

WAYS TO MEASURE VENTRICULAR VOLUMES, MASS, AND EJECTION FRACTION USING CARDIOVASCULAR MAGNETIC RESONANCE

A rapid assessment of global LV size and function can be performed from the long axis views (four- and two-chamber views), and similar to two-dimensional echocardiography (2DE), volume calculations using monoplane or biplane area-length formulas are based on geometric assumptions (elliptical geometry) and are therefore only accurate for normal-shaped ventricles.[28] This approach sacrifices the advantage of CMR to acquire complete volume data sets using multislice short-axis imaging, which represents a far more accurate method for quantification of volume and ejection fraction.[28–30] For the latter, a stack of contiguous short-axis slices is positioned on a diastolic four-chamber-view image at end-expiration, with the first slice positioned at the atrioventricular ring and the last slice covering the apex. When using conventional techniques, each short-axis slice is then acquired during one short breath-hold in expiration, which has been shown to set the diaphragm in a more reproducible position than at any other point in the respiratory cycle.[31] Depending on heart size, usually a total of eight to 13 short-axis slices are needed to encompass the entire left and right ventricle.[32] Although the use of a stack of transverse slices through the ventricle eases the definition of the mitral valve plane,[33] it has been shown to be subject of considerable partial-volume effects, thereby abolishing this advantage.

Image analysis of quality images is relatively straightforward and usually performed using commercial software with semiautomated contour detection or by manual tracing of the RV and LV epicardial and endocardial borders at end-diastole (first cine phase of the R-wave-triggered acquisition) and end-systole (**Fig. 1**). The end-systolic phase is visually determined as being the one with the smallest cavity area. This allows for the calculation of LV mass, LV end-diastolic volume, and LV end-systolic volume, from which

LV stroke volume and ejection fraction are derived. The calculated stroke volume reflects the total stroke volume of the left ventricle, which in case of concomitant mitral or aortic regurgitation does not equal the effective forward stroke volume. Forward stroke volume can be accurately calculated using phase contrast blood flow velocity measurements taken in the ascending aorta just above the aortic valve.

For LV mass calculation, the myocardial volume at end-diastole is multiplied by the specific density of myocardium (approximately 1.05 g/cm^3).[34] The papillary muscles are consistently either included in the mass or included in the volume. Most CMR institutions add the papillary muscles and heavy trabeculations to the myocardial mass. RV parameters are obtained in a manner similar to that used in the left ventricle.

Inclusion of endocardial trabeculations to the myocardial mass in end-systole but not in end-diastole can contribute to small measurement errors. The most difficult task, however, is to correctly identify the most basal short-axis slice. Because of the large area of this basal slice, failure in doing so will result in considerable measurement errors. Advanced analysis software, which traces the ventricular insertion points of the mitral valve in long-axis views during the cardiac cycle, can help to overcome this difficulty. In normally contracting ventricles, a systolic descent of the atrioventricular ring of approximately 10 mm occurs, but in poorly contracting ventricles, this downward motion may be blunted or completely abolished. Another source of error is the misregistration of slices resulting from different diaphragm positions between serial breath-holds. Image artifacts from implanted artificial heart valves and electrocardiographic gating problems can further compromise endocardial and epicardial border delineation.

To enhance the reproducibility, especially in the serial assessment of a single patient over time, the baseline examination should be on screen for direct image comparison and consistency in defining the most basal slice and the endocardial contours.

For many years, ECG-gated gradient recalled echo (GRE)–based pulse sequences were used for cardiac volumetry,[35–37] but in most cases today, steady-state free precession (SSFP) techniques[38] with high spatial and temporal resolution are applied.[39–42] SSFP images provide an excellent contrast-to-noise ratio between blood and myocardium, with a high signal-to-noise ratio, which, in contrast to images in GRE sequences, is independent of inflow of unsaturated blood.[43] Therefore, nowadays, the administration of contrast agents to enhance the signal of blood independent of flow[44] is not needed.

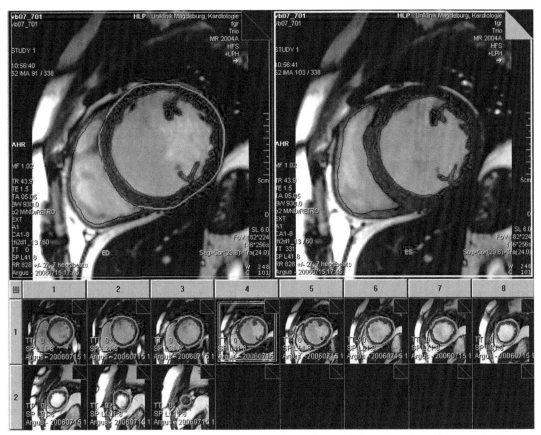

Fig. 1. Volumetric analysis of short-axis SSFP cine images of a patient who has dilated cardiomyopathy. Endocardial (*red* for the LV and *dark red* for the RV) and left epicardial (*green*) borders are traced in end-diastole (*left*) and end-systole (*right*; only endocardial borders). LV end-diastolic and end-systolic volumes amounted to 434 mL and 346 mL, LV ejection fraction was 20%, and left myocardial mass added up to 233 g. RV end-diastolic and end-systolic volumes were 187 mL and 116 mL, which resulted in a RV ejection fraction of 38%.

On 1.5 Tesla systems, a slice thickness of 6 to 8 mm (with a 2- to 4-mm slice gap) seems to represent an adequate compromise between acquisition time, reduction of partial volume effects, and maintenance of a sufficient signal-to-noise ratio. The advent of parallel imaging[45–47] has significantly sped up image acquisition so that even patients who have advanced heart failure are able to cope with the short breath-hold times required.[48–50] Alternatively, the use of a free-breathing navigator technique has also been successful.[51] Nowadays, even real-time imaging with reduced temporal and spatial resolution is feasible, which can be helpful in cases of arrhythmias such as atrial fibrillation.[52]

ACCURACY OF CARDIOVASCULAR MAGNETIC RESONANCE MEASUREMENTS

The accuracy of CMR for LV volume and mass measurements was proved long ago, in ventricular casts,[29,53] animal models,[54–58] and humans,[30,34,59–61] using various forms of the older GRE technique. Likewise, RV volumes[62,63] and mass[64,65] have been validated.

Using the newer SSFP sequence, investigators conducted several animal studies that validated its accuracy in LV and RV mass determination.[66,67] When GRE and SSFP techniques were applied subsequently, in vivo SSFP imaging consistently resulted in larger LV volumes, smaller LV mass, and similar LV ejection fraction.[39,40,68–71] These results have led to separate normal values for SSFP[72–74] and GRE[72,75] techniques.

REPRODUCIBILITY OF CARDIOVASCULAR MAGNETIC RESONANCE MEASUREMENTS

The main strength of CMR is its low intraobserver and interobserver variability.[39,40,54,70,76] Moreover, the interstudy variability is very low, which demonstrates that CMR has the highest reproducibility of all imaging techniques. Also, CMR has shown excellent interstudy reproducibility of LV volumes, function, and mass.[76–84] Several studies have demonstrated the superiority of CMR over 2DE.[59,77,82] For instance, in a direct comparison of 2DE and CMR, considerably lower coefficients of variability were found for end-diastolic (3.7% versus 8.7%, $P = .17$) and end-systolic volumes (6.2% versus 17.3%, $P<.001$), ejection fraction (3.7% versus 11.5%, $P<.001$), and mass (3.9% versus 14.2%, $P<.001$).[77]

Bottini and colleagues[59] were the first to show the impact of a high interstudy reproducibility on planning for sample size in interventional trials. To prove a 10-g decrease in myocardial mass with antihypertensive treatment (80% power, $P = 0.05$) one would require 505 patients with 2DE, compared with only 14 patients using CMR. Similarly, using 2DE and CMR reproducibility data acquired on the same study population, the authors and their colleagues showed a decrease in sample size of 74%, 83%, 87%, and 90% to detect a 10-mL change in end-diastolic and end-systolic volume, a 3% absolute change in ejection fraction, and a 10g change in LV mass, respectively (90% power, $P = 0.05$).[77]

The interstudy reproducibility of quantitative RV measurements was examined in one large study.[85] In comparison with the LV data from the same study population,[77] RV reproducibility values were similar, but generally somewhat lower.

CARDIOVASCULAR MAGNETIC RESONANCE FOR STRUCTURE AND FUNCTION IN HEART FAILURE—WHAT DO THE GUIDELINES SAY?

Several scientific statements have addressed the value of CMR in the evaluation of patients who have heart failure. The 2001 European Society of Cardiology guidelines on heart failure[86] were the first to recommended CMR "if other imaging techniques have not provided a satisfactory diagnostic answer." In that group's 2005 guidelines update, CMR is described as a "versatile, highly accurate, and reproducible imaging technique for the assessment of LV and RV volumes, global function, regional wall motion, myocardial thickness, thickening, myocardial mass, and cardiac valves. . . . However, CMR is expensive, a relatively rare resource and, in term of practical management of most patients with heart failure, it has not been shown to be superior to echocardiography."[87] The Consensus Panel report of the Society of Cardiovascular Magnetic Resonance and the Working Group on Cardiovascular Magnetic Resonance of the European Society of Cardiology[1] have assigned CMR a Class I

indication for the assessment of global ventricular (left and right) function and mass. The newest statement with regard to the appropriateness of CMR in cases of different cardiac pathologies was jointly published in 2006 by eight different societies.[88] Although the general role of CMR was judged as uncertain in the evaluation of LV function following myocardial infarction or in patients who had heart failure, CMR was found to be an appropriate imaging technique in patients from whom technically limited images were obtained using echocardiographic techniques and in cases in which there is discordant information that is clinically significant from prior tests.[88] Likewise, the 2006 Heart Failure Society of America's practice guidelines[89] state that "in patients whose echocardiographic imaging is unsatisfactory, other techniques such as radionuclide ventriculography, cardiac magnetic resonance imaging or computed tomography may be used."

CARDIOVASCULAR MAGNETIC RESONANCE AND LEFT VENTRICULAR REMODELING POST INFARCTION

The term "ventricular remodeling" is generally used for the description of changes in ventricular function and structure related to various causes. A more detailed definition has been proposed by a consensus panel as the "genomic expression resulting in molecular, cellular and interstitial changes that are manifested clinically as changes in size, shape and function of the heart after cardiac injury."[90] LV remodeling after myocardial infarction occurs in response to the ischemic injury, with subsequent loss of myocytes (**Fig. 2**). During the repair phase after the initial injury, infarct expansion with thinning of the affected myocardial segment and increase in its endocardial surface area can occur.[91] The resultant increase in ventricular size also affects the remote myocardium because of increased wall stress, with hypertrophy of mycoytes.[92,93] The degree of dilation in remote regions has been shown to correlate to initial infarct size,[94] and late increase in cardiac size is mainly due to elongation of the noninfarcted segments rather than due to further infarct expansion.[95] As mentioned previously, the left ventricle (end-diastolic and end-systolic volumes) increase in size after myocardial infarction increases the risk of heart failure and correlates with increased rates of mortality.[8]

Hence, an accurate quantification of LV size and function is of importance in determining the prognosis and monitoring the patient's response to medical and interventional therapy. Investigators have stated that CMR is the ideal technique to

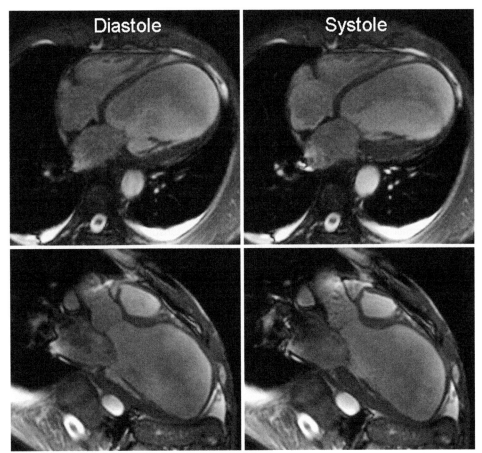

Fig. 2. CMR of a patient who had extensive ventricular remodeling several years after a large anterior myocardial infarction with occlusion of the proximal left anterior descending artery leading to considerable LV enlargement and highly impaired ejection fraction. SSFP cine images in the four-chamber view (*upper panel*) and three-chamber view (*lower panel*) in diastole and systole are shown.

monitor this remodeling process in a serial manner, both in animal models[96–98] and in humans.[99,100]

Of special importance in cases of ischemic cardiomyopathy, CMR allows a qualitative (visual inspection of cines) and accurately quantitative (measurement of wall motion and thickening)[101–105] assessment of regional LV contractile function, in addition to global measures of ventricular size and function. By the use of the tagging technique,[106] which has been validated against invasive sonomicrometer studies,[107] myocardial strain as a measure of contractility can be evaluated.[106,108] Tagging data can be fully resolved in three dimensions to cover the entire heart[109,110] and allow a comprehensive evaluation of circumferential and longitudinal function. Tagging was used in the evaluation of postinfarction remodeling[97,100,111,112] and was used to discriminate infarcted from remote myocardium.[113] Because

analysis of tagging images is cumbersome and requires dedicated software, its use so far has been mainly limited to research purposes.

CMR spectroscopy can be used to study metabolic alterations within remodeled myocardium,[114] but a further discussion of this technique is beyond the scope of this article. The increasing role of contrast-enhanced imaging of myocardial infarction,[115] its potential in assessing the remodeling process, and its prognostic relevance are discussed elsewhere in this issue.

ROLE OF CARDIOVASCULAR MAGNETIC RESONANCE FOR THE EVALUATION OF THERAPEUTIC MEASURES

As mentioned earlier in this article, because its superior interstudy reproducibility, CMR is ideally suited for the evaluation of pharmacologic and interventional therapies in clinical and animal studies of heart failure or postinfarction remodeling. Up to now, numerous experimental[98,116–121] and clinical[122–133] studies have been conducted that have used CMR measurements as surrogate endpoints in such settings. Whereas past clinical trials using 2DE have needed to include several hundred subjects to demonstrate significant treatment effects, when using CMR relatively small-sized study groups were able to be used to generate such results. For example, Groenning and colleagues[131] proved the reverse remodeling effects of the β-blocker metoprolol using only 41 patients in a randomized, placebo-controlled, and double-blind substudy to the Metoprolol CR/XL Randomized Intervention Trial in Heart Failure (MERIT-HF). The small sample size needed when using CMR is of utmost importance, especially in circumstances in which rare pathologies and gene interactions are to be studied[134,135] or in which the therapeutic regimen is expensive and complex, as in stem cell therapy.[129,130]

For pharmaceutical companies conducting clinical trials, the reduced sample size when using CMR translates into substantial cost savings because of reduced hospital and physician fees and fewer internal monitoring and organizing costs. Adding to this, enrollment in smaller-sized trials can be completed faster and drugs might be brought to market earlier.

ALTERNATIVE IMAGING METHODS IN HEART FAILURE
Two-Dimensional Echocardiography

The most frequently used technique for assessment of heart size and function is 2DE. It is widely available, relatively cheap, safe, and mobile, and is performed in real time,[136] but image acquisition depends on the operator and the acoustic window. The quantification of LV volumes, mass, and ejection fraction relies on geometric assumptions that do not apply to ventricles undergoing asymmetric cardiac remodeling, such as in cases of cardiomyopathies.[137–139] Both the area-length method and the modified Simpson's rule rely on good definition of the entire endocardial border, which can be impossible in up to 31% of patients.[139] Therefore, in clinical settings, LV ejection fraction is often visually estimated and an experienced examiner can provide clinically valid estimates.[140]

Although reproducibility of quantitative 2DE measurements is reasonably good in cases of normal ventricles,[141] it is often inadequate in cases of dilated and deformed hearts.[77] In one study that assessed myocardial mass measurements using the older M-mode echocardiography for 74 patients that resulted in interpretable images,

Gottdiener and colleagues[142] found a 95% confidence interval (59 g), which in their opinion "precludes its use to measure changes in mass of the magnitude likely to occur with therapy" because the average change of mass in most antihypertensive therapy trials is from 20 to 40 g/y. In a similar study by Myerson and colleagues,[143] in 212 male army recruits, 95% confidence intervals were ± 46.3 g using 2DE with the area-length formula and ± 57.6 g using the M-mode technique. Using the LV ejection fraction, the coefficient of variation was between 11.5% and 15%.[77,144] Nonetheless, current guidelines list repeated 2DE as a class I indication for patients who have heart failure.[145]

In comparison, the left-heart quantification of RV size and function parameters is even more limited when using 2DE because the complex shape of the right ventricle makes geometric modeling based on formulas barely impossible.

Three-Dimensional Echocardiography

Transthoracic three-dimensional echocardiography (3DE) is a promising imaging modality that resolves some limitations of the two-dimensional approach by removing the need for geometric assumptions.[28,146–148] Validation has been performed against autopsy volumes[149] and CMR,[146–148,150–152] and it showed a good correlation with those techniques. Likewise, cross-sectional comparisons of 3DE, 2DE, and CMR showed less interobserver variability[151] and less variation between repeated studies for 3DE than for 2DE.[150,153] In a longitudinal study of 50 patients who had healed infarction, both CMR and 3DE detected a significant change in LV end-diastolic volumes over time that was unrecognized using 2DE.[154] Moreover, in a study of biplane 2DE and volumetric echocardiography and CMR, results of the biplane method assigned up to 40% of patients to different categories according to the LV ejection fraction when compared with results of CMR. However, the results of 3DE and CMR were in correlation and produced similar results with regard to patient stratification according to LV ejection fraction.[28]

Despite advances in 3DE, problems with image quality persist in a subset of patients and the field of view of a "full-volume" dataset may be insufficient to cover the LV of enlarged hearts. Imaging and quantification of the RV remains challenging.[155]

CT

CT uses the same volumetric approach as CMR and offers a comparable level of accuracy for quantitative measurements.[156–159] The need for intravenous contrast agents and the radiation exposure are major drawbacks and limit its use for patients who have impaired renal function, allergies to iodine, hyperthyroid function, and for patients who have to undergo serial testing. However, in patients with contraindications for CMR (eg, having a pacemaker or ICD), it may constitute a useful alternative imaging modality.

Nuclear Cardiology

Measurement of LV and RV function has previously been performed using radionuclide ventriculography, but relatively low spatial and temporal resolution, problems in measuring volumes, and the impossibility of measuring mass present major limitations. In most cases today, gated-perfusion single-photon-emission CT (SPECT) data are used. Although they can provide additional information for myocardial perfusion studies,[160,161] sole-ventricular function studies are rarely performed. They have been shown to have good accuracy[162] and reproducibility.[163] However, low spatial resolution, attenuation, and border definition in thinned, infarcted regions with low radionuclide counts remain problematic, especially in patients who have had heart failure. Furthermore, ejection fraction is most often determined after stress, and persistent stunning of ischemic segments can lead to an underestimation of resting ejection fraction.[163] Adding to this, the repeated radiation exposure makes serial follow-up studies in the individual patient and their use in research trials problematic. PET[164] offers no advantages with regard to functional studies of the LV, is less widely available, and is more expensive.

LIMITATIONS OF CARDIOVASCULAR MAGNETIC RESONANCE

CMR used to suffer from long scanning times in the past, but improved scanner technology and the advent of faster scanning techniques such as parallel imaging have shortened acquisition times considerably. In conjunction with refinements of analysis software, today a quantitative assessment of cardiac shape, size, and function can be performed in less than 20 minutes. Still, especially in comparison with 2DE, CMR is a more expensive and less widely available imaging technique. However, experience with CMR is growing fast, and cost is expected to fall. The increase in the number of patients who have implanted devices such as cardiac pacemakers and ICDs poses an incremental challenge for those using CMR. Although patients who have had heart failure and who use ICDs or CRT devices are members of a target population who need accurate and reproducible serial follow-up of cardiac size and function, patients in this population should at present not be examined using CMR. Although recent reports suggest a relaxation of this contraindication in the future,[165,166] such a change will necessitate the development of magnetic resonance–safe electrical cardiac devices that can be used to safely study this growing patient population by using CMR.

Arrhythmias such as ventricular ectopic beats or atrial fibrillation are frequent among patients who have had heart failure and can hinder high-quality image acquisition. Faster scanning sequences, up to real-time imaging techniques, can help to overcome this problem.

The examination of patients who have claustrophobia requires sedation, but their anxiety may be alleviated by the use of open-bore MRI scanners that are now available with field strengths up to 1.0 Tesla. Patients who have orthopnea are still difficult to image, and certainly CMR will never become a bedside technique.

SUMMARY

CMR is an accurate, highly reproducible, and well-validated technique for measuring LV and RV volumes, function, and mass, and thus represents the widely accepted current reference standard. The high interstudy reproducibility of measurements makes CMR an ideal tool for monitoring therapeutic effects in interventional trials. In patients who have had heart failure, it is helpful for the initial assessment and longitudinal follow-up. In addition to global function, regional myocardial function can also be studied. Information on structural changes can provide a first hint to the etiology of heart failure, and a functional study can be complemented with the use of additional techniques such as tissue characterization using contrast agents for further clarification within the same scanning session. It is this versatility that makes CMR favored for the study of heart failure and ventricular remodeling compared with the competing modalities of CT and 3DE.

REFERENCES

1. Pennell DJ, Sechtem UP, Higgins CB, et al. Clinical indications for cardiovascular magnetic resonance (CMR): consensus panel report. Eur Heart J 2004; 25(21):1940–65.
2. Kannel WB. Incidence and epidemiology of heart failure. Heart Fail Rev 2000;5(2):167–73.

3. Levy D, Kenchaiah S, Larson MG, et al. Long-term trends in the incidence of and survival with heart failure. N Engl J Med 2002;347(18):1397–402.

4. Spencer FA, Meyer TE, Goldberg RJ, et al. Twenty year trends (1975–1995) in the incidence, in-hospital and long-term death rates associated with heart failure complicating acute myocardial infarction: a community-wide perspective. J Am Coll Cardiol 1999;34(5):1378–87.

5. Spencer FA, Meyer TE, Gore JM, et al. Heterogeneity in the management and outcomes of patients with acute myocardial infarction complicated by heart failure: the National Registry of Myocardial Infarction. Circulation 2002;105(22):2605–10.

6. Ho KK, Anderson KM, Kannel WB, et al. Survival after the onset of congestive heart failure in Framingham Heart Study subjects. Circulation 1993; 88(1):107–15.

7. Muiesan ML, Salvetti M, Monteduro C, et al. Left ventricular concentric geometry during treatment adversely affects cardiovascular prognosis in hypertensive patients. Hypertension 2004;43(4): 731–8.

8. White HD, Norris RM, Brown MA, et al. Left ventricular end-systolic volume as the major determinant of survival after recovery from myocardial infarction. Circulation 1987;76(1):44–51.

9. Otterstad JE, St. John Sutton MG, Froeland GS, et al. Prognostic value of two-dimensional echocardiography and N-terminal proatrial natriuretic peptide following an acute myocardial infarction. Eur Heart J 2002;23(13):1011–20.

10. Schillaci G, Verdecchia P, Porcellati C, et al. Continuous relation between left ventricular mass and cardiovascular risk in essential hypertension. Hypertension 2000;35(2):580–6.

11. Levy D, Garrison R, Savage D, et al. Prognostic implications of echocardiographically determined left ventricular mass in Framingham Heart Study. N Engl J Med 1990;322(22):1561–6.

12. Haider AW, Larson MG, Benjamin EJ. Increased left ventricular mass and hypertrophy are associated with increased risk for sudden death. J Am Coll Cardiol 1998;32(5):1454–9.

13. Koren MJ, Devereux RB, Casale PN, et al. Relation of left ventricular mass and geometry to morbidity and mortality in uncomplicated essential hypertension. Ann Intern Med 1991;114(5):345–52.

14. Bristow MR, Saxon LA, Boehmer J, et al. Cardiac-resynchronization therapy with or without an implantable defibrillator in advanced chronic heart failure. N Engl J Med 2004;350(21): 2140–50.

15. Cleland JG, Daubert JC, Erdmann E, et al. The effect of cardiac resynchronization on morbidity and mortality in heart failure. N Engl J Med 2005; 352(15):1539–49.

16. Moss AJ, Hall WJ, Cannom DS, et al. Improved survival with an implanted defibrillator in patients with coronary disease at high risk for ventricular arrhythmia. N Engl J Med 1996;335(26):1933–40.

17. Moss AJ, Zareba W, Hall WJ, et al. Prophylactic implantation of a defibrillator in patients with myocardial infarction and reduced ejection fraction. N Engl J Med 2002;346(12):877–83.

18. Bardy GH, Lee KL, Mark DB, et al. Amiodarone or an implantable cardioverter-defibrillator for congestive heart failure. N Engl J Med 2005; 352(3):225–37.

19. Mahmud M, Champion HC. Right ventricular failure complicating heart failure: pathophysiology, significance, and management strategies. Curr Cardiol Rep 2007;9(3):200–8.

20. Zakir RM, Al-Dehneh A, Maher J, et al. Right ventricular failure in patients with preserved ejection fraction and diastolic dysfunction: an underrecognized clinical entity. Congest Heart Fail 2007; 13(3):164–9.

21. Polak JF, Holman BL, Wynne J, et al. Right ventricular ejection fraction: an indicator of increased mortality in patients with congestive heart failure associated with coronary artery disease. J Am Coll Cardiol 1983;2(2):217–24.

22. Di Salvo TG, Mathier M, Semigran MJ, et al. Preserved right ventricular ejection fraction predicts exercise capacity and survival in advanced heart failure. J Am Coll Cardiol 1995; 25(5):1143–53.

23. de Groote P, Millaire A, Foucher-Hossein C, et al. Right ventricular ejection fraction is an independent predictor of survival in patients with moderate heart failure. J Am Coll Cardiol 1998;32(4):948–54.

24. Lewis JF, Webber JD, Sutton LL, et al. Discordance in degree of right and left ventricular dilation in patients with dilated cardiomyopathy: recognition and clinical implications. J Am Coll Cardiol 1993; 21(3):649–54.

25. Sun JP, James KB, Yang XS, et al. Comparison of mortality rates and progression of left ventricular dysfunction in patients with idiopathic dilated cardiomyopathy and dilated versus nondilated right ventricular cavities. Am J Cardiol 1997; 80(12):1583–7.

26. Ghio S, Gavazzi A, Campana C, et al. Independent and additive prognostic value of right ventricular systolic function and pulmonary artery pressure in patients with chronic heart failure. J Am Coll Cardiol 2001;37(1):183–8.

27. Rominger MB, Bachmann GF, Pabst W, et al. Right ventricular volumes and ejection fraction with fast cine MR imaging in breath-hold technique: applicability, normal values from 52 volunteers, and evaluation of 325 adult cardiac patients. J Magn Reson Imaging 1999;10(6):908–18.

28. Chuang ML, Hibberd MG, Salton CJ, et al. Importance of imaging method over imaging modality in noninvasive determination of left ventricular volumes and ejection fraction: assessment by two- and three-dimensional echocardiography and magnetic resonance imaging. J Am Coll Cardiol 2000;35(2):477–84.

29. Rehr RB, Malloy CR, Filipchuk NG, et al. Left ventricular volumes measured by MR imaging. Radiology 1985;156(3):717–9.

30. Longmore DB, Klipstein RH, Underwood SR, et al. Dimensional accuracy of magnetic resonance in studies of the heart. Lancet 1985;1(8442):1360–2.

31. Taylor AM, Jhooti P, Wiesmann F, et al. MR navigator-echo monitoring of temporal changes in diaphragm position: Implications for MR coronary angiography. J Magn Reson Imaging 1997;7(4):629–36.

32. Bellenger NG, Francis JM, Davies CL, et al. Establishment and performance of a magnetic resonance cardiac function clinic. J Cardiovasc Magn Reson 2000;2(1):15–22.

33. Buser PT, Auffermann W, Holt WW, et al. Noninvasive evaluation of global left ventricular function with use of cine nuclear magnetic resonance. J Am Coll Cardiol 1989;13(6):1294–300.

34. Katz J, Milliken MC, Stray-Gundersen J, et al. Estimation of human myocardial mass with MR imaging. Radiology 1988;169(2):495–8.

35. Frahm J, Haase A, Matthaei D. Rapid NMR imaging of dynamic processes using the FLASH technique. Magn Reson Med 1986;3(2):321–7.

36. Haase A, Matthaei D, Hanicke W, et al. Dynamic digital subtraction imaging using fast low-angle shot MR movie sequence. Radiology 1986;160(2):537–41.

37. Atkinson DJ, Edelman R. Cineangiography of the heart in a single breath hold with a segmented Turbo-FLASH sequence. Radiology 1991;178(2):357–60.

38. Oppelt A, Graumann R, Barfuss H. FISP: a new fast MRI sequence. Elektromedica 1986;54:15–8.

39. Moon JC, Lorenz CH, Francis JM, et al. Breath-hold FLASH and FISP cardiovascular MR imaging: left ventricular volume differences and reproducibility. Radiology 2002;223(3):789–97.

40. Plein S, Bloomer TN, Ridgway JP, et al. Steady-state free precession magnetic resonance imaging of the heart: comparison with segmented k-space gradient-echo imaging. J Magn Reson Imaging 2001;14(3):230–6.

41. Thiele H, Nagel E, Paetsch I, et al. Functional cardiac MR imaging with steady-state free precession (SSFP) significantly improves endocardial boarder delineation without contrast agents. J Magn Reson Imaging 2001;14(4):362–7.

42. Alfakih K, Thiele H, Plein S, et al. Comparison of right ventricular volume measurement between segmented k-space gradient-echo and steady-state free precession magnetic resonance imaging. J Magn Reson Imaging 2002;16(3):253–8.

43. Schär M, Kozerke S, Fischer SE, et al. Cardiac SSFP imaging at 3 Tesla. Magn Reson Med 2004;51(4):799–806.

44. Bunce NH, Moon JC, Bellenger NG, et al. Improved cine cardiovascular magnetic resonance using Clariscan (NC100150 injection). J Cardiovasc Magn Reson 2001;3(4):303–10.

45. Pruessmann KP, Weiger M, Scheidegger MB, et al. SENSE: sensitivity encoding for fast MRI. Magn Reson Med 1999;42(5):952–62.

46. Weiger M, Pruessmann KP, Boesiger P. Cardiac real-time imaging using SENSE, SENSitivity Encoding scheme. Magn Reson Med 2000;43(2):177–84.

47. Sodickson DK, Manning WJ. Simultaneous acquisition of spatial harmonics (SMASH): fast imaging with radiofrequency coil arrays. Magn Reson Med 1997;38(4):591–603.

48. Wintersperger BJ, Nikolaou K, Dietrich O, et al. Single breath-hold real-time cine MR imaging: improved temporal resolution using generalized autocalibrating partially parallel acquisition (GRAPPA) algorithm. Eur Radiol 2003;13(8):1931–6.

49. Reeder SB, Wintersperger BJ, Dietrich O, et al. Practical approaches to the evaluation of signal-to-noise ratio performance with parallel imaging: application with cardiac imaging and a 32-channel cardiac coil. Magn Reson Med 2005;54(3):748–54.

50. Jung BA, Hennig J, Scheffler K. Single-breathhold 3D-trueFISP cine cardiac imaging. Magn Reson Med 2002;48(5):921–5.

51. Bellenger NG, Gatehouse PD, Rajappan K, et al. Left ventricular quantification in heart failure by CMR using prospective respiratory navigator gating: comparison with breath-hold acquisition. J Magn Reson Imaging 2000;11(4):411–7.

52. Bastarrika Alemañ G, Domínguez Echávarri PD, et al. Quantification of ventricular mass and function using real-time free-breathing SSFP sequences. Radiologia 2008;50(1):67–74.

53. Debatin JF, Nadel SN, Paolini JF, et al. Cardiac ejection fraction: phantom study comparing cine MR imaging, radionuclide blood pool imaging, and ventriculography. J Magn Reson Imaging 1992;2(2):135–42.

54. Markiewicz W, Sechtem U, Kirby R, et al. Measurement of ventricular volumes in the dog by nuclear magnetic resonance imaging. J Am Coll Cardiol 1987;10(1):170–7.

55. Heusch A, Koch JA, Krogmann ON, et al. Volumetric analysis of the right and left ventricle in a porcine heart model: comparison of three-dimensional echocardiography, magnetic resonance

imaging and angiocardiography. Eur J Ultrasound 1999;9(3):245–55.

56. Florentine MS, Grosskreutz CL, Chang W, et al. Measurement of left ventricular mass in vivo using gated nuclear magnetic resonance imaging. J Am Coll Cardiol 1986;8(1):107–12.

57. Keller AM, Peshock RM, Malloy CR, et al. In vivo measurement of myocardial mass using nuclear magnetic resonance imaging. J Am Coll Cardiol 1986;8(1):113–7.

58. Shapiro EP, Rogers WJ, Beyar R, et al. Determination of left ventricular mass by magnetic resonance imaging in hearts deformed by acute infarction. Circulation 1989;79(3):706–11.

59. Bottini PB, Carr AA, Prisant M, et al. Magnetic resonance imaging compared to echocardiography to assess left ventricular mass in the hypertensive patient. Am J Hypertens 1995;8(3):221–8.

60. Sechtem U, Pflugfelder PW, Gould RG, et al. Measurement of right and left ventricular volumes in healthy individuals with cine MR imaging. Radiology 1987;163(3):697–702.

61. Møgelvang J, Stokholm KH, Saunamaki K, et al. Assessment of left ventricular volumes by magnetic resonance in comparison with radionuclide angiography, contrast angiography and echocardiography. Eur Heart J 1992;13(12):1677–83.

62. Jauhainen T, Jarvinen VM, Hekali PE, et al. MR gradient echo volumetric analysis of human cardiac casts: focus on the right ventricle. J Comput Assist Tomogr 1998;22(6):899–903.

63. Helbing WA, Rebergen SA, Maliepaard C, et al. Quantification of right ventricular function with magnetic resonance imaging in children with normal hearts and with congenital heart disease. Am Heart J 1995;130(4):828–37.

64. Katz J, Whang J, Boxt LM, et al. Estimation of right ventricular mass in normal subjects and in patients with primary pulmonary hypertension by nuclear magnetic resonance imaging. J Am Coll Cardiol 1993;21(6):1475–81.

65. McDonald KM, Parrish T, Wennberg P, et al. Rapid, accurate and simultaneous noninvasive assessment of right and left ventricular mass with nuclear magnetic resonance imaging using the snapshot gradient method. J Am Coll Cardiol 1992;19(7):1601–7.

66. Fieno DS, Jaffe WC, Simonetti OP, et al. TrueFISP: assessment of accuracy for measurement of left ventricular mass in an animal model. J Magn Reson Imaging 2002;15(5):526–31.

67. Shors SM, Fung CW, Francois CJ, et al. Accurate quantification of right ventricular mass at MR imaging by using cine true fast imaging with steady-state precession: study in dogs. Radiology 2004;230(2):383–8.

68. Barkhausen J, Ruehm SG, Goyen M, et al. MR evaluation of ventricular function: true fast imaging with steady-state precession versus fast low-angle shot cine MR imaging: feasibility study. Radiology 2001; 219(1):264–9.

69. Lee VS, Resnick D, Bundy JM, et al. Cardiac function: MR evaluation in one breath hold with real-time true fast imaging with steady-state precession. Radiology 2002;222(3):835–42.

70. Li W, Stern JS, Mai VM, et al. Assessment of left ventricular function: quantitative comparison of fast imaging employing steady-state acquisition (FIESTA) with fast gradient echo cine technique. J Magn Reson Imaging 2002;16(5):559–64.

71. Grothues F, Boenigk H, Graessner J, et al. Balanced steady-state free precession vs. segmented fast low-angle shot for the evaluation of ventricular volumes, mass, and function at 3 Tesla. J Magn Reson Imaging 2007;26(2):392–400.

72. Alfakih K, Plein S, Thiele H, et al. Normal human left and right ventricular dimensions for MRI as assessed by turbo gradient echo and steady-state free precession imaging sequences. J Magn Reson Imaging 2003;17(3):323–9.

73. Hudsmith LE, Petersen SE, Francis JM, et al. Normal human left and right ventricular and left atrial dimensions using steady state free precession magnetic resonance imaging. J Cardiovasc Magn Reson 2005;7(5):775–82.

74. Maceira AM, Prasad SK, Khan M, et al. Normalized left ventricular systolic and diastolic function by steady state free precession cardiovascular magnetic resonance. J Cardiovasc Magn Reson 2006;8(3):417–26.

75. Lorenz CH, Walker ES, Morgan VL, et al. Normal human right and left ventricular mass, systolic function and gender differences by cine magnetic resonance imaging. J Cardiovasc Magn Reson 1999; 1(1):7–21.

76. Pattynama PM, Lamb HJ, van der Velde EA, et al. Left ventricular measurements with cine and spin-echo MR imaging: a study of reproducibility with variance component analysis. Radiology 1993; 187(1):261–8.

77. Grothues F, Smith GC, Moon JC, et al. Comparison of interstudy reproducibility of cardiovascular magnetic resonance with two-dimensional echocardiography in normal subjects and in patients with heart failure or left ventricular hypertrophy. Am J Cardiol 2002;90(1):29–34.

78. Semelka RC, Tomei E, Wagner S, et al. Normal left ventricular dimensions and function: interstudy reproducibility of measurements with cine MR imaging. Radiology 1990;174(3 Pt 1):763–8.

79. Semelka RC, Tomei E, Wagner S, et al. Interstudy reproducibility of dimensional and functional measurements between cine magnetic resonance studies in the morphologically abnormal left ventricle. Am Heart J 1990;119(6):1367–73.

80. Germain P, Roul G, Kastler B, et al. Interstudy variability in left ventricular mass measurement. Comparison between m-mode echography and MRI. Eur Heart J 1992;13(8):1011–9.

81. Møgelvang J, Lindvig K, Sondergaard L, et al. Reproducibility of cardiac volume measurements including left ventricular mass determined by MRI. Clin Physiol 1993;13(6):587–97.

82. Bellenger NG, Davies LC, Francis JM, et al. Reduction in sample size for studies of remodeling in heart failure by the use of cardiovascular magnetic resonance. J Cardiovasc Magn Reson 2000;2(4):271–8.

83. Dulce MC, Friese K, Albrecht A, et al. Variability and reproducibility in the determination of left ventricular volume by means of cine MR: a comparison of various methods of measurements. Rofo 1991;155(2):99–108.

84. Benjelloun H, Cranney GB, Kirk KA, et al. Interstudy reproducibility of biplane cine nuclear magnetic resonance measurements of left ventricular function. Am J Cardiol 1991;67(16):1413–20.

85. Grothues F, Moon JC, Bellenger NG, et al. Interstudy reproducibility of right ventricular volumes, function and mass with cardiovascular magnetic resonance. Am Heart J 2004;147(2):218–23.

86. Remme WJ, Swedberg K. Guidelines for the diagnosis and treatment of chronic heart failure. Eur Heart J 2001;22(17):1527–60.

87. Swedberg K, Cleland J, Dargie H, et al. Guidelines for the diagnosis and treatment of chronic heart failure: full text (update 2005): The Task Force for the Diagnosis and Treatment of Chronic Heart Failure of the European Society of Cardiology. Eur Heart J 2005;26:1115–40.

88. Hendel RC, Patel MR, Kramer CM, et al. ACCF/ACR/SCCT/SCMR/ASNC/NASCI/SCAI/SIR 2006 appropriateness criteria for cardiac computed tomography and cardiac magnetic resonance imaging. J Am Coll Cardiol 2006;48(7):1475–97.

89. Heart Failure Society Of America. HFSA 2006 Comprehensive Heart Failure Practice Guideline. J Card Fail 2006;12(1):e1–122.

90. Cohn JN, Ferrari R, Sharpe N. Cardiac remodeling—concepts and clinical implications: a consensus paper from an international forum on cardiac remodeling. Behalf of an International Forum on Cardiac Remodeling. J Am Coll Cardiol 2000;35(3):569–82.

91. Schuster EH, Bulkley BH. Expansion of transmural infarction: a pathophysiologic factor in cardiac rupture. Circulation 1979;60(7):1532–8.

92. Pfeffer JM, Pfeffer MA, Fletcher PJ, et al. Progressive ventricular remodeling in rat with myocardial infarction. Am J Physiol 1991;260(5 Pt 2):H1406–14.

93. Olivetti G, Capasso JM, Meggs LG, et al. Cellular basis of ventricular remodeling in rats. Circ Res 1991;68(3):856–69.

94. McKay RG, Pfeffer MA, Paternak RC, et al. Left ventricular remodeling following myocardial infarction: a corollary to infarct expansion. Circulation 1986;74(4):693–702.

95. Mitchell GF, Lamas GA, Vaughan DE, et al. Left ventricular remodeling in the year after first anterior myocardial infarction. J Am Coll Cardiol 1992;19(6):1136–44.

96. Franco F, Thomas GD, Giroir B, et al. Magnetic resonance imaging and invasive evaluation of development of heart failure in transgenic mice with myocardial expression of tumor necrosis factor-alpha. Circulation 1999;99(3):448–54.

97. Kramer CM, Lima JAC, Reichek N, et al. Regional function within noninfarcted myocardium during left ventricular remodeling. Circulation 1993;88(3):1279–88.

98. Nahrendorf M, Aikawa E, Figueiredo J, et al. Transglutaminase activity in acute infarcts predicts healing outcome and left ventricular remodelling: implications for FXIII therapy and antithrombin use in myocardial infarction. Eur Heart J 2008;29(4):445–54.

99. Konermann M, Sanner BM, Hortsmann E, et al. Changes of the left ventricle after myocardial infarction—estimation with cine magnetic resonance imaging during the first six months. Clin Cardiol 1997;20(3):201–12.

100. Kramer CM, Rogers WJ, Theobald TM, et al. Dissociation between changes in intramyocardial function and left ventricular volumes in the 8 weeks after first anterior myocardial infarction. J Am Coll Cardiol 1997;30(7):1625–32.

101. Peshock RM, Rokey R, Malloy GM, et al. Assessment of myocardial systolic wall thickening using nuclear magnetic resonance imaging. J Am Coll Cardiol 1989;14(3):653–9.

102. Azhari H, Sideman S, Weiss JL, et al. Three-dimensional mapping of acute ischemic regions using MRI: wall thickening versus motion analysis. Am J Physiol 1990;259(5 Pt 2):H1492–503.

103. Sechtem U, Sommerhoff BA, Markiewicz W, et al. Regional left ventricular wall thickening by magnetic resonance imaging: evaluation of normal persons and patients with global and regional dysfunction. Am J Cardiol 1987;59(1):145–51.

104. Fisher MR, Von Schulthess GK, Higgins CB. Multiphasic cardiac magnetic resonance imaging: normal regional left ventricular wall thickening. AJR Am J Roentgenol 1985;145(1):27–30.

105. Holman ER, Buller VG, de Roos A, et al. Detection and quantification of dysfunctional myocardium by magnetic resonance imaging: a new three-dimensional method for quantitative wall-thickening analysis. Circulation 1997;95(4):924–31.

106. Zerhouni EA, Parish DM, Rogers WJ, et al. Human heart: tagging with MR imaging—a method for

noninvasive assessment of myocardial motion. Radiology 1988;169(1):59–63.

107. Lima JA, Jeremy R, Guier W, et al. Accurate systolic wall thickening by nuclear magnetic resonance imaging with tissue tagging: correlation with sonomicrometers in normal and ischemic myocardium. J Am Coll Cardiol 1993;21(7): 1741–51.

108. Buchalter MB, Weiss JL, Rogers WJ, et al. Noninvasive quantification of left ventricular rotational deformation in normal humans using magnetic resonance imaging myocardial tagging. Circulation 1990;81(4):1236–44.

109. Young AA, Axel L. Three-dimensional motion and deformation of the heart wall: estimation with spatial modulation of magnetization—a model-based approach. Radiology 1992;185(1):241–7.

110. Rademakers FE, Rogers WJ, Guier WH, et al. Relation of regional cross-fiber shortening to wall thickening in the intact heart. Three-dimensional strain analysis by NMR tagging. Circulation 1994;89(3): 1174–82.

111. Kramer CM, Rogers WJ, Theobald T, et al. Remote noninfarcted region dysfunction soon after first anterior myocardial infarction. A magnetic resonance tagging study. Circulation 1996;94(4):660–6.

112. Moulton MJ, Downing SW, Creswell LL, et al. Mechanical dysfunction in the border zone of an ovine model of left ventricular aneurysm. Ann Thorac Surg 1995;60(4):986–97.

113. Gotte MJ, van Rossum AC, Twisk JWR, et al. Quantification of regional contractile function after infarction: strain analysis superior to wall thickening analysis in discriminating infarct from remote myocardium. J Am Coll Cardiol 2001; 37(3):808–17.

114. McDonald KM, Yoshiyama M, Francis GS, et al. Myocardial bioenergetic abnormalities in a canine model of left ventricular dysfunction. J Am Coll Cardiol 1994;23(3):786–93.

115. Kim RJ, Wu E, Rafael A, et al. The use of contrast-enhanced magnetic resonance imaging to identify reversible myocardial dysfunction. N Engl J Med 2000;343(20):1445–53.

116. Saeed M, Wendland MF, Seelos K, et al. Effect of cilazapril on regional left ventricular wall thickness and chamber dimension following acute myocardial infarction: in vivo assessment using MRI. Am Heart J 1992;123(6):1472–80.

117. Kramer CM, Ferrari VA, Rogers WJ, et al. Angiotensin-converting enzyme inhibition limits dysfunction in adjacent noninfarcted regions during left ventricular remodeling. J Am Coll Cardiol 1996; 27(1):211–7.

118. McDonald KM, Garr M, Carlyle PF, et al. Relative effects of alpha 1-adrenoceptor blockade, converting enzyme inhibitor therapy, and angiotensin II subtype 1 receptor blockade on ventricular remodeling in the dog. Circulation 1994;90(6):3034–46.

119. McDonald KM, Rector T, Carlyle FM, et al. Angiotensin-converting enzyme inhibition and beta-adrenoceptor blockade regress established ventricular remodeling in a canine model of discrete myocardial damage. J Am Coll Cardiol 1994;24(7):1762–8.

120. Mankad S, d'Amato T, Reichek N, et al. Combined angiotensin II receptor antagonism and angiotensin-converting enzyme inhibition further attenuates postinfarction left ventricular remodeling. Circulation 2001;103(23):2845–50.

121. Blom AS, Pilla JJ, Arkles J, et al. Ventricular restraint prevents infarct expansion and improves borderzone function after myocardial infarction: a study using magnetic resonance imaging, three-dimensional surface modeling, and myocardial tagging. Ann Thorac Surg 2007;84(6): 2004–10.

122. Schulman SP, Weiss JL, Becker LC, et al. Effect of early enalapril therapy on left ventricular function and structure in acute myocardial infarction. Am J Cardiol 1995;76(11):764–70.

123. Johnson DB, Foster RE, Barilla F, et al. Angiotensin-converting enzyme inhibitor therapy affects left ventricular mass in patients with ejection fraction >40% after acute myocardial infarction. J Am Coll Cardiol 1997;29(1):49–54.

124. Foster RE, Johnson DB, Barilla F, et al. Changes in left ventricular mass and volumes in patients receiving angiotensin-converting enzyme inhibitor therapy for left ventricular dysfunction after Q-wave myocardial infarction. Am Heart J 1998; 136(2):269–75.

125. Dubach P, Myers J, Dziekan G, et al. Effects of exercise training on myocardial remodeling in patients with reduced left ventricular function after myocardial infarction: application of magnetic resonance imaging. Circulation 1997;95(8):2060–7.

126. Osterziel KJ, Strohm O, Schuler J, et al. Randomised, double-blind, placebo-controlled trial of human recombinant growth hormone in patients with chronic heart failure due to dilated cardiomyopathy. Lancet 1998;351(9111):1233–7.

127. Bellenger NG, Rajappan K, Rahman SL, et al. Effects of carvedilol on left ventricular remodelling in chronic stable heart failure: a cardiovascular magnetic resonance study. Heart 2004;90(7): 760–4.

128. Westenberg JJ, Braun J, Van de Veire NR, et al. Magnetic resonance imaging assessment of reverse left ventricular remodeling late after restrictive mitral annuloplasty in early stages of dilated cardiomyopathy. J Thorac Cardiovasc Surg 2008; 135(6):1247–52.

129. Meyer GP, Wollert KC, Lotz J, et al. Intracoronary bone marrow cell transfer after myocardial

infarction: eighteen months' follow-up data from the randomized, controlled BOOST (BOne marrOw transfer to enhance ST-elevation infarct regeneration) trial. Circulation 2006;113(10):1287–94.

130. Britten MB, Abolmaali ND, Assmus B, et al. Infarct remodeling after intracoronary progenitor cell treatment in patients with acute myocardial infarction (TOPCARE-AMI): mechanistic insights from serial contrast-enhanced magnetic resonance imaging. Circulation 2003;108(18):2212–8.

131. Groenning BA, Nilsson JC, Sondergaard L, et al. Antiremodeling effects on the left ventricle during beta-blockade with metoprolol in the treatment of chronic heart failure. J Am Coll Cardiol 2000; 36(7):2072–80.

132. Prasad SK, Dargie HJ, Smith GC, et al. Comparison of the dual receptor endothelin antagonist enrasentan with enalapril in asymptomatic left ventricular systolic dysfunction: a cardiovascular magnetic resonance study. Heart 2006;92(6):798–803.

133. Chan AK, Sanderson JE, Wang T, et al. Aldosterone receptor antagonism induces reverse remodeling when added to angiotensin receptor blockade in chronic heart failure. J Am Coll Cardiol 2007; 50(7):591–6.

134. Myerson SG, Montgomery HE, Whittingham M, et al. Left ventricular hypertrophy with exercise and ACE gene insertion/deletion polymorphism: a randomized controlled trial with losartan. Circulation 2001;103(2):226–30.

135. Brull D, Dhamrait S, Woods D, et al. The bradykinin B2 receptor and the human left ventricular growth response. Lancet 2001;358(9288):1155–6.

136. Waggoner AD, Harris KM, Bravermann AC, et al. The role of transthoracic echocardiography in the management of patients seen in an outpatient cardiology clinic. J Am Soc Echocardiogr 1996; 9(6):761–8.

137. Kronik G, Slany J, Mosslacher H. Comparatative value of eight M-mode echocardiographic formulas for determining left ventricular stroke volume. Circulation 1979;60(6):1308–16.

138. Teichholz LE, Kreulen T, Herman MV, et al. Problems in echocardiographic volume determinations: echocardiographic–angiographic correlations in the presence or absence of asynergy. Am J Cardiol 1976;37(1):7–11.

139. Bellenger NG, Burgess M, Ray SG, et al. Comparison of left ventricular ejection fraction and volumes in heart failure by echocardiography, radionuclide ventriculography and cardiovascular magnetic resonance; are they interchangeable? Eur Heart J 2000;21(16):1387–96.

140. Amico AF, Lichtenberg GS, Reisner SA, et al. Superiority of visual versus computerized echocardiography estimation of radionuclide left ventricular ejection fraction. Am Heart J 1989;118(6):1259–65.

141. Gordon EP, Schnittger I, Fitzgerald PJ, et al. Reproducibility of left ventricular volumes by two-dimensional echocardiography. J Am Coll Cardiol 1983; 2(3):506–13.

142. Gottdiener JS, Livengood SV, Meyer PS, et al. Should echocardiography be performed to assess effects of antihypertensive therapy? Test–retest reliability of echocardiography for measurement of left ventricular mass and function. J Am Coll Cardiol 1995;25(2):424–30.

143. Myerson SG, Montgomery HE, World MJ, et al. Left ventricular mass: reliability of M-mode and 2-dimensional echocardiographic formulas. Hypertension 2002;40(5):673–8.

144. Otterstad JE. Measuring left ventricular volume and ejection fraction with the biplane Simpson's method. Heart 2002;88(6):559–60.

145. Cheitlin MD, Armstrong WF, Aurigemma GP, et al. ACC/AHA/ASE 2003 Guideline Update for the Clinical Application of Echocardiography: summary article. A report of the American College of Cardiology/American Heart Association Task Force on Practice Guidelines (ACC/AHA/ASE Committee to Update the 1997 Guidelines for the Clinical Application of Echocardiography). J Am Soc Echocardiogr 2003;16(10):1091–110.

146. Gopal AS, Chukwu EO, Iwuchukwu CJ, et al. Normal values of right ventricular size and function by real-time 3-dimensional echocardiography: comparison with cardiac magnetic resonance imaging. J Am Soc Echocardiogr 2007;20(5): 445–55.

147. Sugeng L, Mor-Avi V, Weinert L, et al. Quantitative assessment of left ventricular size and function: side-by-side comparison of real-time three-dimensional echocardiography and computed tomography with magnetic resonance reference. Circulation 2006;114(7):654–61.

148. Gutiérrez-Chico JL, Zamorano JL, Pérez de Isla L, et al. Comparison of left ventricular volumes and ejection fractions measured by three-dimensional echocardiography versus by two-dimensional echocardiography and cardiac magnetic resonance in patients with various cardiomyopathies. Am J Cardiol 2005;95(6):809–13.

149. Gopal AS, Schnellbaecher MJ, Shen Z, et al. Freehand three-dimensional echocardiography for measurement of left ventricular mass: in vivo anatomic validation using explanted human hearts. J Am Coll Cardiol 1997;30(3):802–10.

150. Jenkins C, Bricknell K, Hanekom L, et al. Reproducibility and accuracy of echocardiographic measurements of left ventricular parameters using real-time three-dimensional echocardiography. J Am Coll Cardiol 2004;44(4):878–86.

151. Hibberd MG, Chuang ML, Beaudin RA, et al. Accuracy of three-dimensional echocardiography with

unrestricted selection of imaging planes for measurement of left ventricular volumes and ejection fraction. Am Heart J 2000;140(3):469–75.

152. Nikitin NP, Constantin C, Loh PH, et al. New generation 3-dimensional echocardiography for left ventricular volumetric and functional measurements: comparison with cardiac magnetic resonance. Eur J Echocardiogr 2006;7(5):365–72.

153. Gopal AS, Shen Z, Sapin PM, et al. Assessment of cardiac function by three-dimensional echocardiography compared with conventional noninvasive methods. Circulation 1995;92(4):842–53.

154. Jenkins C, Bricknell K, Chan J, et al. Comparison of two- and three-dimensional echocardiography with sequential magnetic resonance imaging for evaluating left ventricular volume and ejection fraction over time in patients with healed myocardial infarction. Am J Cardiol 2007;99(3):300–6.

155. Jenkins C, Chan J, Bricknell K, et al. Reproducibility of right ventricular volumes and ejection fraction using real-time three-dimensional echocardiography: comparison with cardiac MRI. Chest 2007;131(6):1844–51.

156. Dewey M, Müller M, Eddicks S, et al. Evaluation of global and regional left ventricular function with 16-slice computed tomography, biplane cineventriculography, and two-dimensional transthoracic echocardiography: comparison with magnetic resonance imaging. J Am Coll Cardiol 2006; 48(10):2034–44.

157. Belge B, Coche E, Pasquet A, et al. Accurate estimation of global and regional cardiac function by retrospectively gated multidetector row computed tomography: comparison with cine magnetic resonance imaging. Eur Radiol 2006;16(7):1424–33.

158. Heuschmid M, Rothfuss JK, Schroeder S, et al. Assessment of left ventricular myocardial function using 16-slice multidetector-row computed tomography: comparison with magnetic resonance imaging and echocardiography. Eur Radiol 2006; 16(3):551–9.

159. Bruners P, Mahnken AH, Knackstedt C, et al. Assessment of global left and right ventricular function using dual-source computed tomography (DSCT) in comparison to MRI: an experimental study in a porcine model. Invest Radiol 2007; 42(11):756–64.

160. Sharir T, Germano G, Kavanagh PB, et al. Incremental prognostic value of post-stress left ventricular ejection fraction and volume by gated myocardial perfusion single photon emission computed tomography. Circulation 1999;100(10): 1035–42.

161. Miron SD, Finkelhor R, Penuel JH, et al. A geometric method of measuring the left ventricular ejection fraction on gated Tc-99m sestamibi myocardial imaging. Clin Nucl Med 1996;21(6): 439–44.

162. Iskandrian AE, Germano G, van Decker W, et al. Validation of left ventricular volume measurements by gated SPECT 99mTc-labeled sestamibi imaging. J Nucl Cardiol 1998;5(6):574–8.

163. Johnson LL, Verdesca SA, Aude WY, et al. Postischemic stunning can affect left ventricular ejection fraction and regional wall motion on post-stress gated sestamibi. J Am Coll Cardiol 1997;30(7): 1641–8.

164. Rajappan K, Livieratos L, Camici PG, et al. Measurement of ventricular volumes and function: a comparison of gated PET and cardiovascular magnetic resonance. J Nucl Med 2002;43(6): 806–10.

165. Nazarian S, Roguin A, Zviman MM, et al. Clinical utility and safety of a protocol for noncardiac and cardiac magnetic resonance imaging of patients with permanent pacemakers and implantable-cardioverter defibrillators at 1.5 tesla. Circulation 2006;114(12):1277–84.

166. Roguin A, Schwitter J, Vahlhaus C, et al. Magnetic resonance imaging in individuals with cardiovascular implantable electronic devices. Europace 2008;10(3):336–46.

Evaluation of Ischemic Heart Disease

Dipan J. Shah, MD, FACC[a,b,*], Han W. Kim, MD[c],
Raymond J. Kim, MD[c,d]

KEYWORDS

- Stress cardiac magnetic resonance
- Myocardial ischemia • Ischemic heart disease

Approximately two thirds of patients with heart failure have underlying coronary artery disease (CAD), the presence of which is associated with worse long-term outcomes.[1,2] In addition to providing prognostic information, the detection of CAD in the setting of heart failure also can result in several therapeutic management alterations, including revascularization and the use of statin and antiplatelet drugs.[1] In the setting of ischemic heart disease, cardiovascular magnetic resonance (CMR) has demonstrated usefulness in two manners: first for the detection of CAD and second for the assessment of myocardial viability in consideration for revascularization. In fact, CMR is widely considered the gold standard for the latter, which is addressed in the following section on myocardial viability and revascularization. This article discusses the use of CMR for the detection of CAD.

Currently there are several CMR approaches for the detection of CAD: (1) coronary magnetic resonance angiography (MRA), (2) pharmacologic stress CMR with dobutamine (to assess contractile reserve and inducible wall motion abnormalities), and (3) pharmacologic stress CMR with adenosine (to assess myocardial perfusion reserve). The purpose of this article is to provide the reader with a brief overview of each of the CMR techniques, their relative strengths, and their relative weaknesses. Because adenosine stress CMR is currently the most widely used clinically, it is the primary focus of this article.

CORONARY MAGNETIC RESONANCE ANGIOGRAPHY

Coronary MRA may be used to directly visualize coronary anatomy and morphology; however, it is technically demanding for several reasons. The coronary arteries are small (3–5 mm) and tortuous compared with other vascular beds that are imaged by MRA, and there is nearly constant motion during the respiratory and cardiac cycles. To counter these difficulties, several technical advancements have been made in recent years to improve the reliability of coronary MRA, including the advent of ultrafast steady-state free precession sequences that offer superior signal-to-noise ratio in combination with whole-heart approaches[3,4] analogous to multidetector CT and parallel imaging to reduce scan times. These sequences typically can be run with submillimeter in-plane spatial resolution (0.8 × 1.0 mm) and slice thickness slightly more than 1 mm. With the use of modifications that compensate for respiratory drift,[5] imaging usually can be completed in less than 10 minutes.

ANOMALOUS CORONARY IMAGING

With recent advances, the ability of coronary MRA to reliably identify the major coronary arteries immediately provides for use in the identification and characterization of anomalous coronary anatomy. Although most coronary anomalies are

This work was supported in part by National Institutes of Health grant RO1-HL64726 (RJK).
[a] Weill Cornell Medical College, New York, NY, USA
[b] Methodist DeBakey Heart and Vascular Center, Houston, TX, USA
[c] Duke University Medical Center, Durham, NC, USA
[d] Duke Cardiovascular Magnetic Resonance Center, Durham, NC, USA
* Corresponding author. Cardiovascular Imaging Institute, Methodist DeBakey Heart & Vascular Center, 6550 Fannin Road, #677, Houston, TX 77030.
E-mail address: djshah@tmhs.org (D.J. Shah).

heartfailure.theclinics.com

benign, situations in which the anomalous segment courses anterior to the aorta and posterior to the pulmonary artery (referred to as "intra-arterial course") can result in myocardial ischemia and sudden cardiac death (**Fig. 1**).[6] Multiple published series exist of patients who underwent blinded comparison of coronary MRA with radiographic angiography.[7–10] These studies uniformly reported excellent accuracy, including several studies in which coronary MRA was determined to be superior to radiographic angiography.[8,9] For these reasons and radiation-protection concerns, coronary MRA is the preferred test for patients in whom an anomalous artery origin is suspected or a known anomalous coronary artery origin needs to be clarified further.[11]

Identification of Native Vessel Coronary Stenosis

Although excellent for the evaluation of anomalous coronaries, coronary MRA is still evolving for detection of native vessel stenosis and is not recommended for routinely assessing symptomatic patients or "screening" high-risk populations.[11] A recent multicenter single-vendor study did demonstrate a high sensitivity rate (100%) and negative predictive value (100%) for detection of left main and triple vessel disease.[12] There may be a role for coronary MRA in the evaluation of patients who present with dilated cardiomyopathy/congestive heart failure in the absence of clinical infarction in whom discrimination between ischemic or nonischemic cardiomyopathy is sought.[11,13] This area requires further investigation, however.

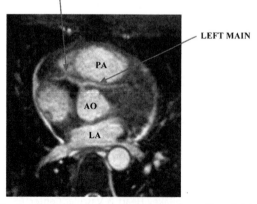

Fig. 1. Anomalous left main arising from the right coronary artery and traveling between the aorta and pulmonary artery (intra-arterial course). AO, aorta; LA, left atrium; PA, pulmonary artery.

Consensus Recommendation for Coronary Magnetic Resonance Angiography

Recently, a consensus document from the American Heart Association addressed the current role of coronary MRA in clinical practice.[11] The panel assigned a Class IIa recommendation (ie, weight of evidence/opinion is in favor of usefulness/efficacy) to use of coronary MRA for identification of coronary anomalies and indicated that radiation protection concerns indicate that coronary MRA is preferred over coronary CT angiography for this indication.

DOBUTAMINE STRESS CARDIOVASCULAR MAGNETIC RESONANCE

Although coronary MRA provides detail concerning anatomy, stress testing with imaging of myocardial contraction can provide information concerning the presence and functional significance of coronary lesions. Dobutamine stress CMR to detect ischemia-induced wall motion abnormalities is an established technique for the diagnosis of coronary disease. It yields higher diagnostic accuracy than dobutamine echocardiography[14] and can be effective in patients not suited for echocardiography because of poor acoustic windows.[15] Since the publication of these studies, MRI quality has improved with the widespread availability of steady-state free precession imaging. Parallel imaging techniques that use spatial information from arrays of radiofrequency detector coils to accelerate imaging are expected to improve image quality further. Logistic issues regarding patient safety and adequate monitoring are nontrivial matters that require thorough planning and experienced personnel.

ADENOSINE STRESS CARDIOVASCULAR MAGNETIC RESONANCE

With recent technical and clinical advances, adenosine stress perfusion CMR has evolved from a promising research tool to an everyday clinical tool that is considered a competitive first-line test for common indications, such as the evaluation of ischemic heart disease. In 2006, a consensus panel from the American College of Cardiology Foundation deemed the following indications as appropriate uses of stress perfusion CMR: (1) evaluating chest pain syndromes in patients with intermediate probability of CAD and (2) ascertaining the physiologic significance of indeterminate coronary artery lesions.[16] In part, this report reflects the growing clinical experience with stress perfusion CMR. In dedicated CMR clinical centers, perfusion stress testing is often the fastest growing component of the clinical volume and can comprise nearly half of all referrals.[17]

Overview

The "goal" of perfusion CMR is to create a movie of the transit of contrast media (typically gadolinium based) with the blood during its initial pass through the left ventricular myocardium ("first-pass contrast-enhancement"). Myocardial perfusion by CMR may be assessed quantitatively or semi-quantitatively by measuring dynamic signal intensities within the myocardium in consecutive images (**Fig. 2**). During pharmacologic vasodilation (eg, adenosine), myocardial blood flow increases four- to fivefold downstream of normal coronary arteries but does not increase downstream of severely diseased arteries because the arteriolar beds are already maximally vasodilated. These physiologic differences result in lower peak myocardial signal intensity and lengthening in the measures of myocardial contrast transit time (eg, signal upslope, arrival time, time to peak signal, mean transit time) in regions supplied by diseased vessels (see **Fig. 2**).[18] Signal intensity parameters can be plotted with respect to time and, with

some assumptions, quantitatively modeled to provide absolute tissue blood flow in milliliters per minutes per gram or used in a semi-quantitative fashion to index relative differences in regional flow.[18] Alternatively, the images can be interpreted visually for the presence or absence of perfusion defects.

Compared with competing technologies such as radionuclide imaging, perfusion CMR has many potential advantages: more than an order of magnitude improvement in spatial resolution (typical voxel dimensions, CMR $3.0 \times 1.8 \times 8$ mm $= 43$ mm^3 versus single photon emission computed tomography (SPECT) $10 \times 10 \times 10$ mm $= 1000$ mm^3); the ability to identify regional differences in flow over the full range of coronary vasodilation (ie, no plateau in signal at high flow rates, as seen with radionuclide tracers);[19,20] the lack of ionizing radiation; and an examination time of 30 to 45 minutes versus 2 to 3 hours.

Preclinical Validation

Several studies have shown a good correlation between semi-quantitative and quantitative CMR indices of perfusion with tissue perfusion in animal

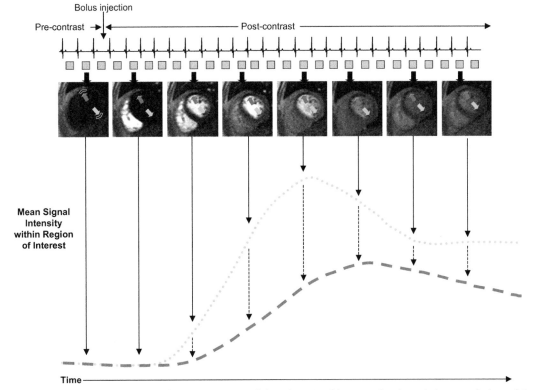

Fig. 2. Signal intensity time curves from two myocardial regions. In this example, there is hypoperfusion of the anterior wall (*red arrow* and *dashed red line*), whereas the perfusion of the inferior wall (*blue arrow* and *dotted blue line*) is normal. From these curves, various parameters can be extracted to derive quantitative measures of blood flow.

models.[21–25] In a porcine model with ligation of the left circumflex (LCx) coronary artery, Wilke and colleagues[21] performed MR perfusion studies at rest and during vasodilation with adenosine. The authors found a linear correlation between relative CMR perfusion indices and true perfusion as measured by radioactive microspheres. Similarly, in a chronically instrumented canine model, Klocke and colleagues[23] produced regional differences in flow with selective LCx infusion of graded doses of adenosine or partial LCx obstruction using a hydraulic occlusion device. Regional differences in the area under the upslope of the CMR signal intensity curve linearly correlated with flow differences measured by fluorescent microspheres (**Fig. 3**). Regional flow differences of twofold or more were consistently discerned by perfusion CMR, which suggests that clinically relevant coronary stenoses of 70% or more could be detected reliably.

Extending these observations are the findings from Lee and colleagues.[24] In their study, perfusion CMR was compared with technetium-99 m (^{99m}Tc) sestamibi and 201-Thallium (^{201}Tl) SPECT imaging in the quantification of regional differences in vasodilated blood flow in viable myocardium. The authors used a canine model in which a hydraulic occluder was placed in the LCx

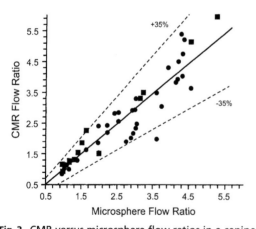

Fig. 3. CMR versus microsphere flow ratios in a canine model. Solid line is linear regression (CMR ratio = 0.96 microsphere +0.07); dotted lines indicate 95% confidence limits for individual values. Solid circle indicates ratios of LCx to remote CMR areas and relative microsphere flows during LCx adenosine infusion. Solid square indicates ratios of remote to LCx CMR areas and relative microsphere flows during LCx constriction in the presence of global left ventricular vasodilation. (*From* Klocke FJ, Simonetti OP, Judd RM, et al. Limits of detection of regional differences in vasodilated flow in viable myocardium by first-pass magnetic resonance perfusion imaging. Circulation 2001;104:2414; with permission.)

coronary artery to produce graded reductions in regional flows. When circumflex microsphere flow was reduced by 50% or more, perfusion defects were apparent on the MR images by visual inspection and analysis of the signal intensity curves. Flows derived from the initial areas under the CMR signal intensity time curves were linearly related to reference microsphere flows over the full range of vasodilation. In contrast, with SPECT imaging, perfusion defects were not evident until flow was reduced by at least 85%, and the relationships between ^{99m}Tc and ^{201}Tl activity and microsphere flows were curvilinear, plateauing as flows increased (**Fig. 4**).

More recently, Christian and colleagues[25] used a Fermi function deconvolution method to quantify absolute perfusion in a canine model of coronary artery stenosis. Vessel occluders or intracoronary adenosine infusion catheters were used to produce a wide range of coronary flows. These authors derived myocardial flow in the endocardial and epicardial layers of the heart by perfusion CMR. They showed that quantitative coronary flow by CMR in both layers was linearly related to flow by fluorescent microspheres (without plateauing at higher flow rates) in the corresponding locations. These findings and those from other researchers[22] demonstrate that perfusion CMR, with its advantage of high spatial resolution, has the potential to discern differences in endocardial and epicardial flow. This may have value in evaluation of three-vessel CAD with "balanced ischemia" or syndrome X or detection of subtle abnormalities such as hypertensive heart disease.

Diagnostic Performance in Patients

The diagnostic performance of stress perfusion CMR has been evaluated in several studies in humans.[26–44] Overall, these studies have shown good correlations with radionuclide imaging and radiographic coronary angiography, although there have been some variable results. **Table 1** summarizes the published stress perfusion CMR studies in humans with coronary angiography comparison. A total of 21 studies have been completed, consisting of 1233 patients with known or suspected CAD. On average, the sensitivity and specificity rates of perfusion CMR for detecting obstructive CAD were 84% (range, 44%–93%) and 80% (range, 60%–100%), respectively. Likely on the basis of these studies, the most recent consensus report on clinical indications for CMR classified perfusion imaging as a Class II indication for the assessment of CAD (ie, provides clinically relevant information and is frequently useful).[45]

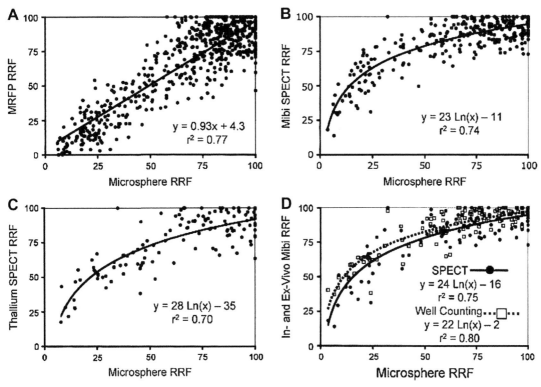

Fig. 4. Comparisons of perfusion CMR, radionuclide, and microsphere flows. CMR signal intensity time curves were linearly related to reference microsphere flows over the full range of vasodilation. Relationships between ^{99m}Tc-sestamibi and ^{201}Thallium activity and microsphere flows were curvilinear, plateauing as flows increased. Data suggest that perfusion CMR, unlike radionuclide imaging, has the potential for detecting stenoses producing only moderate limitations in flow reserve. (A) Normalized magnetic resonance first-pass perfusion (MRFP) imaging and full-thickness microsphere relative regional flows (RRF). (B) Normalized ^{99m}Tc-sestamibi and full-thickness microsphere RRFs. (C) Normalized ^{201}Tl and full-thickness microsphere RRFs. (D) In vivo SPECT and ex vivo well counting values of ^{99m}Tc-sestamibi versus microsphere RRFs. (*From* Lee DC, Simonetti OP, Harris KR, et al. Magnetic resonance versus radionuclide pharmacologic stress perfusion imaging for flow-limiting stenoses of varying severity. Circulation 2004;110:62; with permission.)

Despite the mostly favorable results of these studies, several issues should be considered. Some studies are of limited clinical applicability because they required central venous catheters,[30,34] imaged only one slice per heartbeat,[30] or excluded patients who had diabetes.[39] Many studies had small sample sizes—eight studies had 30 or fewer patients. Most studies included patients already known to have CAD or prior myocardial infarction (MI). In these studies there is pretest referral or "spectrum" bias, which can artificially raise test sensitivity and/or specificity.[46,47] Importantly, in many studies after the data were collected, several methods of analysis were tested and different thresholds for test abnormality were appraised. For these studies, the reported sensitivity and specificity values were optimistic because the endpoints were chosen retrospectively and they represent optimized values.

Two practical issues also limit clinical applicability. First, there is no consensus regarding the optimal pulse sequence or imaging protocol. The studies in **Table 1** are heterogeneous in terms of the techniques and methods used. For example, the dose of gadolinium contrast administered varied sixfold, with doses ranging from 0.025 to 0.15 mmol/kg. The inconsistent results in the literature likely reflect the lack of a standard method for performing perfusion CMR. Second, many of the studies used a quantitative approach for diagnostic assessment. Although a quantitative approach has the potential advantage of allowing absolute blood flow to be measured or parametric maps of perfusion to be generated, the approach is laborious and requires extensive interactive post-processing. Currently, a quantitative approach is not feasible for everyday clinical use.

In contrast, image interpretation by simple visual assessment would be a realistic approach for

Table 1
Stress perfusion CMR studies in humans with coronary angiography comparison

Year	Author	Reference	Patients With Known CAD Excluded	n	CMR Perfusion Protocol[a]	Gadolinium Dose (mmol/kg)	Pluse-Sequence	X-Ray Angiography (CAD Definition)	Analysis Method[b]	Sens	Spec
						Protocol					
1993	Klein	AJR 161(2):257–63	No	5	Stress only	0.05	IR-GRE	>50	Prospective	81*	100*
1994	Hartnell	AJR 163(5):1061–7	No	18	Rest/stress	0.04	IR-GRE	≥70	Prospective	83	100
1994	Eichenberger	JMRI 4(3):425–31	No	10	Rest/stress	0.05	GRE	>75	Retrospective	44*	80*
2000	Al-Saadi	Circ 101(12)1379–83	Yes	34	Rest/stress	0.025	IR-GRE	≥75	Prospective[c]	90	83
2001	Bertschinger	JMRI 14(5):556–62	No	14	Stress only	0.1	SR-EPI	≥50	Retrospective	85	81
2001	Schwitter	Circ 103(18):2230–5	Yes	48	Stress only	0.1	SR-GRE-EPI	≥50	Retrospective	87	85
2001	Panting	JMRI 13(2):192–200	No	22	Rest/stress	0.05	IR Spin Echo-EPI	>50	Retrospective	79	83
2002	Sensky	Int J CV Imaging 18(5):373–83	No	30	Rest/stress	0.025	IR-GRE	>50	Prospective	93*	60*
2002	Ibrahim	JACC 39(5):864–70	No	25	Rest/stress	0.05	SR-GRE-EPI	>75	Retrospective	69*	89*
2003	Chiu	Radiology 226(3):717–22	No[d]	13	Rest/stress	0.05	IR-SSFP	>50	NS	92*	92*
2003	Ishida	Radiology 229(1):209–16	No	104	Stress/rest	0.075	SR-GRE-EPI	≥70	Prospective	90	85
2003	Nagel	Circ 108(4):432–7	No	84	Rest/stress	0.025	SR-GRE-EPI	≥75	Retrospective	88	90
2003	Doyle	JCMR 5(3):475–85	No	138	Rest/stress	0.04	SR-GRE	≥70	Prospective[c]	57	85
2004	Wolff	Circ 110(6):732–7	No	75	Stress/rest	0.05–0.15	SR-GRE-EPI	≥70	Prospective[e]	93	75

Year	Author	Citation	n		Stress		SR	Threshold	Study type	Sens	Spec
2004	Giang	EHJ 25(18):1657–65	80	No	Stress only	0.05–0.15	SR-GRE-EPI	≥50	Retrospective[e]	93	75
2004	Paetsch	Circ 110(7):835–42	79	No	Stress/rest	0.05	SR-GRE-EPI	≥50	Prospective	91	62
2004	Plein	JACC 44(11):2173–81	68	No[d]	Rest/stress	0.05	SR-GRE[f]	≥70	Prospective	88	83
2005	Plein	Radiology 235(2):423–30	92	No	Rest/stress	0.05	SR-GRE[f]	≥70	Retrospective	88	82
2006	Klem	JACC 47(8):1630–8	100	Yes	Stress/rest	0.063	SR-GRE[f]	≥70	Prospective	84**	58**
2006	Cury	Radiology 240(1):39–45	47	No	Stress/rest	0.1	SR-GRE-EPI	≥70	Prospective	81***	87***
2008	Klem	JACCI 2008;1:436–45	147	Yes	Stress only	0.07	SR-GRE[f]	≥70	Prospective	84	88
Total	21		1233								
Weighted average										**84**	**80**

Abbreviations: CMR, cardiovascular magnetic resonance; DE-MRI, delayed enhancement; EPI, echo-planar imaging; GRE, gradient-recalled echo; IR, inversion recovery pre-pulse; MRI; Sens, sensitivity; n, number of patients; NS, not stated; SR, saturation revocery pre-pulse; SSFP, statedy-state free precession

[a] When both rest and stress imaging were performed the order is as listed.
[b] Prospective studies were those in which the criteria for test abnormality were prespecified before data analysis.
[c] Pilot study performed first to determine the best threshold for test abnormality.
[d] At enrollment, all patients had the clinical diagnosis of no-ST elevation MI or acute coronary syndrome.
[e] Reported sensitivity and specificity are from a fraction of the total cohort, a subgroup with the best results.
[f] With parallel imaging acceleration.
* Numbers based on a regional rather than per patient analysis.
** Sensitivity/specificity were higher after incorporating DE-MRI (89% and 87% respectively)
*** Sensitivity/specificity were higher after incorporating DE-MRI (87% and 9%, respectively)
Data from Kim HW, Rehwald W, White JA, et al. Magnetic resonance imaging of the heart. In: Fuster V, Alexander RW, O'Rourke RA, editors. Hurst's The Heart, 12th edition. New York, NY: McGraw-Hill Medical; 2008.

a clinical CMR practice. Unfortunately, the results in the literature regarding visual assessment of perfusion CMR are mixed and generally demonstrate adequate sensitivity but relatively poor specificity for the detection of CAD. In large part, image artifacts are responsible for reduced specificity. In this context, it is noteworthy that recently an interpretation algorithm that combines data from perfusion CMR and delayed enhancement CMR (DE-CMR) was introduced that substantially improves the specificity and accuracy of rapid visual assessment for the detection of CAD.[44,48] Based on these data, we have adopted a multicomponent approach to stress testing that permits rapid visual image interpretation with high diagnostic accuracy.

Multicomponent Cardiovascular Magnetic Resonance Stress Testing Protocol

The multicomponent approach to CMR stress testing includes the following: (1) cine CMR for the assessment of cardiac morphology and regional and global systolic function at baseline, (2) stress perfusion CMR to visualize regions of myocardial hypoperfusion during vasodilation (eg, with adenosine infusion), (3) rest perfusion CMR to aid in distinguishing true perfusion defects from image artifacts, and (4) DE-CMR for the determination of MI (**Fig. 5**). The timeline of the multicomponent CMR stress test is displayed in **Fig. 6**. Details regarding cine CMR and DE-CMR are discussed elsewhere in this issue of *Heart Failure Clinics*.

Stress perfusion imaging is performed after scouting and cine imaging. Typically, before adenosine administration, the patient table is partially pulled out of bore of the magnet to allow direct observation and full access to the patient. Adenosine ($140~\mu g/kg^{-1}/min^{-1}$) is then infused under continuous electrocardiography and blood pressure monitoring for at least 2 minutes. The perfusion sequence is then applied by the scanner operator, which automatically re-centers the

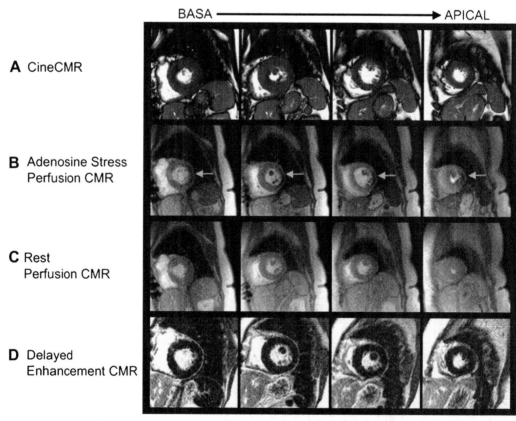

BASA ———————————————➤ APICAL

A CineCMR

B Adenosine Stress Perfusion CMR

C Rest Perfusion CMR

D Delayed Enhancement CMR

Fig. 5. Components of the multicomponent CMR stress test. Cine CMR (*A*), stress (*B*) and rest perfusion (*C*) CMR, and DE-CMR (*D*) are performed at identical short axis locations. During image interpretation, the different components are analyzed side-by-side to facilitate differentiation of perfusion defects caused by infarction, ischemia, or artifact. Arrows points to perfusion defects seen during adenosine infusion but not at rest, which is consistent with the presence of ischemic heart disease.

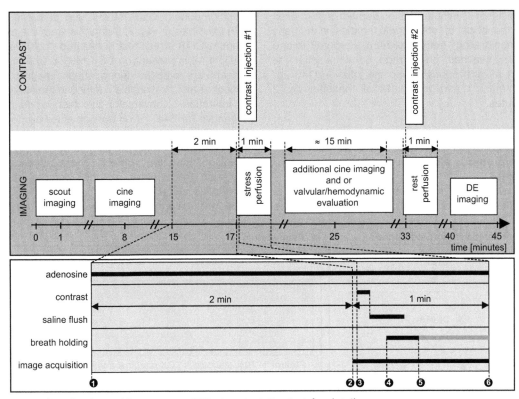

Fig. 6. Timeline for the multicomponent CMR stress test. See text for details.

patient in the scanner bore and commences imaging. Gadolinium contrast (0.075–0.10 mmol/kg body weight) is then administered followed by a saline flush (approximately 50 mL) at a rate of at least 3 mL/s via an antecubital vein. On the console, the perfusion images are observed as they are acquired, with breath-holding starting from the appearance of contrast in the right ventricular cavity. If the scanner software does not provide real-time image display, breath-holding should be started no more than 5 to 6 seconds after beginning gadolinium injection. Breath-holding is performed to ensure the best possible image quality (ie, no artifacts caused by respiratory motion) during the initial wash-in of contrast into the left ventricular myocardium. Once the contrast bolus has transited the left ventricular myocardium, adenosine is stopped and imaging is completed 5 to 10 seconds later. Typically, the total imaging time is 40 to 50 seconds, and the total time of adenosine infusion is 3 to 3.5 minutes. During vasodilation, direct access to the patient is limited only during imaging of the first-pass.

Before the rest perfusion scan, a waiting period of approximately 15 minutes is required for gadolinium to sufficiently clear from the blood pool. During this time, additional cine scans and/or velocity/flow imaging for valvular or hemodynamic

evaluation can be performed. For the rest perfusion scan, an additional dose of 0.075 to 0.10 mmol/kg gadolinium is given, and the imaging parameters are identical to the stress scan. Approximately 5 minutes after rest perfusion, delayed enhancement imaging can be performed. The total scan time for a comprehensive CMR stress test, including cine imaging, stress and rest perfusion, and delayed enhancement is usually well under 45 minutes.

Unlike vasodilator radionuclide imaging, in which adenosine is typically infused for 6 minutes (tracer injection at 3 minutes), stress perfusion CMR is performed using an abbreviated adenosine protocol (approximately 3 minutes total) because the requirements for imaging are different.[44] With radionuclide imaging, maintaining a vasodilated state for 2 to 3 minutes after tracer injection is necessary to allow time for tracer uptake into myocytes. In contradistinction, with CMR currently available gadolinium media are inert, extracellular agents that do not cross sarcolemmal membranes,[49] and vasodilation needs to be maintained only for the initial first-pass through the myocardium. Although severe reactions to adenosine are rare, a shortened protocol is relevant because moderate reactions that affect patient tolerability are relatively commonplace.[50]

A minimum 2-minute infusion duration was chosen on the basis of physiologic studies in humans demonstrating that maximum coronary blood flow is reached, on average, 1 minute after the start of intravenous adenosine infusion (140 μg/kg⁻¹/min⁻¹) and in nearly all patients by 2 minutes.[51]

Image Interpretation

Interpretation algorithm for coronary artery disease

An overview of the interpretation algorithm that facilitates rapid visual interpretation for a multicomponent CMR stress test is presented with examples in **Fig. 7**. Using this stepwise algorithm, a CMR stress test is deemed "positive for CAD" if MI is present on DE-CMR or if perfusion defects are present during stress imaging but absent at rest ("reversible" defect) in the absence of infarction. Conversely, the test is deemed "negative for CAD" if no abnormalities are found (eg, no MI and no stress/rest perfusion defects) or if perfusion defects are seen at stress and rest imaging ("matched" defect) in the absence of infarction. In the latter, matched defects are regarded as artifacts and not suggestive of CAD with rare exceptions (see next section). When

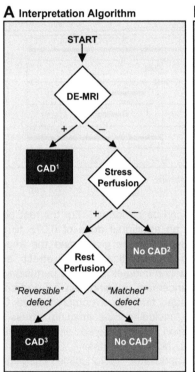

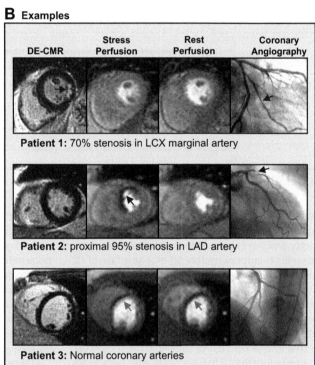

Fig. 7. Interpretation algorithm for incorporating DE-CMR with stress and rest perfusion CMR for the detection of coronary disease. (A) Schema of the interpretation algorithm. (1) Positive DE-CMR study: hyperenhanced myocardium consistent with a prior MI is detected. Does not include isolated midwall or epicardial hyperenhancement, which can occur in nonischemic disorders. (2) Standard negative stress study: no evidence of prior MI or inducible perfusion defects. (3) Standard positive stress study: no evidence of prior MI, but perfusion defects are present with adenosine that are absent or reduced at rest. (4) Artifactual perfusion defect: matched stress and rest perfusion defects without evidence of prior MI on DE-CMR. (B) Patient examples. (*Top row*) Patient with a positive DE-CMR study result demonstrates an infarct in the inferolateral wall (*arrow*), although perfusion CMR is negative. The interpretation algorithm (step 1) classified this patient as positive for CAD. Coronary angiography verified disease in the left circumflex (LCx) marginal artery. Cine CMR demonstrated normal contractility. (*Middle row*) Patient with a negative DE-CMR study but with a prominent reversible defect in the anteroseptal wall on perfusion CMR (*arrow*). The interpretation algorithm (step 3) classified this patient as positive for CAD. Coronary angiography demonstrated a proximal 95% left anterior descending (LAD) stenosis. (*Bottom row*) Patient with a matched stress-rest perfusion defect (*arrows*) but without evidence of prior MI on DE-CMR. The interpretation algorithm (step 4) classified the perfusion defects as artifactual. Coronary angiography demonstrated normal coronary arteries. (*Modified from* Klem I, Heitner JF, Shah DJ, et al. Improved detection of coronary artery disease by stress perfusion cardiovascular magnetic resonance with the use of delayed enhancement infarction imaging. J Am Coll Cardiol 2006;47:1630–8; with permission.)

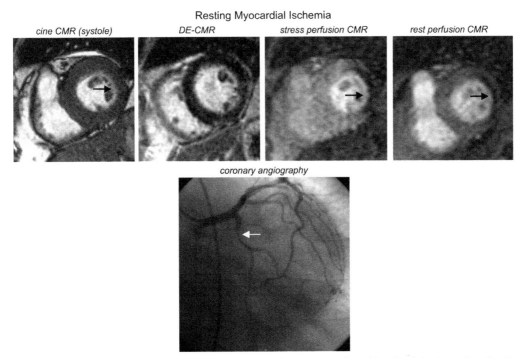

Fig. 8. Example of resting myocardial ischemia. Cine CMR demonstrates hypokinesis of the lateral wall without evidence of MI on DE-CMR. Dense, nearly transmural perfusion defects are present at during stress and rest (although they are larger with stress). Coronary angiography demonstrates a high-grade lesion in the proximal LCx coronary artery. Arrows point to the abnormalities.

DE-CMR and stress perfusion CMR are abnormal, the test is scored positive for ischemia if the perfusion defect is larger than the area of infarction.

The interpretation algorithm is based on two simple principles. First, with perfusion CMR and DE-CMR, there are two independent methods to obtain information regarding the presence or absence of MI. One method could be used to confirm the results of the other. Second, DE-CMR image quality (eg, signal-to-noise ratio) is far better than perfusion CMR because it is less demanding in terms of scanner hardware (DE-CMR images can be built up over several seconds rather than in 0.1 seconds, as is required for first-pass perfusion).[52] DE-CMR should be more accurate for the diagnosis of MI,[52] and the presence of

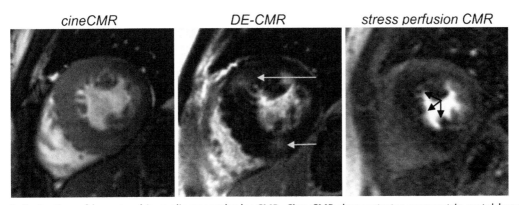

Fig. 9. Evaluation of hypertrophic cardiomyopathy by CMR. Cine CMR demonstrates asymmetric septal hypertrophy. On DE-CMR, there is evidence of scarring in the ventricular septum at the right ventricular insertion sites. The stress perfusion MR images also show a dense perfusion defect in the septum, although the region of ischemia is larger than the area of scarring on DE-CMR. This patient had normal epicardial coronary arteries on angiography. (*Modified from* Shah DJ, Judd RM, Kim RJ. Technology insight: MRI of the myocardium. Nat Clin Pract Cardiovasc Med 2005;2:597–605; with permission.)

Table 2
CMS reimbursement data for 50 United States, District of Columbia, and territories of Puerto Rico and Virgin Islands for 2008

State[c]	SPECT			CMR		
	Technical[a]	Professional[b]	Total	Technical	Professional	Total
Alabama	$1,023.51	$111.26	$1,134.77	$440.73	$147.81	$588.54
Alaska	$1,209.27	$122.99	$1,332.26	$570.12	$163.44	$733.56
Arizona	$1,125.48	$117.25	$1,242.73	$511.45	$155.72	$667.17
Arkansas	$1,008.66	$110.21	$1,118.87	$430.62	$146.49	$577.11
California	$1,332.95	$131.35	$1,464.30	$656.76	$174.75	$831.51
Colorado	$1,137.57	$117.63	$1,255.20	$520.22	$156.32	$676.54
Connecticut	$1,271.40	$128.12	$1,399.52	$613.34	$170.25	$783.59
Delaware	$1,160.75	$119.82	$1,280.57	$536.32	$159.21	$695.53
District of Columbia	$1,312.96	$131.15	$1,444.11	$642.31	$174.26	$816.57
Florida	$1,187.17	$122.06	$1,309.22	$552.85	$161.71	$714.56
Georgia	$1,116.90	$117.06	$1,233.96	$505.53	$155.48	$661.01
Hawaii	$1,233.18	$122.96	$1,356.14	$586.96	$163.45	$750.41
Idaho	$1,037.53	$111.88	$1,149.41	$450.69	$148.69	$599.38
Illinois	$1,170.64	$121.40	$1,292.03	$541.96	$160.98	$702.95
Indiana	$1,063.84	$113.34	$1,177.18	$469.04	$150.64	$619.68
Iowa	$1,032.75	$111.63	$1,144.38	$447.35	$148.34	$595.69
Kansas	$1,046.28	$112.51	$1,158.79	$456.61	$149.50	$606.11
Kentucky	$1,033.90	$112.00	$1,145.90	$447.77	$148.75	$596.52
Louisiana	$1,095.69	$115.72	$1,211.41	$490.53	$153.63	$644.16
Maine	$1,095.99	$115.15	$1,211.14	$491.42	$153.06	$644.48
Maryland	$1,160.29	$119.58	$1,279.87	$535.79	$158.84	$694.63
Massachusetts	$1,286.75	$127.26	$1,414.01	$624.27	$169.18	$793.45
Michigan	$1,166.28	$121.95	$1,288.22	$538.66	$161.65	$700.31
Minnesota	$1,115.07	$115.89	$1,230.96	$505.09	$154.15	$659.24
Mississippi	$1,026.97	$111.63	$1,138.60	$442.93	$148.25	$591.18
Missouri	$1,077.90	$117.63	$1,195.53	$478.13	$152.31	$630.43
Montana	$1,027.04	$111.66	$1,138.70	$442.95	$148.28	$591.23

Nebraska	$1,035.74	$111.57	$449.67	$1,147.31	$598.02	$148.35
Nevada	$1,174.28	$120.24	$545.33	$1,294.52	$705.00	$159.67
New Hampshire	$1,158.17	$118.73	$534.64	$1,276.90	$692.44	$157.80
New Jersey	$1,272.26	$129.18	$613.79	$1,401.44	$785.40	$171.61
New Mexico	$1,065.30	$114.02	$469.35	$1,179.32	$620.72	$151.37
New York	$1,268.27	$127.06	$609.15	$1395.32	$777.87	$168.72
North Carolina	$1,076.34	$114.17	$477.59	$1,190.51	$629.30	$151.71
North Dakota	$1,019.96	$110.90	$438.44	$1,130.86	$585.82	$147.38
Ohio	$1,099.59	$116.03	$493.13	$1,215.62	$647.16	$154.03
Oklahoma	$1,021.19	$110.98	$439.27	$1,132.17	$586.76	$147.49
Oregon	$1,111.19	$115.94	$502.19	$1,227.12	$656.33	$154.14
Pennsylvania	$1,160.05	$120.11	$535.17	$1,280.15	$694.59	$159.43
Puerto Rico	$899.06	$103.97	$354.37	$1,003.03	$492.57	$138.20
Rhode Island	$1,172.39	$122.03	$544.19	$1,294.42	$706.28	$162.09
South Carolina	$1,050.73	$112.48	$460.03	$1,163.21	$609.58	$149.55
South Dakota	$1,028.92	$111.26	$444.84	$1,140.18	$592.75	$147.91
Tennessee	$1,047.76	$112.58	$457.66	$1,160.34	$607.25	$149.59
Texas	$1,121.93	$117.77	$508.62	$1,239.70	$664.94	$156.31
Utah	$1,083.83	$114.84	$482.51	$1,198.67	$635.04	$152.53
Vermont	$1,108.98	$115.78	$500.58	$1,224.76	$654.51	$153.93
Virgin Islands	$1,142.94	$118.28	$523.55	$1,261.22	$680.63	$157.08
Virginia	$1,088.52	$114.81	$486.12	$1,203.33	$638.70	$152.58
Washington	$1,166.55	$119.80	$540.40	$1,286.35	$699.60	$159.20
West Virginia	$1,036.32	$113.01	$448.45	$1,149.33	$598.27	$149.82
Wisconsin	$1,072.63	$113.91	$475.06	$1,186.54	$626.45	$151.39
Wyoming	$1,033.34	$112.16	$447.16	$1,145.50	$596.07	$148.91
NATIONAL AVERAGE	$1,114.58	$117.03	$503.99	$1,231.61	$659.39	$155.39

CMS reimbursement data for 50 United States, District of Columbia, and territories of Puerto Rico and Virgin Islands for 2008. Reimbursement data accessed online from http://www.trailblazerhealth.com/, October 20, 2008. Technical reimbursement rates are for hospital outpatient prospective payment system (HOPPS). In states where reimbursements vary between different localities the average for all localities is listed. SPECT, single photon emission computed tomography; CMR, cardiac magnetic resonance.

a Technical component for SPECT includes CPT (Current Procedure Terminology) descriptor 78465 and 2 doses of radiopharmaceutical (rest and stress imaging).

b Professional component for SPECT includes CPT descriptor 78465 (myocardial perfusion imaging multiple studies) and CPT descriptors 78478 and 78480 (add-on codes for gated study for wall motion and ejection fraction) as per ASNC coding guidelines.

c Both technical and professional components for CMR are billed using CPT descriptor 75563.

Data from Trailblazer Health Enterprises. Available at: http://www.trailblazerhealth.com/. Accessed October 20, 2008.

infarction on DE-CMR favors the diagnosis of CAD, regardless of the perfusion CMR results. Conceptually, it then follows that perfusion defects that have similar intensity and extent during stress and rest ("matched defect") but do not have infarction on DE-CMR are artifactual and should not be considered positive for CAD, with rare exceptions.

Klem and colleagues[44] reported that the determination of CAD using the multicomponent CMR stress test and interpretation algorithm significantly improved diagnostic performance. In that study, the interpretation algorithm yielded a sensitivity rate of 89%, specificity rate of 87%, and diagnostic accuracy rate of 88% for the detection of CAD (major coronary artery with stenosis $\geq$ 70% or left main stenosis $\geq$ 50%). In comparison, when stress/rest perfusion was considered alone (without DE-CMR), the sensitivity, specificity, and diagnostic accuracy rates were 84%, 58%, and 68%, respectively. The interpretation algorithm had markedly higher specificity and diagnostic accuracy than perfusion CMR alone ($P < .0001$ for both). Notably, the higher specificity with the interpretation algorithm was primarily the result of correctly changing the diagnosis from positive to negative for CAD in 12 patients in whom infarction was not observed on DE-CMR, although perfusion CMR demonstrated matched stress-rest perfusion defects. Importantly, in this study, the imaging protocol and interpretation algorithm was prespecified, and all patients were consecutively recruited prospectively from a pool referred for elective coronary angiography. Patients with known CAD (eg, prior MI or revascularization) were excluded to reduce pretest referral or "spectrum" bias. To avoid posttest referral bias, all patients underwent angiography within 24 hours of CMR without regard to the CMR findings. It is likely that these results reflect the actual real world performance of a multicomponent CMR stress test with appropriate image interpretation.

Artifacts

Image artifacts often occur at the interface between the left ventricular cavity and the endocardium (arising from susceptibility effects or rapid cardiac motion) and may mimic true perfusion defects.[53] Characteristics that may be useful in distinguishing between artifact and true perfusion defects include the following: (1) artifacts are more common in the phase-encode direction; true perfusion defects should follow coronary artery distribution territories; (2) artifacts are transitory, varying in signal intensity in consecutive images during the transit of contrast media through the myocardium; true perfusion defects

often linger for multiple image frames and should follow smooth image intensity trajectories; (3) artifacts are generally present at stress and rest imaging; true perfusion defects generally appear only during vasodilator stress.

Concerning this latter point, it is important to recognize that the interpretation of stress/rest perfusion CMR is not analogous to stress/rest SPECT imaging. For instance, matched perfusion defects on perfusion CMR are far more likely to represent artifact than prior MI. We also have observed that severe but matched perfusion defects can occur in the setting of critical resting ischemia (**Fig. 8**). Unlike artifacts, these perfusion defects are transmural (or nearly transmural) and persist for nearly the entire first-pass and are associated with wall motion abnormalities in the same location as the perfusion defects. Although rare, recognition of true perfusion defects occurring at stress and rest with limited or absent MI on DE-CMR is important because they are associated with total or subtotal occlusions and are potentially reversible after revascularization.

Perfusion defects caused by microvascular dysfunction

Data regarding the use of multicomponent CMR stress testing in patients with microvascular dysfunction are limited. The high spatial resolution of perfusion CMR, which allows the identification of perfusion defects that primarily affect the subendocardium, may be useful in patients with potential microvascular dysfunction, such as hypertrophic cardiomyopathy[54] or aortic stenosis, and possibly in cardiac syndrome X,[55] although the latter is somewhat controversial.[56] For example, in patients with hypertrophic cardiomyopathy, we have observed stress-induced perfusion defects in the absence of epicardial coronary disease (**Fig. 9**). These perfusion defects are most apparent in the more hypertrophied portions of the myocardium and co-localize with regions of scarring on DE-CMR (presented elsewhere in this issue of *Heart Failure Clinics*). The clinical significance of these CMR findings has yet to be determined; however, because scarring and ischemia are likely to have prognostic implications, multicomponent CMR stress testing may be useful in risk stratification.

Reporting

At our institutions, CMR stress tests are scored regionally using the American Heart Association 17-segment model.[57] For the determination of the presence of CAD, the components are scored while viewing the images side-by-side (see **Fig. 5**). MI is scored from DE-CMR when hyperenhancement is present, unless the hyperenhancement is isolated to the midwall or subepicardium.[44,58,59] These latter patterns are found in nonischemic rather than ischemic disorders.[60,61] Stress and rest perfusion images are scored for perfusion defects in 16 segments (segment 17 at the apex is usually not visualized) using the interpretation algorithm on a 4-point scale: 0, normal; 1, probably normal; 2, probably abnormal; 3, definitely abnormal.[44] The corresponding coronary artery territory is assigned based on the distribution of abnormal segments.

Stress Cardiovascular Magnetic Resonance as Prognostic Tool

In addition to diagnostic accuracy in comparison to coronary angiography, several studies have evaluated the prognostic value of stress perfusion CMR.[62–64] In a study that evaluated 135 patients who presented to the emergency department with chest pain, Ingkanisorn and colleagues[62] demonstrated that adenosine perfusion abnormalities had 100% sensitivity and 93% specificity rates for detection of significant CAD based on any of the following: coronary artery stenosis less than 50% on angiography, abnormal correlative stress test, new MI, or death. In this study, an abnormal stress CMR added significant prognostic value in predicting future diagnosis of CAD, MI, or death over clinical risk factors.[62] In a more recent study, Jahnke and colleagues[63] performed combined stress perfusion CMR and dobutamine stress CMR in a series of 513 patients with known or suspected CAD. They demonstrated a 97.7% rate of survival free from cardiovascular death or nonfatal MI at 3 years in patients with a normal stress perfusion CMR. These data, along with another series from Bodi and colleagues,[64] demonstrate that stress perfusion CMR is not only useful for detection of CAD but also can provide important prognostic information. Although further confirmatory studies are required, early studies suggest that a normal stress perfusion CMR is associated with a low likelihood of future cardiovascular events, at least in the short-term and intermediate-term.

COST IMPLICATIONS OF CARDIOVASCULAR MAGNETIC RESONANCE

In the current medical environment with rising health care costs, any new cardiac imaging modality would need to be more efficacious and more cost effective than alternative testing. There seems to be a general perception by numerous authors and societies that CMR stress testing is more expensive than current common tests, such as SPECT.[16,45,65,66] To our knowledge, no analyses have compared the direct Center for Medicare & Medicaid Services (CMS) costs of stress CMR to alternative tests. We investigated this by tabulating the CMS reimbursement rates for stress SPECT and stress perfusion CMR, which was performed by visiting the Web site for TrailBlazer Health Enterprises, LLC (a contracted administrator for CMS) at www.trailblazerhealth.com on one given day (October 20, 2008). **Table 2** lists the CMS reimbursement rates for the professional and technical imaging components of a stress SPECT and stress perfusion CMR examination. Although there is considerable variation in the Medicare reimbursement rates from region to region, stress CMR is consistently 40% to 50% less expensive than stress SPECT. A large component of the difference can be explained by the expense for the radiopharmaceutical, which accounts for almost $400 of the expense for stress SPECT and is not required for stress perfusion CMR.

SUMMARY

CMR can play an important role in the evaluation of ischemic heart disease. Although coronary MRA and dobutamine stress CMR may play a role in selected scenarios, most CMR ischemia evaluation is generally performed using adenosine stress perfusion CMR. When combined with DE-CMR, the sensitivity, specificity, and diagnostic accuracy of the multicomponent stress perfusion CMR examination rival other currently available modalities for the evaluation of myocardial ischemia. Importantly, CMR perfusion stress testing has been deemed appropriate for the evaluation of chest pain syndromes in patients with intermediate probability of CAD and for ascertaining the physiologic significance of indeterminate coronary artery lesions. In the future, improvements in parallel imaging and pulse sequence technology, use of higher magnetic field strengths, and protocol optimizations will continue the rapid advance in image quality. Multicenter clinical trials, which are currently ongoing, soon will be available and will establish the diagnostic accuracy and prognostic value of CMR perfusion stress testing in a broad population of patients.

REFERENCES

1. Hunt SA, et al. ACC/AHA 2005 guideline update for the diagnosis and management of chronic heart failure in the adult: a report of the American College of Cardiology/American Heart Association Task Force on Practice Guidelines (Writing Committee to

Update the 2001 Guidelines for the Evaluation and Management of Heart Failure). Circulation 2005; 112(12):e154–235.

2. Gheorghiade M, Sopko G, Luca L, et al. Navigating the crossroads of coronary artery disease and heart failure. Circulation 2006;114(11):1202–13.

3. Weber OM, Martin AJ, Higgins CB. Whole-heart steady-state free precession coronary artery magnetic resonance angiography. Magn Reson Med 2003;50(6):1223–8.

4. Sakuma H, Ichikawa Y, Suzawa N, et al. Assessment of coronary arteries with total study time of less than 30 minutes by using whole-heart coronary MR angiography. Radiology 2005;237(1):316–21.

5. Hackenbroch M, Nehrke K, Gieseke J, et al. 3D motion adapted gating (3D MAG): a new navigator technique for accelerated acquisition of free breathing navigator gated 3D coronary MR-angiography. Eur Radiol 2005;15(8):1598–606.

6. Angelini P. Coronary artery anomalies: an entity in search of an identity. Circulation 2007;115(10): 1296–305.

7. McConnell MV, Ganz P, Selwyn AP, et al. Identification of anomalous coronary arteries and their anatomic course by magnetic resonance coronary angiography. Circulation 1995;92(11): 3158–62.

8. Taylor AM, Thorne SA, Rubens MB, et al. Coronary artery imaging in grown up congenital heart disease: complementary role of magnetic resonance and x-ray coronary angiography. Circulation 2000; 101(14):1670–8.

9. Post JC, van Rossum AC, Bronzwaer JG, et al. Magnetic resonance angiography of anomalous coronary arteries: a new gold standard for delineating the proximal course? Circulation 1995; 92(11):3163–71.

10. Vliegen HW, Doornbos J, de Roos A, et al. Value of fast gradient echo magnetic resonance angiography as an adjunct to coronary arteriography in detecting and confirming the course of clinically significant coronary artery anomalies. Am J Cardiol 1997;79(6):773–6.

11. Bluemke DA, Achenbach S, Budoff M, et al. Noninvasive coronary artery imaging: magnetic resonance angiography and multidetector computed tomography angiography. A scientific statement from the American Heart Association Committee on Cardiovascular Imaging and Intervention of the Council on Cardiovascular Radiology and Intervention, and the Councils on Clinical Cardiology and Cardiovascular Disease in the Young. Circulation 2008;118(5):586–606.

12. Kim WY, Danias PG, Stuber M, et al. Coronary magnetic resonance angiography for the detection of coronary stenoses. N Engl J Med 2001;345(26): 1863–9.

13. Manning WJ, Nezafat R, Appelbaum E, et al. Coronary magnetic resonance imaging. Cardiol Clin 2007;25(1):141–70, vi.

14. Nagel E, Lehmkuhl HB, Bocksch W, et al. Noninvasive diagnosis of ischemia-induced wall motion abnormalities with the use of high-dose dobutamine stress MRI: comparison with dobutamine stress echocardiography. Circulation 1999;99(6):763–70.

15. Hundley WG, Hamilton CA, Thomas MS, et al. Utility of fast cine magnetic resonance imaging and display for the detection of myocardial ischemia in patients not well suited for second harmonic stress echocardiography. Circulation 1999;100(16): 1697–702.

16. Hendel RC, Patel MR, Kramer CM, et al. ACCF/ACR/ SCCT/SCMR/ASNC/NASCI/SCAI/SIR 2006 appropriateness criteria for cardiac computed tomography and cardiac magnetic resonance imaging: a report of the American College of Cardiology Foundation Quality Strategic Directions Committee Appropriateness Criteria Working Group. J Am Coll Cardiol 2006;48(7):1475–97.

17. Rehwald WG, et al. Clinical CMR imaging techniques. In: Manning WJ, Pennell DJ, editors. Cardiovascular magnetic resonance. New York: Churchill Livingstone; in press.

18. Jerosch-Herold M, Seethamraju RT, Swingen CM, et al. Analysis of myocardial perfusion MRI. J Magn Reson Imaging 2004;19(6):758–70.

19. Beller GA, Holzgrefe HH, Watson DD. Effects of dipyridamole-induced vasodilation on myocardial uptake and clearance kinetics of thallium-201. Circulation 1983;68(6):1328–38.

20. Glover DK, Okada RD. Myocardial kinetics of Tc-MIBI in canine myocardium after dipyridamole. Circulation 1990;81(2):628–37.

21. Wilke N, Jerosch-Herold M, Wang Y, et al. Myocardial perfusion reserve: assessment with multisection, quantitative, first-pass MR imaging. Radiology 1997;204(2):373–84.

22. Epstein FH, London JF, Peters DC, et al. Multislice first-pass cardiac perfusion MRI: validation in a model of myocardial infarction. Magn Reson Med 2002;47(3):482–91.

23. Klocke FJ, Simonetti OP, Judd RM, et al. Limits of detection of regional differences in vasodilated flow in viable myocardium by first-pass magnetic resonance perfusion imaging. Circulation 2001; 104(20):2412–6.

24. Lee DC, Simonetti OP, Harris KR, et al. Magnetic resonance versus radionuclide pharmacological stress perfusion imaging for flow-limiting stenoses of varying severity. Circulation 2004;110(1):58–65.

25. Christian TF, Rettmann DW, Aletras AH, et al. Absolute myocardial perfusion in canines measured by using dual-bolus first-pass MR imaging. Radiology 2004;232(3):677–84.

26. Plein S, Greenwood JP, Ridgway JP, et al. Assessment of non-ST-segment elevation acute coronary syndromes with cardiac magnetic resonance imaging. J Am Coll Cardiol 2004;44(11):2173–81.

27. Plein S, Radjenovic A, Ridgway JP, et al. Coronary artery disease: myocardial perfusion MR imaging with sensitivity encoding versus conventional angiography. Radiology 2005;235(2):423–30.

28. Klein MA, Collier BD, Hellman RS, et al. Detection of chronic coronary artery disease: value of pharmacologically stressed, dynamically enhanced turbo-fast low-angle shot MR images. AJR Am J Roentgenol 1993;161(2):257–63.

29. Hartnell G, Cerel A, Kamalesh M, et al. Detection of myocardial ischemia: value of combined myocardial perfusion and cineangiographic MR imaging. AJR Am J Roentgenol 1994;163(5):1061–7.

30. Al-Saadi N, Nagel E, Gross M, et al. Noninvasive detection of myocardial ischemia from perfusion reserve based on cardiovascular magnetic resonance. Circulation 2000;101(12):1379–83.

31. Eichenberger AC, Schuiki E, Kochli VD, et al. Ischemic heart disease: assessment with gadolinium-enhanced ultrafast MR imaging and dipyridamole stress. J Magn Reson Imaging 1994;4(3):425–31.

32. Bertschinger KM, Nanz D, Buechi M, et al. Magnetic resonance myocardial first-pass perfusion imaging: parameter optimization for signal response and cardiac coverage. J Magn Reson Imaging 2001;14(5):556–62.

33. Schwitter J, Nanz D, Kneifel S, et al. Assessment of myocardial perfusion in coronary artery disease by magnetic resonance: a comparison with positron emission tomography and coronary angiography. Circulation 2001;103(18):2230–5.

34. Panting JR, Gatehouse PD, Yang GZ, et al. Echo-planar magnetic resonance myocardial perfusion imaging: parametric map analysis and comparison with thallium SPECT. J Magn Reson Imaging 2001;13(2):192–200.

35. Sensky PR, Samani NJ, Reek C, et al. Magnetic resonance perfusion imaging in patients with coronary artery disease: a qualitative approach. Int J Cardiovasc Imaging 2002;18(5):373–83.

36. Ibrahim T, Nekolla SG, Schreiber K, et al. Assessment of coronary flow reserve: comparison between contrast-enhanced magnetic resonance imaging and positron emission tomography. J Am Coll Cardiol 2002;39(5):864–70.

37. Chiu CW, So NM, Lam WW, et al. Combined first-pass perfusion and viability study at MR imaging in patients with non-ST segment-elevation acute coronary syndromes: feasibility study. Radiology 2003;226(3):717–22.

38. Ishida N, Sakuma H, Motoyasu M, et al. Noninfarcted myocardium: correlation between dynamic first-pass contrast-enhanced myocardial MR imaging and quantitative coronary angiography. Radiology 2003;229(1):209–16.

39. Nagel E, Klein C, Paetsch I, et al. Magnetic resonance perfusion measurements for the noninvasive detection of coronary artery disease. Circulation 2003;108(4):432–7.

40. Doyle M, Fuisz A, Kortright E, et al. The impact of myocardial flow reserve on the detection of coronary artery disease by perfusion imaging methods: an NHLBI WISE study. J Cardiovasc Magn Reson 2003;5(3):475–85.

41. Wolff SD, Schwitter J, Coulden R, et al. Myocardial first-pass perfusion magnetic resonance imaging: a multicenter dose-ranging study. Circulation 2004;110(6):732–7.

42. Giang TH, Nanz D, Coulden R, et al. Detection of coronary artery disease by magnetic resonance myocardial perfusion imaging with various contrast medium doses: first European multi-centre experience. Eur Heart J 2004;25(18):1657–65.

43. Paetsch I, Jahnke C, Wahl A, et al. Comparison of dobutamine stress magnetic resonance, adenosine stress magnetic resonance, and adenosine stress magnetic resonance perfusion. Circulation 2004;110(7):835–42.

44. Klem I, Heitner JF, Shah DJ, et al. Improved detection of coronary artery disease by stress perfusion cardiovascular magnetic resonance with the use of delayed enhancement infarction imaging. J Am Coll Cardiol 2006;47(8):1630–8.

45. Pennell DJ, Sechtem UP, Higgins CB, et al. Clinical indications for cardiovascular magnetic resonance (CMR): consensus panel report. Eur Heart J 2004;25(21):1940–65.

46. Cecil MP, Kosinski AS, Jones MT, et al. The importance of work-up (verification) bias correction in assessing the accuracy of SPECT thallium-201 testing for the diagnosis of coronary artery disease. J Clin Epidemiol 1996;49(7):735–42.

47. Detrano R, Janosi A, Lyons KP, et al. Factors affecting sensitivity and specificity of a diagnostic test: the exercise thallium scintigram. Am J Med 1988;84(4):699–710.

48. Cury RC, Cattani CA, Gabure LA, et al. Diagnostic performance of stress perfusion and delayed-enhancement MR imaging in patients with coronary artery disease. Radiology 2006;240(1):39–45.

49. Weinmann HJ, Brasch RC, Press WR, et al. Characteristics of gadolinium-DTPA complex: a potential NMR contrast agent. AJR Am J Roentgenol 1984;142(3):619–24.

50. Cerqueira MD, Verani MS, Schwaiger M, et al. Safety profile of adenosine stress perfusion imaging: results from the Adenoscan Multicenter Trial Registry. J Am Coll Cardiol 1994;23(2):384–9.

51. Rossen JD, Quillen JE, Lopez AG, et al. Comparison of coronary vasodilation with intravenous dipyridamole and adenosine. J Am Coll Cardiol 1991;18(2): 485–91.

52. Fuster V, Kim RJ. Frontiers in cardiovascular magnetic resonance. Circulation 2005;112(1): 135–44.

53. Di Bella EV, Parker DL, Sinusas AJ. On the dark rim artifact in dynamic contrast-enhanced MRI myocardial perfusion studies. Magn Reson Med 2005; 54(5):1295–9.

54. Shah DJ, Judd RM, Kim RJ. Technology insight: MRI of the myocardium. Nat Clin Pract Cardiovasc Med 2005;2(11):597–605.

55. Panting JR, Gatehouse PD, Yang GZ, et al. Abnormal subendocardial perfusion in cardiac syndrome X detected by cardiovascular magnetic resonance imaging. N Engl J Med 2002;346(25): 1948–53.

56. Vermeltfoort IA, Bondarenko O, Raijmakers PG, et al. Is subendocardial ischaemia present in patients with chest pain and normal coronary angiograms? A cardiovascular MR study. Eur Heart J 2007;28(13):1554–8.

57. Cerqueira MD, Weissman NJ, Dilsizian V, et al. Standardized myocardial segmentation and nomenclature for tomographic imaging of the heart: a statement for healthcare professionals from the Cardiac Imaging Committee of the Council on Clinical Cardiology of the American Heart Association. Circulation 2002;105(4):539–42.

58. Kim RJ, Wu E, Rafael A, et al. The use of contrast-enhanced magnetic resonance imaging to identify reversible myocardial dysfunction. N Engl J Med 2000;343(20):1445–53.

59. Mahrholdt H, Wagner A, Judd RM, et al. Delayed enhancement cardiovascular magnetic resonance assessment of non-ischaemic cardiomyopathies. Eur Heart J 2005; 26(15):1461–74.

60. Choudhury L, Mahrholdt H, Wagner A, et al. Myocardial scarring in asymptomatic or mildly symptomatic patients with hypertrophic cardiomyopathy. J Am Coll Cardiol 2002;40(12):2156–64.

61. McCrohon JA, Moon JC, Prasad SK, et al. Differentiation of heart failure related to dilated cardiomyopathy and coronary artery disease using gadolinium-enhanced cardiovascular magnetic resonance. Circulation 2003;108(1):54–9.

62. Ingkanisorn WP, Kwong RY, Bohme NS, et al. Prognosis of negative adenosine stress magnetic resonance in patients presenting to an emergency department with chest pain. J Am Coll Cardiol 2006;47(7):1427–32.

63. Jahnke C, Nagel E, Gebker R, et al. Prognostic value of cardiac magnetic resonance stress tests: adenosine stress perfusion and dobutamine stress wall motion imaging. Circulation 2007;115(13):1769–76.

64. Bodi V, Sanchis J, Lopez-Lereu MP, et al. Prognostic value of dipyridamole stress cardiovascular magnetic resonance imaging in patients with known or suspected coronary artery disease. J Am Coll Cardiol 2007;50(12):1174–9.

65. Mieres JH, Makaryus AN, Redberg RF, et al. Noninvasive cardiac imaging. Am Fam Physician 2007; 75(8):1219–28.

66. Gani F, Jain D, Lahiri A. The role of cardiovascular imaging techniques in the assessment of patients with acute chest pain. Nucl Med Commun 2007; 28(6):441–9.

Myocardial Viability and Revascularization

Anne S. Kanderian, MD, Rahul Renapurkar, MD,
Scott D. Flamm, MD*

KEYWORDS

- MRI • Myocardium • Viability • Ischemia
- Revascularization

Identification of viable myocardium has become a topic of great interest because evidence has surfaced that ischemic left ventricular dysfunction is potentially reversible.[1,2] Modern drugs and medical therapy have significantly reduced morbidity and mortality associated with ischemic heart disease. Among the most important therapies is surgical revascularization, which has been shown to significantly diminish the mortality rate. Nevertheless, morbidity and mortality associated with ischemic heart disease remains high, and even the success of surgical revascularization is tempered by the high perioperative mortality associated with ischemic heart disease.

Left ventricular dysfunction secondary to coronary artery disease typically is either irreversible, as in transmural myocardial infarction, or potentially reversible, as in states of myocardial ischemia. Potentially reversible ischemic left ventricular dysfunction is felt to arise from one of two pathologic states: myocardial stunning or myocardial hibernation. Myocardial stunning occurs when a transient ischemic insult results in contractile dysfunction that persists for a variable period of time despite adequate restoration of coronary blood flow. Myocardial hibernation occurs as a result of a state of chronic ischemia secondary to reduced coronary blood flow and oxygen supply. In the setting of reduced nutrient supply, myocardial cells reduce their metabolic requirements by adapting in such a way as to decrease contractility, but to otherwise maintain cellular integrity.[3] Hence, with hibernating myocardium, the myocardial cells remain "alive" and viable. Upon restoration of coronary blood flow, left ventricular dysfunction may be reversed.

Because left ventricular function and outcomes can potentially be improved in patients with ischemic left ventricular dysfunction, detecting viable myocardium as a precursor to revascularization is critical. Thus, increasing emphasis is being placed on such detection. Until recently, clinicians relied on thallium scintigraphy and dobutamine echocardiography to identify viable myocardium. Now, however, the focus is shifting toward positron emission tomography (PET) and increasingly to cardiac MRI (CMR) for diagnosis. This article discusses the rationale for this emphasis and reviews the evidence for CMR's role in detection of myocardial viability and therapeutic triage.

IMPORTANCE OF MYOCARDIAL VIABILITY

Over the past 20 years, multiple studies have documented improved survival after revascularization of viable myocardium.[4–10] In 1994, Di Carli and colleagues,[7] after assessing 93 patients (mean ejection fraction of 25%) with PET and following them for 31 months, demonstrated that the annual survival rate of non-revascularized patients with evidence of viability was 50%, compared with 92% in those with no PET mismatch. Eitzman and colleagues,[11] also using PET, found a cardiac event rate of 50% in patients with depressed left ventricular function and evidence of myocardial hibernation. Similarly, in a series of 84 postinfarction patients followed up for a mean of 23 months, Tamaki and colleagues[12]

Cleveland Clinic, Cleveland, OH, USA
* Corresponding author. Cardiovascular Imaging Laboratory, Imaging Institute, J1-4, Cleveland Clinic, 9500 Euclid Avenue, Cleveland, OH 44195.
E-mail address: flamms@ccf.org (S.D. Flamm).

Heart Failure Clin 5 (2009) 333–348
doi:10.1016/j.hfc.2009.02.008

have shown that an increase in uptake of fluorodeoxyglucose F 18 (FDG) was the best predictor of subsequent cardiac events.

Bax and colleagues,[13] reviewing noninvasive techniques for the identification of myocardial viability, reported that 25% to 40% of patients with left ventricular dysfunction and the presence of viable myocardium demonstrate improvement in left ventricular function following revascularization. Other studies have demonstrated that revascularization of viable myocardium in patients with heart failure alleviates symptoms and improves exercise capacity.[14,15] These findings also have been confirmed in a meta-analysis by Allman and colleagues.[16] The investigators pooled 3088 patients from 24 viability studies using thallium perfusion imaging, FDG PET, and dobutamine echocardiography. The mean ejection fraction was 32 ± 8%. Thirty-five percent of patients underwent revascularization while the remainder received medical therapy (16%, P<.0001). In patients without demonstrable myocardial viability, there was no difference in annual mortality between the two groups (7.7% with revascularization versus 6.2% with medical therapy, P not significant). The result of this study provides convincing evidence of the clinical benefit of revascularization in patients with left ventricular dysfunction and viable myocardium as opposed to medical therapy alone.

ALTERNATIVE IMAGING TECHNIQUES TO ASSESS MYOCARDIAL VIABILITY

A number of noninvasive techniques, aside from CMR, have been used to identify and quantify the amount of viable myocardium. These include low-dose dobutamine stress echocardiography (LD-DSE), single photon emission computed tomography (SPECT), PET, and CT.

LD-DSE induces contractility, as a reflection of inotropic reserve, in viable myocardium, whether stunned or hibernating. The value of inotropic reserve in the detection of viable myocardium is well established and has been reviewed.[17] The predictive value of DSE appears greatest when there is a biphasic response: improved contractility at a low dose and then worsening at a higher dose.[18,19] The initial improvement in wall motion reflects recruitment of contractile reserve during low-dose dobutamine (5 μg/kg), and hence indicates viability.[20] Higher doses initially lead to subendocardial ischemia and subsequently to worsening of the wall-motion abnormality as a manifestation of stress-induced ischemia.

Recovery of contractility of akinetic myocardium after revascularization is better predicted by increased contractility on LD-DSE than by SPECT

and PET. In a meta-analysis, Bax and colleagues[13] pooled 925 patients from 28 studies. The determined sensitivity, specificity, and positive and negative predictive values of LD-DSE to detect functional recovery following revascularization were 81%, 80%, 77%, and 85%, respectively.

To assess viability, SPECT imaging depends on myocardial uptake of radiotracers. To identify viable miycardial segments, SPECT imaging makes use of thallium Th 201 to detect intact functional cellular membranes and technetium Tc 99m–based compounds to detect preserved mitochondrial function. Thallium Th 201 is a potassium analog with uptake that is a sodium-potassium-ATPase–dependent active process requiring cell membrane integrity. Uptake of thallium Th 201 is an indicator of both regional perfusion and viability. A variety of protocols have been used for viability assessment using thallium Th 201, including stress-redistribution imaging, late redistribution imaging, and reinjection protocols. With stress imaging protocols, the finding of stress defect reversibility on redistribution or reinjection images is strongly indicative of ischemic, viable myocardium. Likewise, a fixed defect with a severe reduction in thallium Th 201 activity on stress redistribution-reinjection protocols or rest-redistribution protocols strongly implies predominantly nonviable myocardium.

In contrast to thallium Th 201, the uptake of technetium Tc 99m–labeled radiotracers, such as technetium Tc 99m sestamibi and technetium Tc 99m tetrofosmin, is by passive diffusion and depends on intact electrochemical gradients across sarcolemmal and mitochondrial membranes. These agents show minimal redistribution within the myocardium. The development of technetium Tc 99m sestamibi ECG-gated SPECT imaging has enabled the assessment of regional left ventricular function as well as perfusion. Studies comparing viability detection with thallium Th 201 and technetium Tc 99m sestamibi have generally demonstrated good agreement in quantification of viable myocardium and in their ability to predict recovery of function following revascularization.[21,22] In a study by Udelson and colleagues,[21] qualitative and quantitative comparisons of rest and redistribution thallium Th 201 activity and technetium Tc 99m sestamibi activity 1 hour after rest injection were performed in 31 patients with coronary artery disease and left ventricular dysfunction. Positive (75% versus 80% for thallium Th 201 and technetium Tc 99m sestamibi, respectively) and negative (92% versus 96%, respectively) predictive values for recovery of regional ventricular dysfunction after revascularization were similar for the two agents.

PET imaging uses radiotracer-uptake patterns to identify viable myocardium based on evidence of preserved metabolic function. This technique uses positron-emitting isotopes (oxygen 15, carbon 11, nitrogen 13, and fluorine 18) incorporated into physiologically active molecules. Under ischemic conditions, the myocyte metabolism preferentially shifts from using fatty acids to glucose. Therefore, uptake of a glucose analog (FDG) in a region of myocardium indicates metabolic activity, and thus viability. More specifically, the presence of enhanced FDG uptake in a region of decreased flow (known as a PET "mismatch") indicates hibernating myocardium, while a reduction in both the metabolism and flow reflects predominantly nonviable myocardium. In contrast, regional dysfunction in the presence of normal perfusion is suggestive of myocardial stunning. Bax and colleagues[13] demonstrated the value of PET imaging for viability in a meta-analysis. Data for 598 patients from 20 studies revealed that mean sensitivity, specificity, and positive and negative predictive values to detect viability were 93%, 58%, 71%, and 86%, respectively.

CT can assess myocardial viability based on the relative tissue contrast concentrations on postcontrast imaging. Experimental studies have shown that contrast-enhanced CT can accurately depict acute and chronic infarcts as regions of hyperenhancement approximately 5 minutes after contrast injection, whereas areas of microvascular obstruction were characterized by hypoenhancement.[23,24] In a study by Paul and colleagues[25] involving 34 patients, late enhancement on contrast-enhanced CT performed well in defining residual perfusion defects and infarct size in comparison to SPECT (sensitivity and specificity of 93% and 100%, respectively). Nonetheless, this technique remains experimental with only limited human data available.

CARDIAC MRI FOR VIABILITY

As a tool for evaluating structure, function, perfusion, and cellular integrity, CMR can provide a comprehensive assessment of viability. Multiple studies using CMR have demonstrated its value in assessing wall thickness, contractile reserve, perfusion, and transmural extent of necrosis for predicting left ventricular functional recovery.

Wall Thickness and Wall Thickening Measurements

In the setting of acute myocardial infarction, determination of wall thickness and systolic thickening has limited value in assessing viability. Infarct expansion typically is not seen with open infarct-related arteries following early spontaneous

reperfusion, successful interventional revascularization, or thrombolysis. This means wall thickness may be the same in transmural necrosis and nontransmural necrosis early after myocardial infarction. Furthermore, both conditions may be associated with absence of resting function early after the ischemic event.

In chronic myocardial infarction, assessment of the myocardial thickness (using a cut-off of 5.5-mm end-diastolic wall thickness) and systolic thickening by cine-MRI has high sensitivity, but poor specificity and positive predictive value in predicting recovery after revascularization.[26] The likely explanation for this limitation is the inability of cine images to enable direct visualization of viable myocardium.

Low-Dose Dobutamine MRI

Low-dose dobutamine MRI uses the same principles as LD-DSE and has emerged as a technique of comparable accuracy.[27–29] Criteria for viability are a minimal end-diastolic wall thickness of more than 5 mm with resting systolic thickening, or resting akinesis and an improvement in systolic wall thickening of 2 mm or more during low-dose dobutamine infusion (contractile reserve).

Dobutamine MRI has particular advantages over echocardiography in providing better endocardial definition, and is less hindered by acoustic windows, thereby substantially reducing the incidence of poor-quality studies.[28]

Studies using high-dose dobutamine and focusing on the detection of ischemia will not be reviewed here.

CONTRAST-ENHANCED MRI FOR VIABILITY

The concept of delayed enhancement was first described over 20 years ago by Wesbey and colleagues,[30] who performed ECG-gated spin-echo imaging following contrast administration. Regions associated with acute myocardial infarction became bright 1 to 10 minutes after contrast administration. The use of spin-echo techniques did not gain great acceptance secondary to the relatively modest signal enhancement, heterogeneity of enhancement in regions of myocardial infarction, and a tendency to overestimate the area of irreversibly damaged tissue.

In 1999, Kim and colleagues[31] introduced the sequence currently used for viability assessment, and now known as delayed-enhancement MRI (DE-MRI). Simonetti and colleagues,[32] working in the same laboratory with Kim and colleagues, provided a detailed characterization of this imaging sequence. A segmented k-space inversion-recovery gradient-echo pulse sequence where the inversion time is set to null signal from normal myocardium, DE-MRI has the distinct characteristic of providing high contrast for irreversibly damaged myocardium. For example, scar tissue has approximately 10 times the signal of remote normal myocardium (up to 1080%) in animal studies, and nearly five times the signal (485%) in humans (**Fig. 1**). Additional advantages of DE-MRI over the established nuclear imaging methods are lack of radiation exposure and superior spatial resolution (in-plane resolution of 1–2 mm).[31,32]

Kinetics of Delayed-Enhancement MRI

DE-MRI images typically are obtained 10 to 30 minutes following intravenous infusion of gadolinium-chelate (0.1–0.2 mmol/kg). To heighten the contrast between the normal and infarcted myocardium, the signal from normal myocardium must be reduced as much as possible through selection of the appropriate inversion time. The best inversion time can be selected by obtaining a series of two-dimensional DE-MRI images across a range of inversion times. Alternative methods include the use of a Look-Locker sequence, or a lower resolution steady state free precession cine technique incorporating an iteratively adjusted inversion time (**Fig. 2**).

Gadolinium-chelate, considered biologically inert, passively diffuses within the myocardium in the extracellular, interstitial space, with a half-life in blood of approximately 20 minutes.[33] The reason myocardial scars are hyperenhanced relative to normal myocardium is felt to stem from differences in wash-in and wash-out kinetics and volume of distribution.[34–41] Normal myocardium has a relatively rapid wash-in and wash-out rate, while scar tissue has more delayed wash-in and wash-out of contrast. Clinicians can take advantage of the difference between the two with an appropriate delay of approximately 10 to 20 minutes following contrast administration. Furthermore, as a result of an increase in interstitial space, the volume of distribution increases in both chronic and acutely infarcted myocardium. In the former, the presence of fibrotic tissue increases the interstitial space per unit volume, whereas in the latter, the loss of sarcomere integrity due to myocyte death effectively converts much of the intracellular space to interstitial volume. Gadolinium-chelate diffuses rapidly into the interstitial, but not intracellular space. Thus, both chronically and acutely infarcted myocardium have increased concentrations of gadolinium per unit volume, resulting in a greater shortening of T_1 and increased enhancement relative to normal, viable myocardium.[34–37]

Imaging Techniques

DE-MRI was initially performed using a two-dimensional segmented k-space gradient-echo sequence with an inversion recovery preparatory pulse. In the two-dimensional technique, each imaging slice is acquired during a breath hold ranging from 8 to 16 seconds. Coverage of the left ventricle in both long and short axes generally requires a total of 12 to 16 breath holds. DE-MRI images of the left ventricle typically are acquired

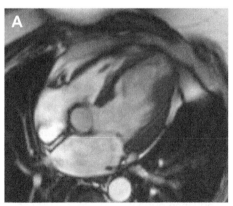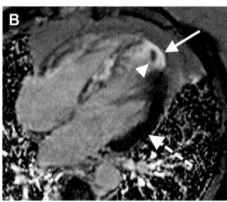

Fig.1. Cine (*A*) and DE-MRI (*B*) four-chamber views in a patient with a left anterior descending artery distribution infarction. The DE-MRI image demonstrates high signal intensity throughout the septum and transmurally in the apex (*arrow*), indicating transmural, nonviable scar tissue. In contrast, the lateral wall (*dashed arrow*) has normal, full-thickness myocardium that is black (or non-hyperenhanced) indicating viable tissue with intact cellular membranes. In addition to differentiating viable from nonviable myocardium, the DE-MRI technique also is well suited for identifying intracavitary thrombus, as noted here in the left ventricular apex (*arrowhead*) and seen as a small black oval lesion.

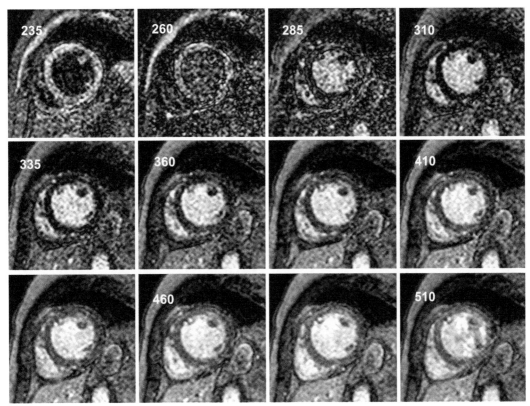

Fig. 2. This image matrix demonstrates use of the Look-Locker sequence for optimizing the inversion time in a DE-MRI sequence. In this series, the inversion time is iteratively advanced during a single breath-hold acquisition of a relatively low spatial-resolution pulse sequence. The corresponding inversion time is noted on each image frame. The optimal nulling time, where the myocardium has the least signal intensity (is black), is seen in the right upper quadrant where the inversion time is noted as 310 ms. Note that the blood pool is nulled earlier in time, on the first image frame, when the inversion time is 235 ms. On later images, the signal intensity of both the blood pool and myocardium increase, and there is loss of contrast between the two tissues.

in the same slice positions as a series of dynamic cine images for direct correlation of function and viability. Successful in both animal and human studies with numerous studies providing robust data, this approach remains a routine method for viability imaging.

Other approaches also have been developed to provide needed flexibility in various clinical scenarios. These alternatives include phase-sensitive inversion recovery, three-dimensional volumetric coverage, and single-shot techniques. The phase-sensitive inversion recovery technique acquires both a magnitude image and a phase-sensitive image, the latter of which can be used to image at a nominal value of the inversion recovery time. This technique achieves a consistent contrast, thus eliminating the need for multiple breath-holds in a sequence with iteratively advanced inversion recovery times to find a precise null time of myocardium[42] (**Fig. 3**). The limitation to the technique is its longer acquisition time. Because of the substantial volume of data that must be acquired, three-dimensional volumetric inversion recovery has been problematic for achieving full coverage of the left ventricle in a single breath-hold. Fortunately, the advancement and incorporation of parallel acquisition techniques (eg, SENSE [sensitivity encoding], SMASH [simultaneous acquisition of spatial harmonics], and GRAPPA [generalized autocalibrating partially parallel acquisitions]) with three-dimensional volumetric inversion recovery provides an opportunity to cover the entire left ventricle in a single breath-hold, dramatically shortening the overall acquisition time compared with sequential two-dimensional techniques (**Fig. 4**). In addition, three-dimensional volumetric techniques eliminate slice misregistration, which may occur when patients perform repeated breath holds. However, the spatial resolution available is less robust than that with current two-dimensional techniques. Finally, single-shot inversion recovery

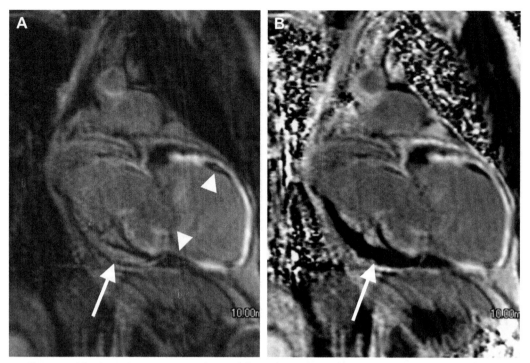

Fig. 3. Phase-sensitive inversion recovery techniques have demonstrated particular utility in DE-MRI. (*A*) Magnitude image. (*B*) Phase-sensitive image. The nulling time chosen was not perfectly optimized, resulting in the myocardium in the anterior and inferior walls (*arrowheads*) being heterogeneous with both black and gray areas. The phase-sensitive image is notable for these same areas of myocardium being uniformly black. One limitation of the technique, evidenced in this example, is the phase-sensitive treatment of some pericardial effusions. In A, the inferior pericardial effusion overlying the left atrium and base of the left ventricle is gray in signal intensity and easily distinguished from adjacent areas of myocardium. In contrast, in B, the pericardial effusion is black in signal intensity and blends with the myocardium at the base of the inferior left ventricle.

sequences have been developed that acquire each image slice within a single heartbeat, reducing or eliminating the need for breath-holding. This technique is particularly valuable in patients who have difficulty in breath-holding or in those with arrhythmias[43] (**Fig. 5**). In addition, these can be combined with parallel imaging to achieve higher spatial resolution.

DE-MRI images are usually interpreted in combination with cine images to assess segmental wall motion. In broad categories, the images may be interpreted as follows:

> The combination of normal wall-motion and lack of hyperenhancement on a segmental basis implies normal or viable tissue.
> Normal wall-motion or segmental dysfunction in combination with a mild degree of hyperenhancement (<25% of the segment) implies normal or viable tissue.
> A segmental wall-motion abnormality in combination with greater than 75% hyperenhancement suggests nonviable tissue.

For these categories, the prognostic value of DE-MRI seems clear. The difficulty, however, lies in segments that are dysfunctional, but have intermediate degrees of hyperenhancement (>25% and <75%). The available data, which will be highlighted, suggest heterogeneity of response to revascularization consistent with the nonbinary gradient of myocardial involvement and resultant spectrum of response.

VIABILITY IMAGING: EVIDENCE FROM ANIMAL STUDIES
Accuracy of Delayed-Enhancement MRI for Irreversible Myocardial Damage

Kim and colleagues[31] published the initial article describing the current DE-MRI technique. In this seminal study, the left anterior descending artery was instrumented in a canine model and occluded either transiently or permanently. DE-MRI of the explanted hearts was compared with 2,3,5-triphenyltetrazolium chloride–stained pathology specimens at 1 day, 3 days, and 8 weeks after

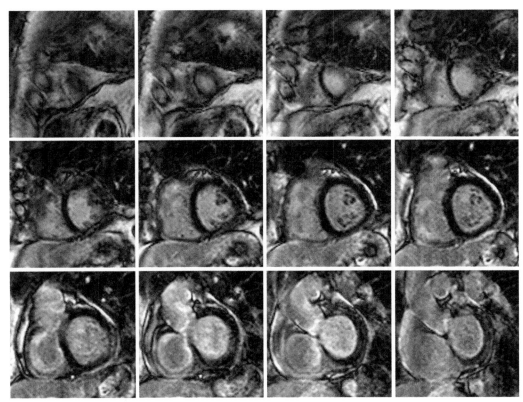

Fig. 4. This image matrix demonstrates a series of 12 short-axis slices obtained through the left ventricle in a single breath-hold of 22 seconds. Because the technique is three-dimensional volumetric and performed in a single breath-hold, there is no slice misregistration. Signal-to-noise and contrast-to-noise ratios are comparable to those of two-dimensional techniques, though the spatial resolution is slightly inferior.

instrumentation, with close correlation demonstrated between hyperenhancement on CMR and irreversible damage at pathology.

Further demonstration of the accuracy of DE-MRI for distinguishing between infarcted and reversibly injured myocardium was provided by Fieno and colleagues,[44] who studied a series of dogs subjected to coronary occlusion with or without reperfusion. In animals that had reperfused infarcts, coronary reocclusion was performed before sacrifice, and fluorescent microparticles were injected into the heart to identify jeopardized areas, but viable myocardium at risk of infarction. In vivo DE-MRI was performed at serial time points (1 day to 8 weeks) before animal sacrifice with ex vivo DE-MRI and subsequent histopathology analysis (2,3,5-triphenyltetrazolium chloride stain) performed for quantification of infarcted and viable myocardium. Consistent with prior studies, in vivo and ex vivo DE-MRI provided near-identical findings for quantification of infarct size (r = 0.99), with near exact agreement between histopathology and DE-MRI–determined infarct size (lowest r = 0.95, largest bias 1.7% of total left ventricular area).

Some studies have suggested overestimation of the area of myocardial infarction by DE-MRI. In one such study, Saeed and colleagues[45] suggested that, although hyperenhanced regions consist predominately of scar tissue, they may also encompass a small area of viable peri-infarct myocardium. This finding was based on a study of rat infarcts employing a necrosis-specific magnetic resonance contrast medium (mesoporphyrin). Overestimation of infarcted tissue is a concern because the amount of irreversibly damaged tissue has prognostic implications. Nonetheless, the variation in contrast uptake is potentially explained by intrinsic differences in kinetics between and among species, and by distinctions in imaging protocols used.

In a compelling study by Rehwald and colleagues,[41] convincing evidence was produced indicating that DE-MRI is highly specific for irreversibly injured myocardium. Reversible and irreversible injuries were studied in 38 rabbits divided into four groups defined by occlusion and reperfusion time. The investigators used an electron probe x-ray microanalysis (EPXMA) to

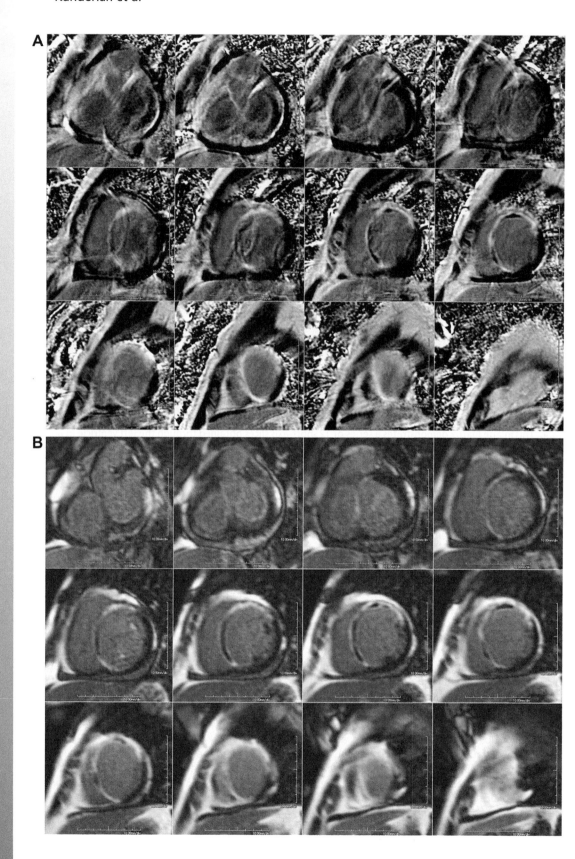

simultaneously examine concentrations of gadolinium, sodium, phosphorus, sulfur, chlorine, potassium, and calcium in myocardium and used histologic staining to define areas of scar. Myocardium was categorized as acute or chronic infarction. The at-risk peri-infarction zones in acute infarctions were analyzed. Compared with remote regions, gadolinium levels measured by EPXMA were more than doubled in acutely infarcted nonviable areas and were fourfold higher in chronically infarcted regions. The concentration of gadolinium was not elevated in regions that were considered at risk but not infarcted, despite being reperfused. This work appears to have solidified the notion that elevations in myocardial gadolinium are confined to regions of histologically defined irreversible ischemic injury.

Relationship of Delayed-Enhancement MRI Transmurality to Functional Recovery in Acute Myocardial Infarction

The above-noted research has clarified the ability of DE-MRI to accurately identify irreversibly damaged myocardium, a critical starting point in determining myocardial viability. Further categorization involves classifying the likelihood of functional myocardial recovery based on the degree of hyperenhancement present. To that end, Hillebrand and colleagues,[46] in an animal model involving 15 canines, evaluated the relationship between the transmural extent of hyperenhancement at 3 days and the contractile recovery at 28 days after myocardial infarction. They found for segments with 25% or less hyperenhancement, the majority (87%) improved function. In contrast, for segments with hyperenhancement of 75% or more, functional recovery was unlikely, while in segments with 100% hyperenhancement, no functional recovery occurred.

Further evidence for the importance of defining the transmural extent of hyperenhancement comes from a study by Gerber and colleagues.[47] In this study, 13 canines were imaged with low-dose dobutamine–tagged MRI and contrast-enhanced DE-MRI within 48 hours of infarction. No significant inotropic reserve was evident in segments with transmural hyperenhancement when assessed with low-dose dobutamine-tagged MRI, while segments with nontransmural hyperenhancement demonstrated contractile reserve, indicating residual viability. These findings, using low-dose dobutamine wall motion to reveal potential recovery of contractile reserve relative to the degree of transmural scarring, emphasizes the independent prognostic power of DE-MRI.

VIABILITY IMAGING: EVIDENCE FROM STUDIES IN HUMANS

Several studies in humans have authenticated the usefulness of DE-MRI in detecting the presence, location, and extent of myocardial scar[48–50] (Fig. 6). The high spatial resolution that DE-MRI offers allows the detection of subendocardial scar and small infarcts, even in the absence of Q waves on ECG.

A wealth of data exists showing that DE-MRI is just as good or better than alternative techniques in identifying viable myocardium, thus explaining why DE-MRI has recently gained in clinical popularity. A study by Wagner and colleagues[51] showed that, in 91 patients, DE-MRI and SPECT were able to detect transmural infarcts at similar rates. However, in detecting subendocardial infarcts, 47% of segments (13% of patients) detected by DE-MRI were missed by SPECT. Similarly, another study that compared DE-MRI to SPECT in the setting of an acute myocardial infarct revealed that DE-MRI was more sensitive than SPECT in detecting all infarcts (97% versus 84%).[52]

An early study, using a precursor technique to DE-MRI (with similar characteristics), evaluated myocardial viability in patients with stable coronary artery disease and left ventricular dysfunction in 24 patients who had thallium imaging, or

Fig. 5. Single-shot techniques are invaluable in patients who are unable to perform breath holds of sufficient length for standard techniques. This example illustrates two-dimensional phase-sensitive short-axis images through the left ventricle (A), with each image requiring an approximately 15-second breath hold. Note that the more basal slices suffer from marked respiratory artifact, while some of the middle and apical images are less marred. The lower set of images (B) are non–breath-hold images using the single-shot technique where each image is acquired in a single heartbeat. The contrast between and among the blood pool, infarcted nonviable tissue (*bright*), and viable tissue (*black*), and the spatial resolution are both inferior to contrast and spatial resolution with the phase-sensitive technique. Nonetheless, the lack of respiratory artifact allows for a complete diagnostic evaluation of myocardial viability throughout the left ventricle with the single-shot technique, which is not possible with the phase-sensitive technique in this patient.

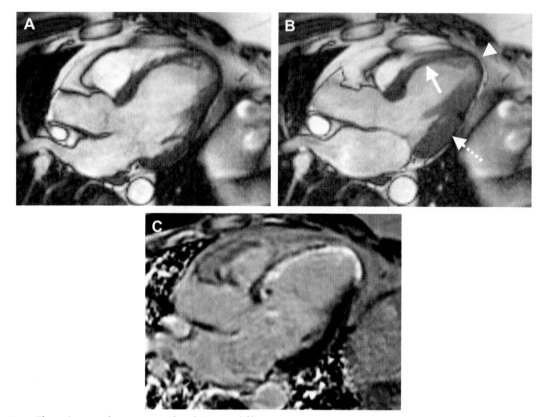

Fig. 6. These images demonstrate the clarity in differentiating normal from nonviable tissue using DE-MRI on a resting, nonstress study. The three images were all obtained at rest in the parasternal long-axis projection: cine MRI in diastole (*A*), and cine MRI in end-systole (*B*), and DE-MRI (*C*). The cine images reveal akinesis of the anteroseptum (*arrow*) and apex (*arrowhead*). The corresponding DE-MRI image reveals near-transmural hyperenhancement in the anteroseptum (>50%) and transmural hyperenhancement in the apex (100%), indicating low likelihood of functional improvement or recovery following revascularization. The inferolateral wall (*dotted arrow*), however, has normal contractility and normal, full-thickness myocardium that is black (or non-hyperenhanced), indicating normal viable tissue.

dobutamine echocardiography, or both.[53] The investigators found that hyperenhanced segments were associated with nonviability on thallium imaging, and also associated with dysfunctional myocardium declared nonviable by dobutamine echocardiography. A more recent study by Nelson and colleagues[54] sought to determine the effect of scar thickness on viability compared with dobutamine echocardiography and thallium SPECT imaging. Segmental hyperenhancement between 25% and 75% thickness was often associated with preserved contractile function in more than 50% of segments. However, there was virtually no contractile function with hyperenhancement greater than 75% thickness. Another study by Baer and colleagues[55] compared low-dose dobutamine transesophageal echocardiography to low-dose dobutamine MRI in 103 patients after myocardial infarction. The study demonstrated

similar results for both techniques to accurately predict recovery of left ventricular function after revascularization.

PET is often considered the gold standard technique for determining myocardial viability. Multiple studies are now available comparing DE-MRI to myocardial PET. All show similar findings, indicating a close correlation between the two techniques in defining myocardial viability. Klein and colleagues,[56] in a study involving 31 patients with severe ischemic left ventricular dysfunction, were the first to demonstrate that DE-MRI as a marker of myocardial scar correlated well with PET data (r = 0.81, *P*<.0001). DE-MRI areas of hyperenhancement closely reflected areas of decreased flow and metabolism seen on PET, yet DE-MRI, because of superior spatial resolution, also identified myocardial scar, in the form of subendocardial scar, significantly more frequently than PET did.

Kuhl and colleagues[57] obtained similar results after studying the use of DE-MRI, PET, and SPECT in examining 26 patients with chronic coronary artery disease and severe left ventricular dysfunction. At a defined optimal cutoff value of 37% segmental hyperenhancement, DE-MRI's ability to detect nonviable myocardium, as defined by PET, had a sensitivity and specificity of 96% and 84%, respectively. In a third study, Knuesel and colleagues[58] studied 19 patients with remote myocardial infarctions by CMR and PET. They concluded that using PET characterization of various classes of dysfunctional myocardium, DE-MRI segments with nontransmural hyperenhancement were metabolically viable, while those with near-transmural hyperenhancement demonstrated low potential for recovery of contractile function.

Myocardial Viability by Delayed-Enhancement MRI Following Revascularization

Several recent studies have also confirmed DE-MRI's ability to provide prognostic information in detecting reversible dysfunctional myocardium. The first such work was presented in a landmark study from Kim and colleagues[59] where the investigators performed CMR examinations with DE-MRI on 41 patients with mild left ventricular dysfunction and regional wall-motion abnormalities. These patients were imaged before and after surgical or percutaneous revascularization. Each myocardial segment was evaluated for the extent of hyperenhancement using the following categorizations: 0%, 1% to 25%, 26% to 50%, 51% to 75%, and 76% to 100%. Follow-up scans were performed 79 ± 36 days after revascularization. The mean ejection fraction improved from 43 ± 13% to 47 ± 12% following revascularization, and an improvement of at least 5% in ejection fraction was observed in 44% of patients. A full 53% of myocardial segments classified as having abnormal contractility improved after revascularization.

The study demonstrated for the first time in humans, that the likelihood of improvement in contractility after revascularization was significantly and inversely related to the extent of hyperenhanced myocardium per segment. From the broad perspective, 78% of myocardial segments with no hyperenhancement improved in contractility after revascularization compared with only 2% of segments with hyperenhancement greater than 75%. More specifically, 60% of segments with 1% to 25% hyperenhancement, 42% of segments with 26% to 50% hyperenhancement, and 10% of segments with 51% to 75%

hyperenhancement improved contractility after revascularization.

In a subsequent study by Schvartzman and colleagues,[60] 29 patients with severe ischemic left ventricular dysfunction (mean ejection fraction 28 ± 10%) underwent DE-MRI before surgical revascularization. This study similarly revealed that 82% of segments with abnormal contraction and no evidence of hyperenhancement recovered function after revascularization, as compared with an 18% recovery of segments with abnormal contraction and hyperenhancement of 50% or more (P<.001). The investigators' data suggested that segmental hyperenhancement of 50% or more constituted an optimal threshold for discriminating segments with failure of functional recovery after revascularization (positive predictive value 81%, specificity 95%) (**Fig. 7**).

Extending these findings, Selvanayagam and colleagues[61] studied 52 patients with CMR, including DE-MRI, before multivessel coronary artery bypass grafting and again 6 months afterwards. This group of patients had normal pre-revascularization global function, but demonstrated improved function following revascularization (62 ±12% to 67 ± 10%). Only 50% of patients had evidence of hyperenhancement preoperatively. This single-center study confirmed that the transmural extent of hyperenhancement correlated well with recovery of function at 6 months (P<.001). The trend in functional recovery of segments after revascularization was comparable to that seen in Kim and colleagues' and Schvartzman and colleagues' work: Eighty-two percent of segments with no hyperenhancement improved function after revascularization versus only 4% of segments with hyperenhancement greater than 75%.

Finally, Knuesel and colleagues[58] studied 10 patients with remote myocardial infarctions pre-revascularization and 11 ± 2 months post-revascularization using both DE-MRI and PET. The investigators used a different segmental categorization system, yet achieved results comparable to those of the previously mentioned studies. Specifically, by PET, segments described as thick (>4.5 mm) and metabolically viable corresponding to nontransmural hyperenhancement on DE-MRI demonstrated functional recovery in 85%, whereas thin and metabolically nonviable segments corresponding to near-transmural hyperenhancement on DE-MRI demonstrated functional recovery in only 13% (P<.0005).

The data presented above represent compelling evidence for expanding the role of DE-MRI in determining myocardial viability. However, these data were all collected as single-center trials,

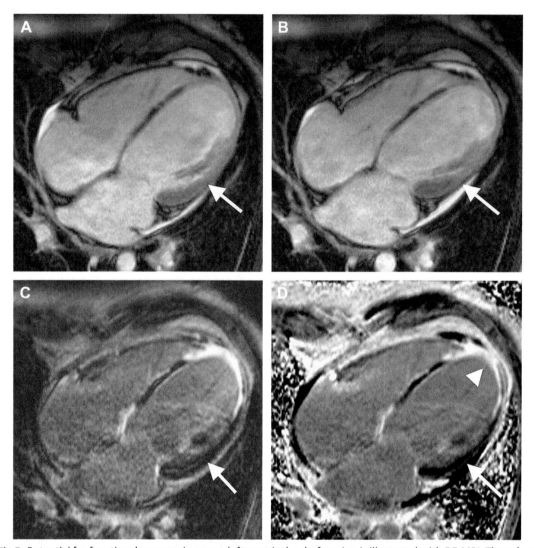

Fig. 7. Potential for functional recovery in severe left ventricular dysfunction is illustrated with DE-MRI. These four images were obtained in the four-chamber long-axis projection: cine MRI in diastole (*A*) and end-systole (*B*), and magnitude (*C*) and phase-sensitive (*D*) DE-MRI. The cine images reveal severe global hypokinesis. The corresponding DE-MRI images reveal transmural hyperenhancement of the apex (*arrowhead*) and the expectation of a near-zero likelihood of functional improvement following revascularization. The basal two thirds of the lateral wall (*arrows*) also have severe segmental wall-motion abnormality, but the myocardium is uniformly "nulled," indicating viable myocardium. Available data suggest that this myocardial distribution, despite being thinned, has good potential for functional improvement or recovery after revascularization.

which could limit the usefulness of the results. For example, it is uncertain how the data from a series of single centers, each expert in the performance of CMR and DE-MRI, can be extrapolated to more generalized clinical use. There clearly is a need for larger, multicenter trials using DE-MRI, as well as for randomized studies comparing DE-MRI with other techniques to gain a fuller understanding of its broader clinical implications. While the latter designs are not yet in place, an international, multicenter trial of DE-MRI has been

completed and recently presented.[62] This study emulated the design of Kim and colleagues[59] but expanded the scope to nine centers on three continents. The study included 183 patients (167 men, age 59.1 ± 9.7 years), each with angiographically confirmed coronary artery disease and resting wall-motion abnormality, and each scheduled for coronary bypass grafting or angioplasty. Cine MRI and DE-MRI were acquired within 30 days before and 5.6 ± 2.4 months after revascularization. The investigators analyzed 12,274 segments, 46% of which had abnormal contractility at baseline, and 24% had hyperenhancement. Like the data from the single-center trials, data from this study showed a significant inverse relationship between the transmural extent of hyperenhancement and improvement in contractility of impaired segments following revascularization ($r^2 = 0.9$). Seventy-two percent of dysfunctional segments without evidence of hyperenhancement at baseline demonstrated improvement in contractility after revascularization, and 52% of these segments had complete recovery of function ($P<.001$). Compared to the single-center trials, however, there was a higher, though still modest, rate of functional improvement after revascularization (18%) in segments with more than 75% hyperenhancement.

SUMMARY

The ability to detect viable myocardium and the transmural extent of scar accurately has important implications in the clinical decision-making process for potential revascularization in ischemic left ventricular dysfunction. Such information is critical in that revascularization of viable myocardium has been documented to reduce cardiac mortality by as much as fourfold compared with medical therapy alone. Because of the greater spatial resolution that DE-MRI provides, this technique is superior to all other noninvasive techniques available for not only revealing the presence of scar seen as hyperenhancement, but also for quantifying the transmural extent of scar. Additional, practical advantages of DE-MRI include the absence of radiation exposure, as well as the additional information easily gleaned, such information for global and regional wall-motion assessment.

A wealth of clinical data, including data from at least one multicenter trial, now substantiates the contention that DE-MRI accurately characterizes pathophysiologic states. Mild degrees of segmental hyperenhancement in the setting of normal wall-motion or segmental dysfunction portend a high likelihood of contractile recovery. Meanwhile, a segmental wall-motion abnormality in the setting of near-transmural or transmural hyperenhancement (>75%) indicates a strong unlikelihood of contractile improvement following revascularization. However, intermediate degrees of hyperenhancement are less straightforward and correspondingly demonstrate intermediate rates of response. The use of DE-MRI technique may be disconcerting to some clinicians because it fails to provide an unambiguous yes-or-no response. Even so, the technique demonstrates

a continuum of response that clearly reflects the heterogeneity of myocardial substrate. Greater clarification will no doubt be revealed as more details are gained as the spatial resolution of DE-MRI improves, as true volumetric approaches become routine, and as larger studies across the spectrum of ischemic left ventricular dysfunction are performed. These advances will continue to increase the clinical utility of DE-MRI in the analysis of dysfunctional myocardium, and promote the integration of DE-MRI into the diagnostic and therapeutic algorithm.

REFERENCES

1. Shan K, Constantine G, Sivananthan M, et al. Role of cardiac magnetic resonance imaging in the assessment of myocardial viability. Circulation 2004; 109(11):1328–34.
2. Wagner A, Mahrholdt H, Kim RJ, et al. Use of cardiac magnetic resonance to assess viability. Curr Cardiol Rep 2005;7(1):59–64.
3. Braunwald E, Kloner RA. The stunned myocardium: prolonged, postischemic ventricular dysfunction. Circulation 1982;66(6):1146–9.
4. Tillisch J, Brunken R, Marshall R, et al. Reversibility of cardiac wall-motion abnormalities predicted by positron tomography. N Engl J Med 1986;314(14):884–8.
5. Dilsizian V, Perrone-Filardi P, Arrighi JA, et al. Concordance and discordance between stress-redistribution-reinjection and rest-redistribution thallium imaging for assessing viable myocardium. Comparison with metabolic activity by positron emission tomography. Circulation 1993;88(3):941–52.
6. Meluzin J, Cerny J, Frelich M, et al. Prognostic value of the amount of dysfunctional but viable myocardium in revascularized patients with coronary artery disease and left ventricular dysfunction. Investigators of this multicenter study. J Am Coll Cardiol 1998;32(4):912–20.
7. Di Carli MF, Davidson M, Little R, et al. Value of metabolic imaging with positron emission tomography for evaluating prognosis in patients with coronary artery disease and left ventricular dysfunction. Am J Cardiol 1994;73(8):527–33.
8. Pagley PR, Beller GA, Watson DD, et al. Improved outcome after coronary bypass surgery in patients with ischemic cardiomyopathy and residual myocardial viability. Circulation 1997;96(3):793–800.
9. Beanlands RS, Ruddy TD, deKemp RA, et al. Positron emission tomography and recovery following revascularization (PARR-1): the importance of scar and the development of a prediction rule for the degree of recovery of left ventricular function. J Am Coll Cardiol 2002;40(10):1735–43.
10. Nagueh SF, Mikati I, Weilbaecher D, et al. Relation of the contractile reserve of hibernating myocardium to

myocardial structure in humans. Circulation 1999; 100(5):490–6.

11. Eitzman D, al-Aouar Z, Kanter HL, et al. Clinical outcome of patients with advanced coronary artery disease after viability studies with positron emission tomography. J Am Coll Cardiol 1992;20(3):559–65.

12. Tamaki N, Kawamoto M, Takahashi N, et al. Prognostic value of an increase in fluorine-18 deoxyglucose uptake in patients with myocardial infarction: comparison with stress thallium imaging. J Am Coll Cardiol 1993;22(6):1621–7.

13. Bax JJ, Poldermans D, Elhendy A, et al. Sensitivity, specificity, and predictive accuracies of various noninvasive techniques for detecting hibernating myocardium. Curr Probl Cardiol 2001;26(2):147–86.

14. Di Carli MF, Asgarzadie F, Schelbert HR, et al. Quantitative relation between myocardial viability and improvement in heart failure symptoms after revascularization in patients with ischemic cardiomyopathy. Circulation 1995;92(12):3436–44.

15. Marwick TH, Zuchowski C, Lauer MS, et al. Functional status and quality of life in patients with heart failure undergoing coronary bypass surgery after assessment of myocardial viability. J Am Coll Cardiol 1999;33(3):750–8.

16. Allman KC, Shaw LJ, Hachamovitch R, et al. Myocardial viability testing and impact of revascularization on prognosis in patients with coronary artery disease and left ventricular dysfunction: a meta-analysis. J Am Coll Cardiol 2002;39(7):1151–8.

17. Shan K, Nagueh SF, Zoghbi WA. Assessment of myocardial viability with stress echocardiography. Cardiol Clin 1999;17(3):539–53.

18. Cornel JH, Bax JJ, Elhendy A, et al. Biphasic response to dobutamine predicts improvement of global left ventricular function after surgical revascularization in patients with stable coronary artery disease: implications of time course of recovery on diagnostic accuracy. J Am Coll Cardiol 1998;31(5):1002–10.

19. Afridi I, Kleiman NS, Raizner AE, et al. Dobutamine echocardiography in myocardial hibernation. Optimal dose and accuracy in predicting recovery of ventricular function after coronary angioplasty. Circulation 1995;91(3):663–70.

20. Sawada SG, Lewis SJ, Foltz J, et al. Usefulness of rest and low-dose dobutamine wall motion scores in predicting survival and benefit from revascularization in patients with ischemic cardiomyopathy. Am J Cardiol 2002;89(7):811–6.

21. Udelson JE, Coleman PS, Metherall J, et al. Predicting recovery of severe regional ventricular dysfunction. Comparison of resting scintigraphy with 201Tl and 99mTc-sestamibi. Circulation 1994;89(6):2552–61.

22. Marzullo P, Parodi O, Reisenhofer B, et al. Value of rest thallium-201/technetium-99m sestamibi scans and dobutamine echocardiography for detecting myocardial viability. Am J Cardiol 1993;71(2):166–72.

23. Hoffmann U, Millea R, Enzweiler C, et al. Acute myocardial infarction: contrast-enhanced multidetector row CT in a porcine model. Radiology 2004;231(3):697–701.

24. Lardo AC, Cordeiro MA, Silva C, et al. Contrast-enhanced multidetector computed tomography viability imaging after myocardial infarction: characterization of myocyte death, microvascular obstruction, and chronic scar. Circulation 2006;113(3):394–404.

25. Paul JF, Wartski M, Caussin C, et al. Late defect on delayed contrast-enhanced multi-detector row CT scans in the prediction of SPECT infarct size after reperfused acute myocardial infarction: initial experience. Radiology 2005;236(2):485–9.

26. Baer FM, Theissen P, Schneider CA, et al. Dobutamine magnetic resonance imaging predicts contractile recovery of chronically dysfunctional myocardium after successful revascularization. J Am Coll Cardiol 1998;31(5):1040–8.

27. Baer FM, Voth E, Deutsch HJ, et al. Predictive value of low dose dobutamine transesophageal echocardiography and fluorine-18 fluorodeoxyglucose positron emission tomography for recovery of regional left ventricular function after successful revascularization. J Am Coll Cardiol 1996;28(1):60–9.

28. Nagel E, Lehmkuhl HB, Bocksch W, et al. Noninvasive diagnosis of ischemia-induced wall motion abnormalities with the use of high-dose dobutamine stress MRI: comparison with dobutamine stress echocardiography. Circulation 1999;99(6):763–70.

29. Sandstede JJ, Bertsch G, Beer M, et al. Detection of myocardial viability by low-dose dobutamine cine MR imaging. Magn Reson Imaging 1999;17(10):1437–43.

30. Wesbey G, Higgins CB, Lanzer P, et al. Imaging and characterization of acute myocardial infarction in vivo by gated nuclear magnetic resonance. Circulation 1984;69(1):125–30.

31. Kim RJ, Fieno DS, Parrish TB, et al. Relationship of MRI delayed contrast enhancement to irreversible injury, infarct age, and contractile function. Circulation 1999;100(19):1992–2002.

32. Simonetti OP, Kim RJ, Fieno DS, et al. An improved MR imaging technique for the visualization of myocardial infarction. Radiology 2001;218(1):215–23.

33. Weinmann HJ, Laniado M, Mutzel W. Pharmacokinetics of GdDTPA/dimeglumine after intravenous injection into healthy volunteers. Physiol Chem Phys Med NMR 1984;16(2):167–72.

34. Kim RJ, Chen EL, Lima JA, et al. Myocardial Gd-DTPA kinetics determine MRI contrast enhancement and reflect the extent and severity of myocardial injury after acute reperfused infarction. Circulation 1996;94(12):3318–26.

35. Lima JA, Judd RM, Bazille A, et al. Regional heterogeneity of human myocardial infarcts demonstrated by contrast-enhanced MRI. Potential mechanisms. Circulation 1995;92(5):1117–25.

36. Arheden H, Saeed M, Higgins CB, et al. Reperfused rat myocardium subjected to various durations of ischemia: estimation of the distribution volume of contrast material with echo-planar MR imaging. Radiology 2000;215(2):520–8.

37. Flacke SJ, Fischer SE, Lorenz CH. Measurement of the gadopentetate dimeglumine partition coefficient in human myocardium in vivo: normal distribution and elevation in acute and chronic infarction. Radiology 2001;218(3):703–10.

38. Judd RM, Lugo-Olivieri CH, Arai M, et al. Physiological basis of myocardial contrast enhancement in fast magnetic resonance images of 2-day-old reperfused canine infarcts. Circulation 1995;92(7):1902–10.

39. Klein C, Nekolla SG, Balbach T, et al. The influence of myocardial blood flow and volume of distribution on late Gd-DTPA kinetics in ischemic heart failure. J Magn Reson Imaging 2004;20(4):588–93.

40. Klein C, Schmal TR, Nekolla SG, et al. Mechanism of late gadolinium enhancement in patients with acute myocardial infarction. J Cardiovasc Magn Reson 2007;9(4):653–8.

41. Rehwald WG, Fieno DS, Chen EL, et al. Myocardial magnetic resonance imaging contrast agent concentrations after reversible and irreversible ischemic injury. Circulation 2002;105(2):224–9.

42. Kellman P, Arai AE, McVeigh ER, et al. Phase-sensitive inversion recovery for detecting myocardial infarction using gadolinium-delayed hyperenhancement. Magn Reson Med 2002;47(2):372–83.

43. Kellman P, Larson AC, Hsu LY, et al. Motion-corrected free-breathing delayed enhancement imaging of myocardial infarction. Magn Reson Med 2005;53(1):194–200.

44. Fieno DS, Kim RJ, Chen EL, et al. Contrast-enhanced magnetic resonance imaging of myocardium at risk: distinction between reversible and irreversible injury throughout infarct healing. J Am Coll Cardiol 2000;36(6):1985–91.

45. Saeed M, Lund G, Wendland MF, et al. Magnetic resonance characterization of the peri-infarction zone of reperfused myocardial infarction with necrosis-specific and extracellular nonspecific contrast media. Circulation 2001;103(6):871–6.

46. Hillenbrand HB, Kim RJ, Parker MA, et al. Early assessment of myocardial salvage by contrast-enhanced magnetic resonance imaging. Circulation 2000;102(14):1678–83.

47. Gerber BL, Rochitte CE, Bluemke DA, et al. Relation between Gd-DTPA contrast enhancement and regional inotropic response in the periphery and center of myocardial infarction. Circulation 2001;104(9):998–1004.

48. Choi KM, Kim RJ, Gubernikoff G, et al. Transmural extent of acute myocardial infarction predicts long-term improvement in contractile function. Circulation 2001;104(10):1101–7.

49. Ingkanisorn WP, Rhoads KL, Aletras AH, et al. Gadolinium delayed enhancement cardiovascular magnetic resonance correlates with clinical measures of myocardial infarction. J Am Coll Cardiol 2004;43(12):2253–9.

50. Wu E, Judd RM, Vargas JD, et al. Visualisation of presence, location, and transmural extent of healed Q-wave and non-Q-wave myocardial infarction. Lancet 2001;357(9249):21–8.

51. Wagner A, Mahrholdt H, Holly TA, et al. Contrast-enhanced MRI and routine single photon emission computed tomography (SPECT) perfusion imaging for detection of subendocardial myocardial infarcts: an imaging study. Lancet 2003;361(9355):374–9.

52. Ibrahim T, Bulow HP, Hackl T, et al. Diagnostic value of contrast-enhanced magnetic resonance imaging and single-photon emission computed tomography for detection of myocardial necrosis early after acute myocardial infarction. J Am Coll Cardiol 2007;49(2):208–16.

53. Ramani K, Judd RM, Holly TA, et al. Contrast magnetic resonance imaging in the assessment of myocardial viability in patients with stable coronary artery disease and left ventricular dysfunction. Circulation 1998;98(24):2687–94.

54. Nelson C, McCrohon J, Khafagi F, et al. Impact of scar thickness on the assessment of viability using dobutamine echocardiography and thallium single-photon emission computed tomography: a comparison with contrast-enhanced magnetic resonance imaging. J Am Coll Cardiol 2004;43(7):1248–56.

55. Baer FM, Theissen P, Crnac J, et al. Head to head comparison of dobutamine-transoesophageal echocardiography and dobutamine-magnetic resonance imaging for the prediction of left ventricular functional recovery in patients with chronic coronary artery disease. Eur Heart J 2000;21(12):981–91.

56. Klein C, Nekolla SG, Bengel FM, et al. Assessment of myocardial viability with contrast-enhanced magnetic resonance imaging: comparison with positron emission tomography. Circulation 2002;105(2):162–7.

57. Kuhl HP, Beek AM, van der Weerdt AP, et al. Myocardial viability in chronic ischemic heart disease: comparison of contrast-enhanced magnetic resonance imaging with (18)F-fluorodeoxyglucose positron emission tomography. J Am Coll Cardiol 2003;41(8):1341–8.

58. Knuesel PR, Nanz D, Wyss C, et al. Characterization of dysfunctional myocardium by positron emission tomography and magnetic resonance: relation to functional outcome after revascularization. Circulation 2003;108(9):1095–100.

59. Kim RJ, Wu E, Rafael A, et al. The use of contrast-enhanced magnetic resonance imaging to identify reversible myocardial dysfunction. N Engl J Med 2000;343(20):1445–53.

60. Schvartzman PR, Srichai MB, Grimm RA, et al. Non-stress delayed-enhancement magnetic resonance imaging of the myocardium predicts improvement of function after revascularization for chronic ischemic heart disease with left ventricular dysfunction. Am Heart J 2003;146(3):535–41.

61. Selvanayagam JB, Kardos A, Francis JM, et al. Value of delayed-enhancement cardiovascular magnetic resonance imaging in predicting myocardial viability after surgical revascularization. Circulation 2004;110(12):1535–41.

62. Lenge VV, Van den Bosch H, Greenwood J, et al. Delayed-enhancement MRI can predict recovery of LV function after revascularization: results from an international multicenter myocardial viability trial. J Cardiovasc Magn Reson 2008;10(Suppl 1):A25.

Identifying the Etiology: A Systematic Approach Using Delayed-Enhancement Cardiovascular Magnetic Resonance

Annamalai Senthilkumar, MD, Maulik D. Majmudar, MD,
Chetan Shenoy, MBBS, Han W. Kim, MD, Raymond J. Kim, MD*

KEYWORDS

- Heart failure • Cardiomyopathy • Ischemic • Non-ischemic
- Cardiovascular magnetic resonance
- Delayed enhancement imaging

Several classification schemes have been proposed for the various cardiomyopathies. Some are based on the disease phenotype, and others focus on the genetic aspects of disease.[1,2] Although these detailed classification methods are important in the research arena, a practical first step in the clinical setting is to categorize patients as having ischemic or non-ischemic cardiomyopathy. This simple classification is important because it can affect patient management directly. If ischemic cardiomyopathy is identified, there are clearly defined treatment strategies that have proven survival benefit, such as coronary artery bypass grafting in patients who have left main or three-vessel disease.[3] This classification also provides insight into patient prognosis: ischemic cardiomyopathy is associated with reduced survival compared with non-ischemic cardiomyopathy (**Fig. 1**).[4] As a second step, within the broad category of non-ischemic cardiomyopathy, a specific cause must be determined. Again, the importance of determining the cause is related to patient treatment and survival. For instance, beta-blockers are beneficial in some forms of non-ischemic cardiomyopathy (eg. idiopathic dilated cardiomyopathy) but not others (eg. cardiac amyloidosis),[5] and the prognosis is quite variable depending on the underlying cause of non-ischemic cardiomyopathy. Patients who have peripartum cardiomyopathy have significantly better survival than those who have idiopathic dilated cardiomyopathy, who in turn have better survival than those who have infiltrative myocardial diseases.[6]

Clinically, identifying the presence or absence of obstructive epicardial coronary artery disease (CAD), by coronary angiography or stress testing, has been the cornerstone in differentiating ischemic from non-ischemic cardiomyopathy. Delayed-enhancement cardiovascular magnetic resonance (DE-CMR) may provide a novel approach to determining the origin of the cardiomyopathy by allowing a direct assessment of myopathic processes. Comparative studies with histopathology have shown that the presence, extent, and location of hyperenhancement by DE-CMR is a precise indicator of nonviable myocardium in both ischemic[7] and non-ischemic

This work was supported in part by National Institutes of Health Grant RO1-HL64726 (RJK).
Duke University Medical Center, Durham, NC, USA
* Corresponding author. Duke Cardiovascular Magnetic Resonance Center, Duke University Medical Center, P.O. Box 3934, Durham, NC 27710.
E-mail address: raymond.kim@duke.edu (R.J. Kim).

Heart Failure Clin 5 (2009) 349–367
doi:10.1016/j.hfc.2009.02.009

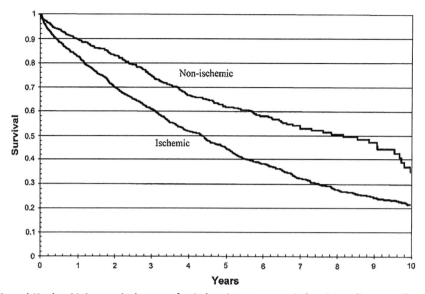

Fig. 1. Unadjusted Kaplan-Meier survival curves for ischemic versus non-ischemic cardiomyopathy. (*From* Felker GM, Shaw LK, O'Connor CM. A standardized definition of ischemic cardiomyopathy for use in clinical research. J Am Coll Cardiol 2002;39(2):212; with permission.)

heart disease.[8,9] Although nonviable myocardium can be identified by several imaging modalities, DE-CMR may be particularly suited to evaluating the myocardial processes in cardiomyopathy. DE-CMR offers significantly higher spatial resolution (40-fold greater than radionuclide imaging[10]), can systematically detect subendocardial infarcts that are missed by single-photon emission computed tomography,[11] and even may identify micro scars that cannot be detected by other imaging techniques (**Fig. 2**).[12]

This article presents an overall imaging approach for the diagnosis of cardiomyopathy that is based fundamentally on DE-CMR. It describes how this approach is based on the underlying myocardial pathophysiology that is present in ischemic and non-ischemic cardiomyopathy. It also discusses how a DE-CMR–based approach may provide insight into the conundrums that can occur when coronary artery disease coexists with non-ischemic cardiomyopathy.

TRADITIONAL APPROACH TO ETIOLOGY

Ischemic cardiomyopathy usually is diagnosed by identifying the presence of obstructive CAD. The coronary anatomy can be assessed either directly (ie, by invasive coronary angiography) or indirectly by stress-testing, depending on the pretest probability of disease as derived from a combination of historical, clinical, electrocardiographic, and laboratory data. An individual who has few risk factors and atypical symptoms may undergo stress

testing (or simple reassurance, if the risk is deemed particularly low), whereas an individual who has multiple risk factors and classic symptoms of angina may proceed directly to the catheterization laboratory. Likewise, the broad diagnosis of non-ischemic cardiomyopathy usually is made by assessing the coronary anatomy, either directly or indirectly. Once significant CAD has been excluded, a comprehensive evaluation, possibly including endomyocardial biopsy, may allow a specific cause to be determined.

The traditional approach has several drawbacks, however. For one, many patients do not undergo definitive testing (ie, invasive coronary angiography), and the accuracy of diagnosing CAD indirectly is only moderate. Autopsy data from patients enrolled in the Assessment of Treatment with Lisinopril and Survival (ATLAS) Trial,[13] a large multicenter, randomized trial of patients who had moderate to severe heart failure, underscores this concern. Of the 171 patients who had autopsy, 70% (n = 120) were diagnosed in life as having ischemic cardiomyopathy, and 30% (n = 51) were diagnosed as having non-ischemic cardiomyopathy. Autopsy documented that 17% of those diagnosed as having ischemic cardiomyopathy did not have CAD, whereas 31% of those diagnosed as having non-ischemic cardiomyopathy had significant CAD. Overall, 21% had an incorrect clinical diagnosis.

One possible reason for the high rate of misdiagnosis may be an over-reliance on certain

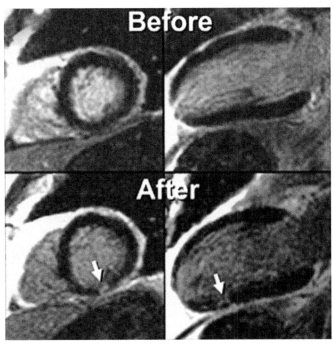

Fig. 2. Images before and after coronary stenting demonstrate the ability of DE-CMR to identify microinfarcts. Arrows point to new discrete regions of hyperenhancement in the inferior wall related to the procedure. (*Adapted from* Ricciardi MJ, Wu E, Davidson CJ, et al. Visualization of discrete microinfarction after percutaneous coronary intervention associated with mild creatine kinase-MB elevation. Circulation 2001;103(23):2782; with permission.)

findings from noninvasive imaging. Initially, it was thought that ventricular dysfunction caused by non-ischemic cardiomyopathy was primarily global rather than segmental, as in ischemic cardiomyopathy, and that this characteristic could be used to distinguish these disorders by echocardiography.[14] It is now recognized, however, that abnormalities in segmental wall motion are evident in up to 60% of patients who have non-ischemic dilated cardiomyopathy, even when patients who have left bundle branch block are excluded.[15] Furthermore, it is known that radionuclide scintigraphy with either dipyridamole or exercise testing is unreliable in differentiating ischemic heart disease from non-ischemic cardiomyopathy, because both groups of patients may have evidence of reversible and fixed perfusion abnormalities.[16]

Additionally, when a specific cause of non-ischemic cardiomyopathy is being explored, classic imaging features such as "granular sparkling" on echocardiography in cardiac amyloidosis are limited to a few rare diseases and may be less accurate than first reported. In fact, in a recent study of 196 patients clinically suspected of having cardiac amyloidosis, this finding had a sensitivity of only 26%.[17] Endomyocardial biopsy, the presumed reference standard, has limitations as

well. Because of sampling error, test sensitivity may be low,[18,19] and, especially in the chronic setting, many patients who have cardiomyopathy may show only nonspecific changes on biopsy (eg, cell loss and fibrosis). Not surprisingly, Felker and colleagues[6] reported that the biopsy provided a specific histologic diagnosis in only 15% of 1230 patients who underwent endomyocardial biopsy as part of an evaluation for unexplained cardiomyopathy.

Finally, simple distinctions between cardiomyopathies based on the presence or absence of CAD can be problematic. For instance, a patient who has non-ischemic cardiomyopathy also may have CAD that is incidental and does not contribute to contractile dysfunction. The quandary is that coronary atherosclerosis is common, especially in elderly patients and patients who have diabetes mellitus, even if the patients are asymptomatic and do not have myocardial dysfunction.[20] A recent study in 1921 patients who had symptomatic heart failure and left ventricular (LV) dysfunction (LV ejection fraction [LVEF] < 40%) undergoing diagnostic coronary angiography highlights this issue.[4] The prognosis for patients who had LV dysfunction "out of proportion" to their degree of CAD (ie, those who had single-vessel disease) was more similar to the prognosis of patients who had non-ischemic cardiomyopathy than to the prognosis of the remaining group of patients who had ischemic cardiomyopathy. The authors concluded that even though obstructive CAD is present, patients who have single-vessel disease should be reclassified as non-ischemic for prognostic purposes.

Another problem with the traditional approach is the inherent assumption that ischemic and non-ischemic cardiomyopathy cannot coexist. It is plausible that both ischemic and non-ischemic myopathic processes can be present simultaneously and may contribute independently or synergistically to systolic dysfunction (mixed cardiomyopathy). Thus, the presence of obstructive coronary atherosclerosis does not mandate an ischemic origin, and, even with objective information such as that obtained from invasive coronary angiography, the appropriate classification for a given patient is not always clear.

PATHOPHYSIOLOGIC BASIS OF A NEW APPROACH USING DELAYED-ENHANCEMENT CARDIOVASCULAR MAGNETIC RESONANCE

Because the cardiomyopathies represent diseases of the myocardium with attendant ventricular dysfunction, one could expect that focusing on the myocardium, rather than on the coronary arteries, might provide added diagnostic insight. The importance of assessing myocardial viability is readily evident in patients who have ischemic heart disease and who may undergo coronary revascularization.[21] The assessment of viability or, conversely, the detection of necrosis or scarring also may be important in many patients in whom coronary revascularization is not an issue, such as those who have non-ischemic cardiomyopathy. The usefulness of DE-CMR in the setting of cardiomyopathy is based on the understanding that, rather than simply measuring viability, the presence and pattern of hyperenhancement (nonviable myocardium) provides additional information. This section first explores the mechanism of myocardial hyperenhancement in the setting of acute and chronic myocardial infarction and reviews the spatial progression of cell death that occurs over time following coronary occlusion. This discussion provides the basis for understanding the DE-CMR findings that can occur in the setting of ischemic cardiomyopathy. Next, it reviews the initial studies comparing the presence and pattern of hyperenhancement in ischemic cardiomyopathy with that found in idiopathic dilated cardiomyopathy. A brief description of findings in other forms of non-ischemic cardiomyopathy follows, along with a summary of the current understanding of the pathophysiological basis of hyperenhancement in non-ischemic cardiomyopathy.

Mechanism of Hyperenhancement in Myocardial Infarction

Both acute and chronic myocardial infarction are depicted accurately by DE-CMR as hyperenhanced regions, independent of wall motion and reperfusion status.[7] The gadolinium chelates that are used for DE-CMR are biologically inert, however, and are not transported actively by any cells or tissues. Moreover, the tissue composition of acute myocardial infarction (necrotic myocytes and acute inflammation) is completely different from that of chronic myocardial infarction (dense collagenous scar). Thus, it is difficult to understand how a "nonspecific" contrast agent can distinguish between viable and infarcted myocardium, especially across the wide range of tissue environments that occur during infarct healing.

Although the mechanism of myocardial hyperenhancement in the setting of infarction has not been elucidated fully, one mechanism has been proposed that accounts for the variety of tissues that can characterize nonviable myocardium.[22,23] The proposed mechanism is based on two simple facts. First, gadolinium chelates are extracellular contrast agents that cannot cross myocyte cell membranes.[24] Second, in normal myocardium, myocytes are densely packed, and thus myocyte intracellular space forms the majority (78%) of the volume.[25] Conceptually, it then follows that the volume of distribution of gadolinium in a hypothetical voxel of normal myocardium is small, and the overall number of gadolinium molecules is low (**Fig. 3**). In acute myocardial infarction, rupture of myocyte membranes allows additional gadolinium to diffuse into what previously was intracellular space, resulting in increased gadolinium concentration,[26] shortened T1 relaxation times, and therefore hyperenhancement. Loss of sarcolemmal membrane integrity is thought to be very closely related to cell death, and the idea that an event specific to cell death is related to hyperenhancement would explain the nearly one-to-one relationship of hyperenhancement to necrotic tissue found in acute myocardial infarction.[7]

In chronic myocardial infarction, myocytes have been replaced with collagenous scar tissue. In this situation, the interstitial space is expanded, again leading to increased gadolinium concentration and hyperenhancement.[26] In both acute and chronic myocardial infarction

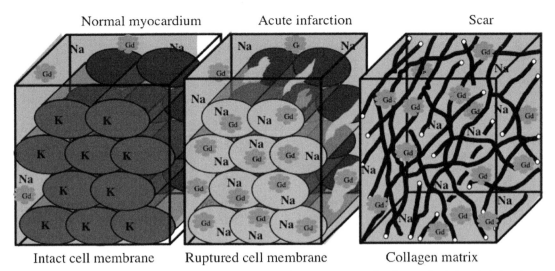

Fig. 3. Mechanisms of hyperenhancement in myocardial infarction: scar may be the result of chronic infarction or non-ischemic damage (see text for details). Gd, gadolinium; K, potassium; Na, sodium. (*Adapted from* Kim RJ, Elliott MD, Judd RM. Assessment of myocardial viability by contrast enhancement. In: Higgins CB, de Roos A, editors. MRI and CT of the cardiovascular system. 2nd edition. Philadelphia: Lippincott Williams & Wilkins; 2005. p. 244; with permission.)

(and in all intermediate stages), one can consider viable myocytes as actively excluding the gadolinium contrast medium. Thus, the unifying mechanism for the hyperenhancement of nonviable myocardium may be the absence of viable myocytes rather than any inherent properties that are specific for acutely necrotic tissue, collagenous scar, or other forms of nonviable tissue.

The "Wavefront" of Ischemic Necrosis

The typical pattern of hyperenhancement that occurs in patients who have prior myocardial infarction and thus in those who have ischemic cardiomyopathy can be explained by the pathophysiology of ischemia. Following a coronary occlusion, myocardial contractility falls within seconds throughout the "area at risk," which is the ischemic zone with reduced perfusion. Although blood begins to flow by way of pre-existing collaterals (vascular channels that interconnect ordinary arteries), collateral flow is lowest and myocardial oxygen consumption is highest in the subendocardium. As a consequence, ischemia is most severe and necrosis begins first in the subendocardium starting about 15 to 20 minutes after total occlusion.[27] Necrosis then progresses as a "wavefront" toward the epicardium over the next few hours. During this period the size of the area at risk remains the same, but the size of the infarcted region within the area at risk increases continuously towards a transmural infarction

(**Fig. 4**). Another facet of the wavefront phenomenon is that increasing the duration or severity of ischemic injury generally increases the transmurality of infarction, but the circumferential extent of infarction does not increase appreciably because the lateral margins are established relatively early in the ischemic period.[27] Therefore, an "ischemic-type" or "CAD-type" pattern of hyperenhancement always should involve the subendocardium (ie, be subendocardial or transmural) and should be located in a region that is consistent with the perfusion territory of an epicardial coronary artery. Conversely, a "non–CAD-type" pattern of hyperenhancement is one that spares the subendocardium and is secondary to non-ischemic disorders.

Ischemic Versus Idiopathic Dilated Cardiomyopathy

Several studies have compared the presence and patterns of hyperenhancement on DE-CMR in patients who have various forms of cardiomyopathy. Wu and colleagues[10] were the first to report that DE-CMR may hold promise in differentiating ischemic from non-ischemic, idiopathic dilated cardiomyopathy. In this study, nearly all patients who had CAD and prior myocardial infarction had myocardial hyperenhancement, whereas none of the patients who had idiopathic dilated cardiomyopathy or the normal volunteers had hyperenhancement. In another study, Bello and colleagues[28] evaluated a cohort of patients who

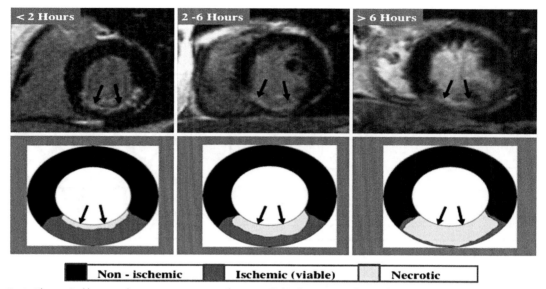

Fig. 4. The typical hyperenhancement pattern of myocardial infarction can be explained by the pathophysiology of ischemia. Little or no cellular necrosis is found until about 15 minutes after occlusion. Over the next few hours a wavefront of necrosis begins in the subendocardium and moves progressively towards the epicardium. During this period, the infarcted region (*arrows*) within the ischemic zone increases continuously and ultimately can become transmural. (*From* Mahrholdt H, Wagner A, Judd RM, et al. Delayed-enhancement cardiovascular magnetic resonance assessment of non-ischaemic cardiomyopathies. Eur Heart J 2005;26(15):1464; with permission.)

had severe LV systolic dysfunction (mean EF was 26 ± 11%); hyperenhancement was found in 100% of patients who had ischemic cardiomyopathy but in only 12% of those who had idiopathic dilated cardiomyopathy. In a group of ambulatory patients seen at a heart failure clinic, Casolo and colleagues[29] noted myocardial hyperenhancement in 98% of patients who had CAD, as compared with 16% in those who did not have CAD. Other recent studies showed similar findings.[30] These data indicate that myocardial hyperenhancement consistent with gross myocardial scarring almost always is present in patients who have chronic ischemic cardiomyopathy but is relatively rare in patients who have idiopathic dilated cardiomyopathy. This conclusion is consistent with previous pathology studies.[31,32] Schuster and Bulkley[31] demonstrated that virtually all patients who had congestive heart failure and significant CAD have gross myocardial scarring at autopsy, even in those who did not have a clinical history of myocardial infarction, angina, or Q-waves. Conversely, Roberts and colleagues[33] found visible scars at necropsy in only 14% of patients who had idiopathic dilated cardiomyopathy.

Recently, McCrohon and colleagues[34] performed DE-CMR in 90 patients diagnosed as having ischemic (n = 27) or idiopathic dilated (n = 63) cardiomyopathy on the basis of coronary angiography. All the patients who had ischemic cardiomyopathy had myocardial hyperenhancement, but 41% of the patients who had idiopathic dilated cardiomyopathy also had hyperenhancement. Although the prevalence of hyperenhancement in patients who had idiopathic dilated cardiomyopathy seems to be significantly higher in this study than in the reports by Wu and colleagues[10] and Bello and colleagues,[28] there were differences in how these studies defined hyperenhancement. For instance, in the earlier studies, only hyperenhancement patterns consistent with regions of prior myocardial infarction were included in the analysis. Taking into account the pattern of hyperenhancement (CAD-type versus non–CAD-type), McCrohon and colleagues[34] found that 13% of patients who had idiopathic dilated cardiomyopathy had CAD-type hyperenhancement, whereas 28% had non–CAD-type. These findings now are consistent with those of Bello and colleagues,[28] in that among patients who had idiopathic dilated cardiomyopathy the rate of CAD-type hyperenhancement was quite low in both studies (13% and 12%, respectively). Additionally, these rates are nearly identical to the rate of chronic infarcts found at autopsy in patients who had idiopathic dilated cardiomyopathy by Roberts and colleagues[33] and in the ATLAS substudy by Uretsky and colleagues[13] (14% and 12%, respectively).

The clinical interpretation of CAD-type hyperenhancement in patients who have idiopathic dilated cardiomyopathy is unclear. Certainly the occurrence of recanalization after an occlusive coronary event or embolization from minimally stenotic but unstable plaque is well documented.[35,36] Therefore, McCrohon and colleagues[34] believed that these patients were incorrectly diagnosed by coronary angiography as having idiopathic dilated cardiomyopathy. On the other hand, 28% of the patients in the study by McCrohon and colleagues[34] had patchy or linear striae of hyperenhancement limited to the mid-myocardium of the ventricular wall and were classified as having non–CAD-type scar. In the authors' experience, linear mid-wall hyperenhancement usually is found in the basal interventricular septum. It is observed more frequently in patients who have long-standing LV dysfunction and in those who have a possible prior history of myocarditis. Current studies in patients who have idiopathic dilated cardiomyopathy suggest that the presence of mid-wall hyperenhancement is associated with worsened prognosis, even after adjustment for LVEF.[37]

Hyperenhancement Patterns in Non-Ischemic Cardiomyopathy

The studies described in the previous section evaluated only patients who had ischemic or idiopathic dilated cardiomyopathy. Patients who had hypertrophic cardiomyopathy, myocarditis, infiltrative disorders, or other forms of non-ischemic cardiomyopathy were excluded. Some of these diseases are addressed in detail in other articles in this issue, but a brief summary of DE-CMR findings in several cardiomyopathies is provided in **Table 1**.

The locations and patterns of scarring on DE-CMR are often quite distinct, and a pattern-recognition approach based on the visualization of hyperenhancement can provide useful diagnostic information about the likely cause. **Fig. 5** illustrates potential hyperenhancement patterns that may be encountered in clinical practice with a partial list of their differential diagnoses. Importantly, emerging data suggest that certain non-ischemic cardiomyopathies have a predilection for specific scar patterns. For instance, in the setting of LV hypertrophy, the presence of mid-wall hyperenhancement in one or both junctions of the interventricular septum and right ventricular free wall is highly suggestive of hypertrophic cardiomyopathy,[38] whereas mid-wall or epicardial hyperenhancement in the inferolateral wall is consistent with Anderson-Fabry disease.[39] Likewise, in a patient who has the appropriate demographic profile, the involvement of both the LV basal lateral wall and apex seems to be relatively specific for Chagas disease.[40] Moreover, instead of an infinite

variety of patterns, a general classification into a limited number of common hyperenhancement phenotypes seems to be possible. In some disorders, however, more than one pattern can occur or coexist in the same patient. For example, three patterns of hyperenhancement are encountered commonly in patients who have myocarditis (**Fig. 6**). Certain patterns of hyperenhancement seem to be related to the type of virus causing myocarditis and, importantly, to the clinical course.[41]

Pathophysiologic Basis of Hyperenhancement in Non-Ischemic Cardiomyopathy

Currently, two lines of evidence indicate that areas of gadolinium hyperenhancement represent regions of nonviable myocardium. First, the locations and patterns of hyperenhancement seen in vivo in patients who have various forms of non-ischemic cardiomyopathy seem to match the locations and patterns of scarred or necrotic myocardium seen in gross pathology specimens of autopsy studies. In patients who have hypertrophic cardiomyopathy, scarring often is prominent at the site of the right ventricular insertion into the ventricular septum and neatly matches the pattern of hyperenhancement.[42] In patients who had fatal myocarditis, a common location for necrosis with inflammatory infiltrates is the epicardial portion of the LV free wall,[43] again matching in vivo DE-CMR observations. Second, there now are data, although limited, comparing in vivo hyperenhancement patterns with gross pathology findings in the same patient. In a case report of a patient who had hypertrophic cardiomyopathy, there was a direct relationship between the presence and location of hyperenhancement on DE-CMR and the presence and location of replacement scarring on pathology performed 49 days later after cardiac transplantation.[9] Similarly, in a patient who had Anderson-Fabry disease, nearly exact concordance was seen between in vivo DE-CMR and whole-heart histologic validation performed 22 months later after witnessed sudden cardiac death.[44]

Grossly visible scarring, however, represents only one type of myocardial fibrosis. Diffuse fine interstitial fibrosis is common in many cardiomyopathies, including idiopathic dilated cardiomyopathy,[33] and one important question is whether this form of fibrosis also leads to focal hyperenhancement on delayed-enhancement imaging. This possibility is unlikely for two reasons. First, DE-CMR is sensitive to regional differences in gadolinium accumulation rather than to an overall increase, because the technique depends on the

Table 1
Scar characteristics in non-ischemic cardiomyopathies by DE-CMR

Disease	Hyperenhancement Patterns	Reported Prevalence	References
Idiopathic dilated cardiomyopathy	Linear mid-wall, typically in the basal septum	10%–35%	30,34,37,60
Hypertrophic cardiomyopathy	Patchy, multifocal, predominantly mid-wall More common in hypertrophied areas and the interventricular septum If HE is present, RV insertion sites of the septum are almost always involved	48%–89%; nearly 100% in patients who have severe hypertrophy (wall thickness >30 mm)	38,53–63
Infiltrative			
Amyloidosis	Diffuse HE often with global subendocardial involvement HE also may be localized	69%–80%	64–67
Sarcoidosis	May have CAD-type HE (subendocardial and transmural) Non–CAD-type HE is also common (mid-wall or epicardial) Involvement of RV side of the basal septum seems to be relatively specific for sarcoidosis	33%–50%; almost 100% in known cardiac sarcoidosis	52,68–70
Infectious/inflammatory			
Myocarditis	Three different patterns: (1) linear mid-wall striae in the basal septum; (2) lateral epicardial HE; and (3) multiple, focal mid-wall HE globally More than one pattern can coexist in the same patient (**Fig. 6**)	75%–100%	8,41,71–73
Chagas disease	Preferentially affects basal lateral wall and apex Involvement of both areas concomitantly is relatively specific for Chagas disease	20% in seropositive asymptomatic patients; 86% in clinical Chagas disease; 100% in patients who have VT	40
Genetic/miscellaneous			
Anderson–Fabry disease	HE in the basal inferolateral wall, often epicardial or intramural	31%–50%	39,74,75
Muscular dystrophy	Epicardial or mid-wall HE in the basal inferolateral wall	32%–75%	76–78
Pulmonary hypertension	Right ventricular insertion sites of the interventricular septum	97%	79

Systemic sclerosis	Can be poorly defined/patchy or well-defined/focal	15%–66%	80–82
Takotsubo cardiomyopathy	Predominantly mid-wall and in the basal segments HE typically absent		83,84
Uremic cardiomyopathy	CAD-type HE in patients who have LV systolic dysfunction Regions of diffuse fibrosis in patients who have normal function and severe concentric hypertrophy	14% and 14% (in patients with ESRD)	85
Limited data from single reports with few patients			
Aortic stenosis	Focal, patchy HE in patients who have severe hypertrophy	27% (6 of 22 patients)	86
Churg-Strauss syndrome	Narrow rim of subendocardial HE, not confined to a single coronary territory	82% (9 of 11 patients who had suspected cardiac involvement)	87
HIV cardiomyopathy	No specific HE pattern for HIV cardiomyopathy Myocarditis pattern or MI pattern may be present	33% (4 of 12 in patients with elevated BNP)	88
Lamin A/C cardiomyopathy	Mid-myocardial fibrosis in basal interventricular septum	45% (5 of 11 patients)	89
Peripartum cardiomyopathy	HE absent	8 patients studied	90
Postchemotherapy (trastuzumab) cardiomyopathy	Epicardial pattern often involving the lateral wall	100% (in 10 patients who had an LV ejection fraction < 40%)	91
Primary desminopathies	Mid-wall	36% (4 of 11 patients)	92
SLE	Inferolateral segment with subendocardial sparing	38% (in 3 of 8 patients)	93

Abbreviations: CAD, coronary artery disease; ESRD, end-stage renal disease; HE, hyperenhancement; LV, left ventricle; MI, myocardial infarction; RV, right ventricle; SLE, systemic lupus erythematosus; VT, ventricular tachycardia.

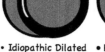

Ischemic

A. Subendocardial Infarct

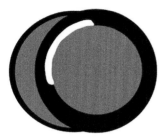

B. Transmural Infarct

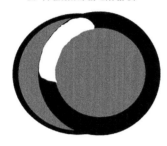

Nonischemic

A. Mid-wall HE

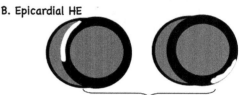

- Idiopathic Dilated Cardiomyopathy
- Myocarditis

- Hypertrophic Cardiomyopathy
- Right ventricular pressure overload (eg. congenital heart disease, pulmonary HTN)

- Sarcoidosis
- Myocarditis
- Anderson–Fabry
- Chagas Disease

B. Epicardial HE

- Sarcoidosis, Myocarditis, Anderson–Fabry, Chagas Disease

C. Global Endocardial HE

- Amyloidosis, Systemic Sclerosis, Post cardiac transplantation

Fig. 5. Hyperenhancement (HE) patterns encountered in clinical practice. If hyperenhancement is present, the endocardium should be involved in patients who have ischemic disease. Isolated mid-wall or epicardial hyperenhancement strongly suggests a non-ischemic cause. (*From* Shah DJ, Judd RM, Kim RJ. Myocardial Viability. In: Edelman RR, Hesselink JR, Zlatkin MB, et al, eds. Clinical magnetic resonance imaging. 3rd edition. New York: Elsevier; 2006. p. 992; with permission.)

ability to "null" signal from "remote" (presumably normal) myocardium.[45,46] Therefore, cardiac disorders that lead to focal regions of fibrosis enhance, and disorders that lead to global changes do not. Second, one should remember that the voxel resolution of DE-CMR is approximately 1.8 mm × 1.3 mm × 6 mm. A region of hyperenhancement that is visible on DE-CMR will comprise several voxels, and the pathology analogue would be a macroscopic scar that is visible to the naked eye. Thus, DE-CMR depicts regions of replacement scarring in vivo that previously could be detected at only autopsy, but DE-CMR currently is unable to identify the presence of diffuse reticular interstitial fibrosis.

A STEPWISE APPROACH INCORPORATING DELAYED-ENHANCEMENT CARDIOVASCULAR MAGNETIC RESONANCE

Recently, a systematic approach to interpreting DE-CMR images in patients who have heart failure

or cardiomyopathy has been proposed (**Fig. 7**).[22,47] In clinical practice, DE-CMR almost never is performed or interpreted in isolation, and a slightly modified approach to determining the cause of cardiomyopathy is shown in **Fig. 8**. Cine imaging almost always is part of an initial evaluation of heart failure and is part of the core CMR examination. As discussed in other articles in this issue, cine CMR is arguably the reference-standard technique for evaluating myocardial structure and function. Small changes in ejection fraction and cardiac mass are detected more readily (and with greater precision) with cine CMR than with echocardiography,[48,49] and therapeutic interventions for patients who have heart failure may be assessed best using CMR. Thus, the first step is to assess the severity and regionality of LV dysfunction, chamber sizes, wall thickness, and valvular function, using cine CMR.

The second step is to determine the presence or absence of hyperenhancement on DE-CMR. Almost all patients who have longstanding ischemic

Linear Midwall Striae

Lateral Epicardial and
Linear Midwall Striae

Multiple Focal Midwall

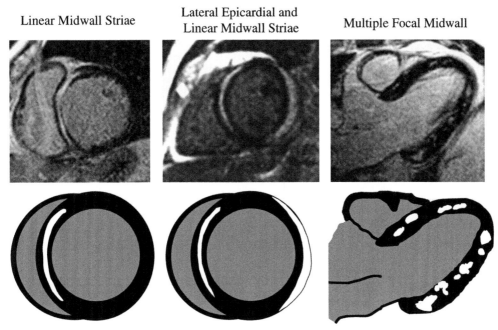

Fig. 6. The top row displays delayed-enhancement images of three commonly encountered patterns of hyperenhancement in patients who have myocarditis. The bottom row is a schematic representation of the respective hyperenhancement patterns.

cardiomyopathy have evidence of prior myocardial infarction (as discussed previously). The implication is that the diagnosis of non-ischemic cardiomyopathy should be considered strongly in patients who have severe cardiomyopathy but not hyperenhancement. Common conditions in which hyperenhancement frequently is absent include idiopathic dilated, alcoholic, Takotsubo, and peripartum cardiomyopathy (see **Table 1**).

If hyperenhancement is present, the third step is to classify the location and distribution of hyperenhancement as CAD-type or non–CAD-type hyperenhancement. For this determination, the concept that ischemic injury progresses as a "wavefront" from the subendocardium to the epicardium is crucial. Correspondingly, hyperenhancement patterns that spare the subendocardium and are limited to the middle or epicardial portion of the LV wall are clearly non–CAD-type hyperenhancement. It is important to remember, however, that in a given patient both CAD-type and non–CAD-type hyperenhancement may be present. This finding does not necessarily indicate a mixed cardiomyopathy, because both patterns are present commonly in certain non-ischemic cardiomyopathies (eg, cardiac sarcoidosis). As a second part of this step, further classification should be considered if hyperenhancement is present in

a non-CAD pattern. Depending on the clinical history and associated data, a specific cause may be entertained as described in **Table 1** and **Fig. 5**.

In some patients, additional testing might aid in the interpretation of DE-CMR findings and would represent a fourth step. These data may be acquired during the same CMR imaging session (eg, coronary MR angiography, stress perfusion CMR), or by other modalities before or after CMR. In a patient who has an ischemic myopathic process (CAD-type scarring), knowledge of the coronary anatomy and/or presence of ischemia will be valuable for decisions regarding treatment, including revascularization. In a patient who has a non-ischemic myopathic process (non–CAD-type scarring), additional testing may reveal the precise cause or causes of cardiomyopathy. If coronary angiography demonstrates no atherosclerosis, the ventricular dysfunction is caused solely by non-ischemic cardiomyopathy. Anatomic evidence of coronary atherosclerosis without evidence of ischemia on functional testing suggests the presence of non-ischemic cardiomyopathy with incidental CAD. On the other hand, a patient who has coronary lesions and inducible ischemia is likely to have a mixed disorder and

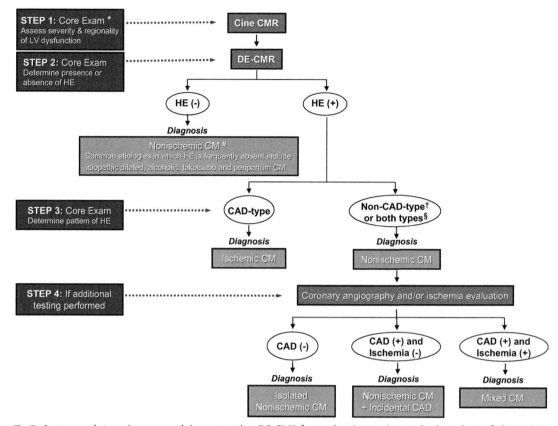

Fig. 7. A proposed stepwise approach incorporating DE-CMR for evaluating patients who have heart failure. CAD, coronary artery disease; CM, cardiomyopathy; CMR, cardiac magnetic resonance; DE, delayed enhancement; HE, hyperenhancement; LV, left ventricle. *Core examination typically consists of cine followed by delayed-enhancement imaging. #Presumes long-standing, chronic cardiomyopathy and severe ventricular dysfunction. †See **Table 1** and **Fig. 5** for details of non-CAD–type patterns of hyperenhancement in various non-ischemic cardiomyopathies. §Patients who have non-ischemic cardiomyopathy often can have both non-CAD and CAD-type hyperenhancement (eg, sarcoidosis).

to have ischemic and non-ischemic cardiomyopathy concomitantly.

Potential Complexities

Several issues may complicate the clinical interpretation of DE-CMR. Although the absence of hyperenhancement suggests a non-ischemic process, this interpretation presumes longstanding, chronic cardiomyopathy and severe ventricular dysfunction. If the LV ejection fraction is reduced only mildly (eg, LVEF > 40%), or if the cardiomyopathy is of recent onset, an ischemic process may be operative, and dysfunctional regions without hyperenhancement may represent areas of stunned or hibernating myocardium.

Occasionally CAD-type hyperenhancement may be present along with normal-appearing coronary arteries on radiographic angiography. There are several possible explanations for this scenario. One possibility is that coronary artery disease is present but was missed by angiography. In authors' experience this situation is rare but can occur when there is a flush, ostial occlusion of a secondary coronary branch. The infarct-related artery usually is small and, correspondingly, the size of hyperenhancement is small also. A second scenario is that coronary artery disease is present but represents a dynamic process, and a ruptured plaque with acute thrombotic occlusion—although leading to acute myocardial infarction—may have healed without residual stenosis.[50] In this case intravascular ultrasound may demonstrate substantial coronary atherosclerosis with remodeling and preserved luminal patency. A third possibility is that a non-ischemic cardiomyopathy is present, but coronary vasospasm or emboli may have led to a myocardial infarction. Tests for abnormal coronary reactivity or the appropriate clinical scenario (eg, the presence of intracardiac thrombus) may be helpful in this situation. A fourth possibility is that a non-ischemic cardiomyopathy is present, but the hyperenhancement pattern mimics that of myocardial infarction. Examples are shown in **Fig. 8**, and it is worthwhile to remember that certain non-ischemic disorders (ie. infiltrative cardiomyopathy) are more likely than others to present with CAD-type hyperenhancement.

Finally, some caveats should be mentioned regarding the pattern of hyperenhancement. Novices should be cautioned against making a quick decision in favor of non–CAD-type

hyperenhancement. Additionally it is important to distinguish carefully between patterns that are clearly non-CAD type (such as often found in myocarditis; see **Fig. 6**), and one or two patchy lesions that vaguely seem to spare the subendocardium. In the latter case (and when in doubt), one should opt for CAD-type hyperenhancement. In nearly 70% of patients, the cause of heart failure is ischemic heart disease,[51] and in these patients effective therapy, including revascularization, may change the outcome substantially. Other common sources of error in interpreting hyperenhancement patterns are listed in **Table 2** and are shown in **Figs. 9** and **10**.

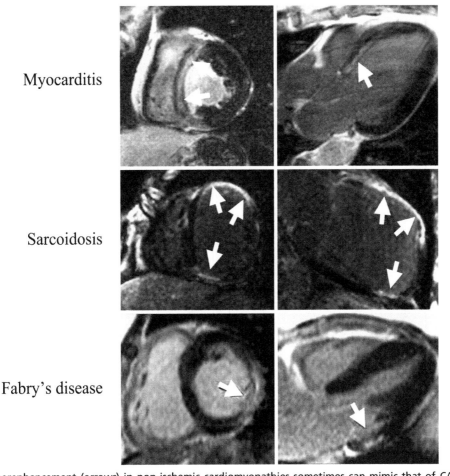

Fig. 8. Hyperenhancement (*arrows*) in non-ischemic cardiomyopathies sometimes can mimic that of CAD. (*Top row*) The patient had biopsy-proven HHV6 myocarditis and no CAD by angiography. (*Middle row*) Like myocardial infarction, cardiac sarcoidosis can cause transmural scarring resulting in wall thinning. (*Bottom row*) The lesions of Anderson-Fabry disease usually are intramural, but, rarely, the subendocardium can be affected also. (*Bottom row modified from* Moon JC, Sachdev B, Elkington AG, et al. Gadolinium enhanced cardiovascular magnetic resonance in Anderson-Fabry disease. Evidence for a disease specific abnormality of the myocardial interstitium. Eur Heart J 2003;24(23):2153; with permission.)

Table 2
Common sources of error in interpreting hyperenhancement patterns

Pitfalls	Comments/Teaching Points
Patients who have ischemic cardiomyopathy who seem to have non–CAD-type HE	
The most basal aspect of a myocardial infarction can spare the subendocardium (**Fig. 9**)	The coronary artery is epicardial, and the most basal (proximal) aspect of its perfusion territory can involve only the epicardial portion of the LV wall. When deciding that HE is of non-CAD type (ie, "spares the subendocardium"), note that this sparing refers to the entire extent of HE and not merely a part of the HE.
No-reflow zone can mimic normal myocardium (ie, appear black), thus suggesting that HE does not involve the subendocardium (**Fig. 10**)	Use DE-CMR with a long inversion time (600 ms); with this technique, the no-reflow zone will appear black, and normal myocardium will be gray. Repeat imaging at a later time point; the no-reflow zone should fill in at least partly, and normal myocardium should appear unchanged.
Patients who have non-ischemic cardiomyopathy who seem to have CAD-type HE	
In many non-ischemic cardiomyopathies, in addition to non–CAD-type HE, subendocardial or transmural HE (eg. sarcoidosis) is common	Search for definite non–CAD-type HE (ie, epicardial HE). If definite non–CAD-type HE coexists with other regions that have CAD-type HE, the diagnosis probably is non-ischemic cardiomyopathy rather than mixed cardiomyopathy.
Miscellaneous	
Mid-wall striae of HE at the base of the LV may be found in myocarditis or idiopathic dilated cardiomyopathy but may also be a nonspecific finding	Obtain DE-CMR images in orthogonal planes to delineate the scar adequately; nonspecific fibrosis tends to be contiguous with the fibrous skeleton of the heart. In the authors' experience, this finding can have multiple causes.
In amyloidosis it may be difficult to find the null point of normal myocardium	Use TI scout images; the finding that the majority of myocardium nulls at a shorter time than blood in LV cavity (ie, myocardium has shorter T1 relaxation time) is pathognomonic for cardiac amyloidosis.

Abbreviations: CAD, coronary artery disease; DE-CMR, delayed-enhancement cardiac magnetic resonance; HE, hyperenhancement; LV, left ventricle; RV, right ventricle; TI, inversion time.

A Animal model of acute MI: Pathology

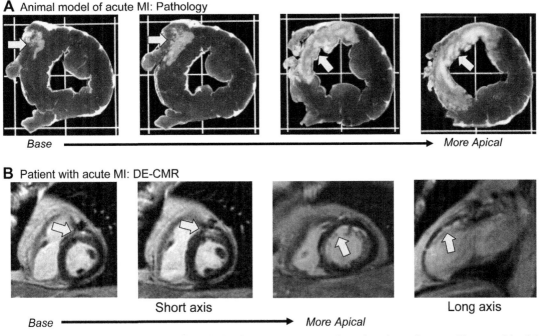

Base ⟶ *More Apical*

B Patient with acute MI: DE-CMR

Short axis   Long axis

Base ⟶ *More Apical*

Fig. 9. The most basal aspect of a myocardial infarction can spare the subendocardium, as illustrated by (*A*) gross pathology in a canine heart with acute myocardial infarction (*Modified from* Kim RJ, Fieno DS, Parrish TB, et al. Relationship of MRI delayed contrast enhancement to irreversible injury, infarct age, and contractile function. Circulation 1999;100(19):1996; with permission) and (*B*) in vivo delayed-enhancement images from a patient who has acute infarction. Arrows point to infarcted myocardium. The more distal contiguous slices and orthogonal views demonstrate the subendocardial involvement by the infarction. Thus, before deciding that hyperenhancement is non–CAD-type (ie, spares the subendocardium), one should note that subendocardial sparing refers to the entire extent of hyperenhancement and not merely a small portion.

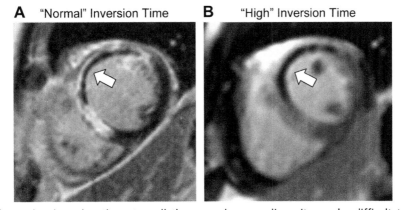

A   "Normal" Inversion Time   **B**   "High" Inversion Time

Fig. 10. (*A*) When using inversion times to null the normal myocardium, it may be difficult to differentiate normal myocardium from no-reflow zones within the core of an acute myocardial infarction, because both regions appear black (*arrow*). (*B*) With higher inversion times (∼600 ms), however, the no-reflow region, which remains black, may be reliably differentiated from normal myocardium, which is now gray in appearance.

SUMMARY

In conclusion, DE-CMR may be a valuable tool in evaluating the cause of cardiomyopathy. Because it provides direct assessment of myopathic processes, it represents a fundamentally different approach than that traditionally undertaken (ie, tests to determine the presence or absence of CAD). This article has presented a stepwise algorithm for interpreting CMR images that accounts for differences among cardiomyopathies in the presence, locations, and patterns of myocardial hyperenhancement. Additionally, a combination of DE-CMR with assessment of coronary anatomy and/or functional testing for ischemia may allow the identification of patients who have non-ischemic cardiomyopathy and incidental CAD and patients who have mixed cardiomyopathy. In the future, this approach should be evaluated in larger populations for diagnostic accuracy and cost effectiveness and, ultimately, to determine whether patient outcomes can be improved.

REFERENCES

1. Richardson P, McKenna W, Bristow M, et al. Report of the 1995 World Health Organization/International Society and Federation of Cardiology Task Force on the Definition and Classification of cardiomyopathies. Circulation 1996;93(5):841–2.
2. Maron BJ, Towbin JA, Thiene G, et al. Contemporary definitions and classification of the cardiomyopathies: an American Heart Association Scientific Statement from the Council on Clinical Cardiology, Heart Failure and Transplantation Committee; Quality of Care and Outcomes Research and Functional Genomics and Translational Biology Interdisciplinary Working Groups; and Council on Epidemiology and Prevention. Circulation 2006; 113(14):1807–16.
3. Alderman EL, Fisher LD, Litwin P, et al. Results of coronary artery surgery in patients with poor left ventricular function (CASS). Circulation 1983;68(4):785–95.
4. Felker GM, Shaw LK, O'Connor CM. A standardized definition of ischemic cardiomyopathy for use in clinical research. J Am Coll Cardiol 2002;39(2):210–8.
5. Packer M, Coats AJ, Fowler MB, et al. Effect of carvedilol on survival in severe chronic heart failure. N Engl J Med 2001;344(22):1651–8.
6. Felker GM, Thompson RE, Hare JM, et al. Underlying causes and long-term survival in patients with initially unexplained cardiomyopathy. N Engl J Med 2000;342(15):1077–84.
7. Kim RJ, Fieno DS, Parrish TB, et al. Relationship of MRI delayed contrast enhancement to irreversible injury, infarct age, and contractile function. Circulation 1999;100(19):1992–2002.
8. Mahrholdt H, Goedecke C, Wagner A, et al. Cardiovascular magnetic resonance assessment of human myocarditis: a comparison to histology and molecular pathology. Circulation 2004;109(10):1250–8.
9. Moon JC, Reed E, Sheppard MN, et al. The histologic basis of late gadolinium enhancement cardiovascular magnetic resonance in hypertrophic cardiomyopathy. J Am Coll Cardiol 2004;43(12):2260–4.
10. Wu E, Judd RM, Vargas JD, et al. Visualisation of presence, location, and transmural extent of healed Q-wave and non-Q-wave myocardial infarction. Lancet 2001;357(9249):21–8.
11. Wagner A, Mahrholdt H, Thomson L, et al. Effects of time, dose, and inversion time for acute myocardial infarct size measurements based on magnetic resonance imaging-delayed contrast enhancement. J Am Coll Cardiol 2006;47(10):2027–33.
12. Ricciardi MJ, Wu E, Davidson CJ, et al. Visualization of discrete microinfarction after percutaneous coronary intervention associated with mild creatine kinase-MB elevation. Circulation 2001;103(23):2780–3.
13. Uretsky BF, Thygesen K, Armstrong PW, et al. Acute coronary findings at autopsy in heart failure patients with sudden death: results from the assessment of treatment with lisinopril and survival (ATLAS) trial. Circulation 2000;102(6):611–6.
14. Corya B, Feigenbaum H, Rasmussen S, et al. Echocardiographic features of congestive cardiomyopathy compared with normal subjects and patients with coronary artery disease. Circulation 1974; 49(6):1153–9.
15. Wallis DE, O'Connell JB, Henkin RE, et al. Segmental wall motion abnormalities in dilated cardiomyopathy: a common finding and good prognostic sign. J Am Coll Cardiol 1984;4(4):674–9.
16. Glamann DB, Lange RA, Corbett JR, et al. Utility of various radionuclide techniques for distinguishing ischemic from non-ischemic dilated cardiomyopathy. Arch Intern Med 1992;152(4):769–72.
17. Rahman JE, Helou EF, Gelzer-Bell R, et al. Noninvasive diagnosis of biopsy-proven cardiac amyloidosis. J Am Coll Cardiol 2004;43(3):410–5.
18. Kubo N, Morimoto S, Hiramitsu S, et al. Feasibility of diagnosing chronic myocarditis by endomyocardial biopsy. Heart Vessels 1997;12(4):167–70.
19. Hauck AJ, Kearney DL, Edwards WD. Evaluation of postmortem endomyocardial biopsy specimens from 38 patients with lymphocytic myocarditis: implications for role of sampling error. Mayo Clin Proc 1989;64(10):1235–45.
20. Kronmal RA, McClelland RL, Detrano R, et al. Risk factors for the progression of coronary artery calcification in asymptomatic subjects: results from the Multi-Ethnic Study of Atherosclerosis (MESA). Circulation 2007;115(21):2722–30.

21. Kim RJ, Wu E, Rafael A, et al. The use of contrast-enhanced magnetic resonance imaging to identify reversible myocardial dysfunction. N Engl J Med 2000;343(20):1445–53.

22. Shah DJ, Judd RM, Kim RJ. Myocardial viability. In: Edelman RR, Hesselink JR, Zlatkin MB, editors. Clinical magnetic resonance imaging. 3rd edition. New York: Elsevier; 2006.

23. Kim RJ, Elliott MD, Judd RM. Assessment of myocardial viability by contrast enhancement. In: Higgins CB, de Roos A, editors. MRI and CT of the cardiovascular system. 2nd edition. Philadelphia: Lippincott Williams & Wilkins; 2005.

24. Koenig SH, Spiller M, Brown RD III, et al. Relaxation of water protons in the intra- and extracellular regions of blood containing Gd(DTPA). Magn Reson Med 1986;3(5):791–5.

25. Polimeni PI. Extracellular space and ionic distribution in rat ventricle. Am J Physiol 1974;227(3):676–83.

26. Rehwald WG, Fieno DS, Chen EL, et al. Myocardial magnetic resonance imaging contrast agent concentrations after reversible and irreversible ischemic injury. Circulation 2002;105(2):224–9.

27. Reimer KA, Lowe JE, Rasmussen MM, et al. The wavefront phenomenon of ischemic cell death. 1. Myocardial infarct size vs duration of coronary occlusion in dogs. Circulation 1977;56(5):786–94.

28. Bello D, Shah DJ, Farah GM, et al. Gadolinium cardiovascular magnetic resonance predicts reversible myocardial dysfunction and remodeling in patients with heart failure undergoing beta-blocker therapy. Circulation 2003;108(16):1945–53.

29. Casolo G, Minneci S, Manta R, et al. Identification of the ischemic etiology of heart failure by cardiovascular magnetic resonance imaging: diagnostic accuracy of late gadolinium enhancement. Am Heart J 2006;151(1):101–8.

30. Soriano CJ, Ridocci F, Estornell J, et al. Noninvasive diagnosis of coronary artery disease in patients with heart failure and systolic dysfunction of uncertain etiology, using late gadolinium-enhanced cardiovascular magnetic resonance. J Am Coll Cardiol 2005; 45(5):743–8.

31. Schuster EH, Bulkley BH. Ischemic cardiomyopathy: a clinicopathologic study of fourteen patients. Am Heart J 1980;100(4):506–12.

32. Boucher CA, Fallon JT, Johnson RA, et al. Cardiomyopathic syndrome caused by coronary artery disease. III: Prospective clinicopathological study of its prevalence among patients with clinically unexplained chronic heart failure. Br Heart J 1979;41(5):613–20.

33. Roberts WC, Siegel RJ, McManus BM. Idiopathic dilated cardiomyopathy: analysis of 152 necropsy patients. Am J Cardiol 1987;60(16):1340–55.

34. McCrohon JA, Moon JC, Prasad SK, et al. Differentiation of heart failure related to dilated cardiomyopathy and coronary artery disease using gadolinium-enhanced cardiovascular magnetic resonance. Circulation 2003;108(1):54–9.

35. Topol EJ, Yadav JS. Recognition of the importance of embolization in atherosclerotic vascular disease. Circulation 2000;101(5):570–80.

36. Arroyo LH, Lee RT. Mechanisms of plaque rupture: mechanical and biologic interactions. Cardiovasc Res 1999;41(2):369–75.

37. Assomull RG, Prasad SK, Lyne J, et al. Cardiovascular magnetic resonance, fibrosis, and prognosis in dilated cardiomyopathy. J Am Coll Cardiol 2006; 48(10):1977–85.

38. Choudhury L, Mahrholdt H, Wagner A, et al. Myocardial scarring in asymptomatic or mildly symptomatic patients with hypertrophic cardiomyopathy. J Am Coll Cardiol 2002;40(12):2156–64.

39. Moon JC, Sachdev B, Elkington AG, et al. Gadolinium enhanced cardiovascular magnetic resonance in Anderson-Fabry disease. Evidence for a disease specific abnormality of the myocardial interstitium. Eur Heart J 2003;24(23):2151–5.

40. Rochitte CE, Oliveira PF, Andrade JM, et al. Myocardial delayed enhancement by magnetic resonance imaging in patients with Chagas' disease: a marker of disease severity. J Am Coll Cardiol 2005;46(8): 1553–8.

41. Mahrholdt H, Wagner A, Deluigi CC, et al. Presentation, patterns of myocardial damage, and clinical course of viral myocarditis. Circulation 2006; 114(15):1581–90.

42. Kim RJ, Judd RM. Gadolinium-enhanced magnetic resonance imaging in hypertrophic cardiomyopathy: in vivo imaging of the pathologic substrate for premature cardiac death? J Am Coll Cardiol 2003; 41(9):1568–72.

43. Shirani J, Freant LJ, Roberts WC. Gross and semiquantitative histologic findings in mononuclear cell myocarditis causing sudden death, and implications for endomyocardial biopsy. Am J Cardiol 1993; 72(12):952–7.

44. Moon JC, Sheppard M, Reed E, et al. The histological basis of late gadolinium enhancement cardiovascular magnetic resonance in a patient with Anderson-Fabry disease. J Cardiovasc Magn Reson 2006;8(3):479–82.

45. Simonetti OP, Kim RJ, Fieno DS, et al. An improved MR imaging technique for the visualization of myocardial infarction. Radiology 2001;218(1):215–23.

46. Kim RJ, Shah DJ, Judd RM. How we perform delayed enhancement imaging. J Cardiovasc Magn Reson 2003;5(3):505–14.

47. Mahrholdt H, Wagner A, Judd RM, et al. Delayed enhancement cardiovascular magnetic resonance assessment of non-ischaemic cardiomyopathies. Eur Heart J 2005;26(15):1461–74.

48. Bellenger NG, Burgess MI, Ray SG, et al. Comparison of left ventricular ejection fraction and volumes

in heart failure by echocardiography, radionuclide ventriculography and cardiovascular magnetic resonance; are they interchangeable? Eur Heart J 2000; 21(16):1387–96.

49. Bellenger NG, Davies LC, Francis JM, et al. Reduction in sample size for studies of remodeling in heart failure by the use of cardiovascular magnetic resonance. J Cardiovasc Magn Reson 2000;2(4):271–8.

50. Kotani J, Mintz GS, Castagna MT, et al. Intravascular ultrasound analysis of infarct-related and non-infarct-related arteries in patients who presented with an acute myocardial infarction. Circulation 2003;107(23):2889–93.

51. Hunt SA, Abraham WT, Chin MH, et al. ACC/AHA 2005 Guideline update for the diagnosis and management of chronic heart failure in the adult: a report of the American College of Cardiology/ American Heart Association Task Force on Practice Guidelines (Writing Committee to Update the 2001 Guidelines for the Evaluation and Management of Heart Failure): developed in collaboration with the American College of Chest Physicians and the International Society for Heart and Lung Transplantation: endorsed by the Heart Rhythm Society. Circulation 2005;112(12):e154–235.

52. Matoh F, Satoh H, Shiraki K, et al. The usefulness of delayed enhancement magnetic resonance imaging for diagnosis and evaluation of cardiac function in patients with cardiac sarcoidosis. J Cardiol 2008; 51(3):179–88.

53. Wilson JM, Villareal RP, Hariharan R, et al. Magnetic resonance imaging of myocardial fibrosis in hypertrophic cardiomyopathy. Tex Heart Inst J 2002; 29(3):176–80.

54. Moon JC, McKenna WJ, McCrohon JA, et al. Toward clinical risk assessment in hypertrophic cardiomyopathy with gadolinium cardiovascular magnetic resonance. J Am Coll Cardiol 2003;41(9):1561–7.

55. Amano Y, Takayama M, Takahama K, et al. Delayed hyper-enhancement of myocardium in hypertrophic cardiomyopathy with asymmetrical septal hypertrophy: comparison with global and regional cardiac MR imaging appearances. J Magn Reson Imaging 2004;20(4):595–600.

56. Teraoka K, Hirano M, Ookubo H, et al. Delayed contrast enhancement of MRI in hypertrophic cardiomyopathy. Magn Reson Imaging 2004;22(2):155–61.

57. Moon JC, Mogensen J, Elliott PM, et al. Myocardial late gadolinium enhancement cardiovascular magnetic resonance in hypertrophic cardiomyopathy caused by mutations in troponin I. Heart 2005;91(8):1036–40.

58. Soler R, Rodriguez E, Monserrat L, et al. Magnetic resonance imaging of delayed enhancement in hypertrophic cardiomyopathy: relationship with left ventricular perfusion and contractile function. J Comput Assist Tomogr 2006;30(3):412–20.

59. Dumont CA, Monserrat L, Soler R, et al. [Clinical significance of late gadolinium enhancement on cardiovascular magnetic resonance in patients with hypertrophic cardiomyopathy]. Rev Esp Cardiol 2007;60(1):15–23 [in Spanish].

60. Matoh F, Satoh H, Shiraki K, et al. Usefulness of delayed enhancement magnetic resonance imaging to differentiate dilated phase of hypertrophic cardiomyopathy and dilated cardiomyopathy. J Card Fail 2007;13(5):372–9.

61. Melacini P, Corbetti F, Calore C, et al. Cardiovascular magnetic resonance signs of ischemia in hypertrophic cardiomyopathy. Int J Cardiol 2008;128(3): 364–73.

62. Paya E, Marin F, Gonzalez J, et al. Variables associated with contrast-enhanced cardiovascular magnetic resonance in hypertrophic cardiomyopathy: clinical implications. J Card Fail 2008;14(5):414–9.

63. Suk T, Edwards C, Hart H, et al. Myocardial scar detected by contrast-enhanced cardiac magnetic resonance imaging is associated with ventricular tachycardia in hypertrophic cardiomyopathy patients. Heart Lung Circ 2008;17(5):370–4.

64. Maceira AM, Joshi J, Prasad SK, et al. Cardiovascular magnetic resonance in cardiac amyloidosis. Circulation 2005;111(2):186–93.

65. Perugini E, Rapezzi C, Piva T, et al. Non-invasive evaluation of the myocardial substrate of cardiac amyloidosis by gadolinium cardiac magnetic resonance. Heart 2006;92(3):343–9.

66. Hosch W, Libicher M, Ley S, et al. [MR imaging in cardiac amyloidosis–morphology, function and late enhancement]. Rofo 2008;180(7):639–45 [in German].

67. Vogelsberg H, Mahrholdt H, Deluigi CC, et al. Cardiovascular magnetic resonance in clinically suspected cardiac amyloidosis: noninvasive imaging compared to endomyocardial biopsy. J Am Coll Cardiol 2008;51(10):1022–30.

68. Shimada T, Shimada K, Sakane T, et al. Diagnosis of cardiac sarcoidosis and evaluation of the effects of steroid therapy by gadolinium-DTPA-enhanced magnetic resonance imaging. Am J Med 2001; 110(7):520–7.

69. Smedema JP, Snoep G, van Kroonenburgh MP, et al. Evaluation of the accuracy of gadolinium-enhanced cardiovascular magnetic resonance in the diagnosis of cardiac sarcoidosis. J Am Coll Cardiol 2005; 45(10):1683–90.

70. Tadamura E, Yamamuro M, Kubo S, et al. Effectiveness of delayed enhanced MRI for identification of cardiac sarcoidosis: comparison with radionuclide imaging. AJR Am J Roentgenol 2005;185(1):110–5.

71. Laissy JP, Hyafil F, Feldman LJ, et al. Differentiating acute myocardial infarction from myocarditis: diagnostic value of early- and delayed-perfusion cardiac MR imaging. Radiology 2005;237(1):75–82.

72. Yelgec NS, Dymarkowski S, Ganame J, et al. Value of MRI in patients with a clinical suspicion of acute myocarditis. Eur Radiol 2007;17(9):2211–7.

73. Gutberlet M, Spors B, Thoma T, et al. Suspected chronic myocarditis at cardiac MR: diagnostic accuracy and association with immunohistologically detected inflammation and viral persistence. Radiology 2008;246(2):401–9.

74. Weidemann F, Breunig F, Beer M, et al. The variation of morphological and functional cardiac manifestation in Fabry disease: potential implications for the time course of the disease. Eur Heart J 2005;26(12):1221–7.

75. Beer M, Weidemann F, Breunig F, et al. Impact of enzyme replacement therapy on cardiac morphology and function and late enhancement in Fabry's cardiomyopathy. Am J Cardiol 2006;97(10):1515–8.

76. Silva MC, Meira ZM, Gurgel Giannetti J, et al. Myocardial delayed enhancement by magnetic resonance imaging in patients with muscular dystrophy. J Am Coll Cardiol 2007;49(18):1874–9.

77. Yilmaz A, Gdynia HJ, Baccouche H, et al. Cardiac involvement in patients with Becker muscular dystrophy: new diagnostic and pathophysiological insights by a CMR approach. J Cardiovasc Magn Reson 2008;10(1):50.

78. Puchalski MD, Williams RV, Askovich B, et al. Late gadolinium enhancement: precursor to cardiomyopathy in Duchenne muscular dystrophy? Int J Cardiovasc Imaging 2009;25(1):57–63.

79. Sanz J, Dellegrottaglie S, Kariisa M, et al. Prevalence and correlates of septal delayed contrast enhancement in patients with pulmonary hypertension. Am J Cardiol 2007;100(4):731–5.

80. Tzelepis GE, Kelekis NL, Plastiras SC, et al. Pattern and distribution of myocardial fibrosis in systemic sclerosis: a delayed enhanced magnetic resonance imaging study. Arthritis Rheum 2007;56(11):3827–36.

81. Kobayashi H, Yokoe I, Hirano M, et al. Cardiac magnetic resonance imaging with pharmacological stress perfusion and delayed enhancement in asymptomatic patients with systemic sclerosis. J Rheumatol 2009;36(1):106–12.

82. Nassenstein K, Breuckmann F, Huger M, et al. Detection of myocardial fibrosis in systemic sclerosis by contrast-enhanced magnetic resonance imaging. Rofo 2008;108(12):1054–60.

83. Mitchell JH, Hadden TB, Wilson JM, et al. Clinical features and usefulness of cardiac magnetic resonance imaging in assessing myocardial viability and prognosis in Takotsubo cardiomyopathy (transient left ventricular apical ballooning syndrome). Am J Cardiol 2007;100(2):296–301.

84. Eitel I, Behrendt F, Schindler K, et al. Differential diagnosis of suspected apical ballooning syndrome using contrast-enhanced magnetic resonance imaging. Eur Heart J 2008;29(21):2651–9.

85. Mark PB, Johnston N, Groenning BA, et al. Redefinition of uremic cardiomyopathy by contrast-enhanced cardiac magnetic resonance imaging. Kidney Int 2006;69(10):1839–45.

86. Debl K, Djavidani B, Buchner S, et al. Delayed hyperenhancement in magnetic resonance imaging of left ventricular hypertrophy caused by aortic stenosis and hypertrophic cardiomyopathy: visualisation of focal fibrosis. Heart 2006;92(10):1447–51.

87. Wassmuth R, Gobel U, Natusch A, et al. Cardiovascular magnetic resonance imaging detects cardiac involvement in Churg-Strauss syndrome. J Card Fail 2008;14(10):856–60.

88. Breuckmann F, Nassenstein K, Kondratieva J, et al. MR characterization of cardiac abnormalities in HIV+ individuals with increased BNP levels. Eur J Med Res 2007;12(5):185–90.

89. Raman SV, Sparks EA, Baker PM, et al. Mid-myocardial fibrosis by cardiac magnetic resonance in patients with lamin A/C cardiomyopathy: possible substrate for diastolic dysfunction. J Cardiovasc Magn Reson 2007;9(6):907–13.

90. Mouquet F, Lions C, de Groote P, et al. Characterisation of peripartum cardiomyopathy by cardiac magnetic resonance imaging. Eur Radiol 2008;18(12):2765–9.

91. Fallah-Rad N, Lytwyn M, Fang T, et al. Delayed contrast enhancement cardiac magnetic resonance imaging in trastuzumab induced cardiomyopathy. J Cardiovasc Magn Reson 2008;10(1):5.

92. Strach K, Sommer T, Grohe C, et al. Clinical, genetic, and cardiac magnetic resonance imaging findings in primary desminopathies. Neuromuscul Disord 2008;18(6):475–82.

93. Abdel-Aty H, Siegle N, Natusch A, et al. Myocardial tissue characterization in systemic lupus erythematosus: value of a comprehensive cardiovascular magnetic resonance approach. Lupus 2008;17(6):561–7.

Cardiovascular Magnetic Resonance in the Evaluation of Hypertrophic and Infiltrative Cardiomyopathies

Rory O'Hanlon, MRCPI[a], Dudley J. Pennell, MD, FRCP, FACC[a,b],*

KEYWORDS
- Cardiomyopathy • Cardiovascular imaging
- Cardiovascular magnetic resonance
- Hypertrophic cardiomyopathy • Infiltrative cardiomyopathies

Thanks to significant advances in recent years, imaging technologies are now able to characterize a much wider number of cardiomyopathies than ever before in a noninvasive manner. The most significant developments have without doubt been those related to cardiovascular magnetic resonance (CMR) scanners, sequences, and software. In a single-scan setting, it is now possible to provide for both ischemic and nonischemic cardiomyopathies a comprehensive assessment that includes cardiac anatomy, function, tissue characterization, epicardial and microvascular perfusion, valvular flows, and coronary and peripheral angiography (**Fig. 1**). This comprehensive examination can be completed in a short time, typically 45 minutes, without prolonged breath-holds (~10 seconds). The information obtained helps establish diagnoses with a high degree of clarity, aids in guiding and monitoring therapeutic response, and assists in optimal risk stratification. Furthermore, CMR is well tolerated. Follow-up imaging to monitor progression and response to interventions can be performed safely and, because there is no ionizing radiation, without any concern regarding cumulative radiation exposure. Gadolinium-based contrast agents are remarkably safe and the incidence of adverse reactions is exceedingly low.

Hypertrophic and infiltrative cardiomyopathies represent an important challenge to clinical cardiologists. They are considered rare conditions and reaching a definitive diagnosis using routine invasive or noninvasive imaging modalities is often difficult. With considerable overlap in the phenotypic cardiac morphology and presentation, clinicians frequently require patients to undergo an array of detailed investigations to reach the diagnosis. This is especially true when the clinician is trying to differentiate constrictive from restrictive cardiomyopathic processes. A considerable number of diseases can lead to a common restrictive cardiomyopathy phenotype, such as hypertrophic cardiomyopathy (HCM), amyloidosis, sarcoidosis, iron overload, endomyocardial fibrosis, and storage diseases (Fabry, glycogen storage diseases). Clearly, a single imaging modality to differentiate one disease from another would be very useful. In patients with various degrees of left ventricular (LV) hypertrophy or increased wall thickening, deciding if there is a sarcomeric abnormality or simple essential hypertension is often not straightforward. Furthermore, such conditions as

a Royal Brompton Hospital, London, UK
b Imperial College London, London, UK
* Corresponding author. CMR Unit, Royal Brompton Hospital, Sydney Street, London SW3 6NP.
E-mail address: dj.pennell@rbht.nhs.uk (D.J. Pennell).

Heart Failure Clin 5 (2009) 369–387
doi:10.1016/j.hfc.2009.02.003

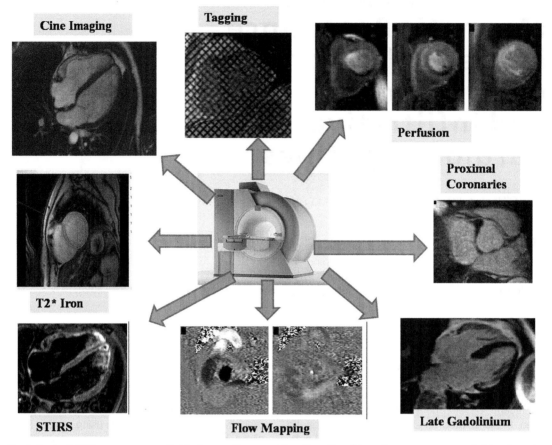

Fig. 1. Typical CMR sequences available for routine use. The diversity of imaging sequences available allow for a comprehensive assessment of both ischemic and nonischemic cardiomyopathies in a single-scan setting and without the need for ionizing radiation. STIRS, short tau inversion recovery images.

cardiac amyloidosis, sarcoidosis, Fabry, and HCM may all be considered in the differential of a hypertrophic LV (**Fig. 2**). With a single CMR scan exploiting the wide field of view, delivering superior spatial resolution, and revealing varied disease tissue characteristics, it is now possible to arrive at a diagnosis with a great degree of certainty and possibly without the need for other investigations. Each of these conditions shall be discussed separately in this review.

HYPERTROPHIC CARDIOMYOPATHY

HCM, the most common genetic cardiomyopathy, is caused by mutations in at least 14 sarcomeric genes. It occurs in 0.2% of the general population and is inherited in an autosomal-dominant manner. The pathologic hallmark is a triad of myocyte hypertrophy, disarray, and myocardial fibrosis.[1–4] With marked heterogeneity with respect to clinical manifestations, natural history, and prognosis, HCM remains the commonest

cause of sudden cardiac death (SCD) and an important cause of morbidity at any age. The tasks of diagnosing and managing HCM present a number of challenging issues. Improvement is needed in determining the risk of sudden death in individuals with HCM. CMR can help in risk assessment by offering a complete and complementary evaluation of patients with known or suspected HCM in a single-scan setting and by providing an ideal imaging modality to follow up patients over time.

Diagnosis

Two-dimensional echocardiography is still regarded as the gold standard test to diagnose HCM. By echocardiography, a maximal LV wall thickness greater than or equal to 15 mm is compatible with the condition, but genotype–phenotype correlations have shown that virtually any wall thickness (including those within normal range) is compatible with the presence of an HCM mutant gene.[5–7] The quality of images

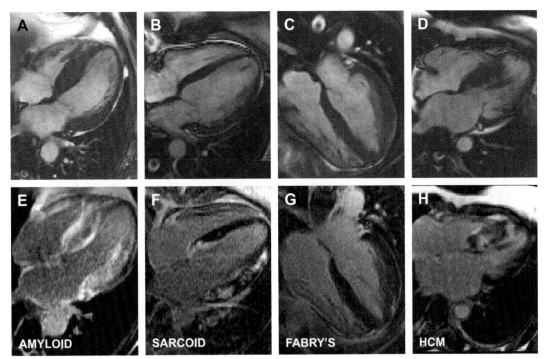

Fig. 2. (*A–D*) Four-chamber steady state free procession images of different patterns of LV hypertrophy. (*A* and *E*) Cardiac amyloidosis showing diffuse subendocardial LGE pattern with "sparing" of the epicardium and septum, characteristically referred to as a "zebra" pattern. (*B* and *F*) Sarcoidosis typically shows focal LGE patterns of scars, which are typically patchy and involving the basal and lateral segments. (*C* and *G*) Fabry shows midwall LGE patterns in the basal lateral wall. (*D* and *H*) Septum HCM typically shows patchy midwall LGE patterns in the regions of maximal hypertrophy.

obtained by echocardiography is limited by the available acoustic windows and the orientation of the heart in the mediastinum to ensure adequate cross-sectional images and to avoid oblique views. Furthermore, because of poor lateral resolution and substantial image distortion, certain areas of the myocardium are not visualized well with echocardiography, especially the anterolateral free wall in the parasternal short axis view, and detection of subtle areas of abnormal hypertrophy can be missed. Given that CMR images can be acquired in any given plane, oblique views are avoided and hypertrophied areas can be visualized and measured with confidence. In a study comparing the incremental benefit of CMR over echocardiography in the evaluation of patients with HCM, the degree of LV wall thickness was underestimated by echocardiography compared with CMR in the anterolateral free wall. Furthermore, in those with severe LV hypertrophy (>30 mm), echocardiography appeared to underestimate the magnitude of wall thickness to a significant degree in 10% of patients.[8] This may have important prognostic implications regarding SCD risk stratification and the need for implantable cardioverter defibrillator (ICD) implantation.

With transthoracic echocardiogram, the apical variant of HCM can often be difficult to diagnose because of signal dropout. By contrast, the apex is easily visualized by CMR. In a series of 10 patients who had nondiagnostic echocardiography and abnormal ECGs, Moon and colleagues[9] used CMR to diagnose apical HCM. Conventional assessment algorithms used when assessing patients with abnormal ECGs or suspected HCM may be missing apical or indeed anterolateral HCM with important prognostic implications. Hence, CMR should be considered as the new gold standard imaging modality and diagnostic test of choice in all patients with suspected HCM or abnormal ECG patterns (**Fig. 3**).[10]

As part of a complete single-scan comprehensive assessment of HCM with CMR, in-plane and through-plane velocity flow mapping is useful to quantify LV outflow tract obstruction and is comparable to values achieved using Doppler echocardiography.[11] The presence of systolic anterior motion of the mitral valve can also be easily visualized with standard cine imaging or, to an even better degree, with high temporal resolution imaging. The amount of mitral regurgitation can be calculated by the difference in aortic output

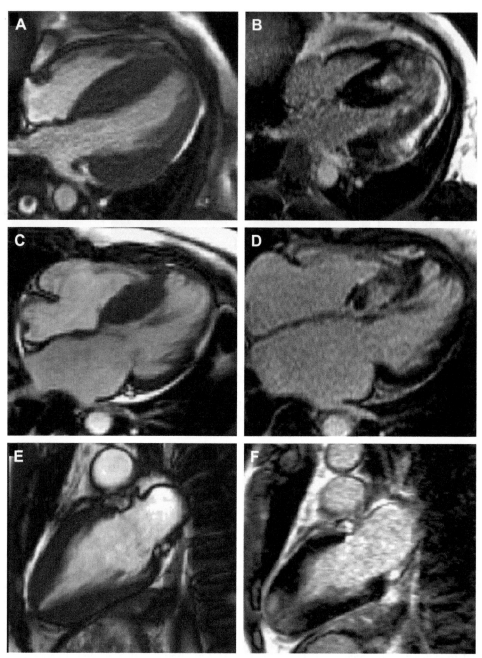

Fig. 3. Various hypertrophy and LGE patterns in HCM. (*A* and *B*) Marked global hypertrophy with extensive LGE patterns in the midwall of the anterolateral LV. (*C* and *D*) Typical case of HCM with marked asymmetrical hypertrophy and patchy midwall fibrosis in the region of maximum wall thickness. (*E* and *F*) Apical HCM with diffuse LGE patterns in the apex. The signal intensity of the LGE pattern in HCM is frequently markedly heterogenous.

measured by phase-velocity flow mapping and the LV stroke volume.

Risk Stratification

There are several challenges in the clinical management of HCM. For SCD, risk stratification can be difficult. Current American College of Cardiology/European Society of Cardiology criteria are effective in defining those at highest risk and for whom there is clear benefit from prophylactic ICD therapy. The wide field of view and quality of images make it possible to avoid obliquity, and thus more reliably define peak wall thickness. A potentially more relevant marker of risk may be the total LV mass index. The assessment of LV mass by echocardiography is unreliable because of the asymmetric distribution of hypertrophy. Olivotto and colleagues[12] demonstrated in a recent study that LV mass index was a more sensitive indicator of risk of death than peak wall thickness. Other potential prognostic markers evaluated by CMR could be the presence of right ventricular (RV) hypertrophy or even the presence of myocardial edema.[13,14]

A more challenging group clinically is the intermediate risk cohort with one or two risk factors who do not meet conventional criteria for ICD deployment.[15–17] Postmortem studies have shown that the majority of patients with HCM who die suddenly have none or only a single identifiable risk factor based on current criteria.[18] ICD implantation is expensive, often has important psychological impact on patients, and carries a risk of around 10% for complications.[19] Hence the decision to implant a primary prophylactic ICD is a major one for patient and physician. In one major study of ICD implantation in HCM patients, inappropriate ICD discharge events occurred in 25% of the studied population, at a rate of approximately 7% per year.[15] A more recent study has suggested that a single risk factor for SCD in HCM patients may warrant ICD implantation.[20] Hence, better risk stratification is needed. CMR as described is the gold standard method to image the heart and allows for more accurate diagnosis of HCM as described above. It is unique in its ability to determine myocardial tissue characteristics in vivo using the late gadolinium enhancement (LGE) technique. The pattern of replacement fibrosis in HCM is distinct from that seen in coronary artery disease or that seen in patients with dilated cardiomyopathy, and is unlike patterns seen in HCM phenocopies in the majority of cases. The typical patterns of LGE described are patchy, mid-wall with multiple foci, and most commonly found in regions of hypertrophy. Several patterns of LGE are seen. At one end of the spectrum is a diffuse transseptal or RV septal pattern. At the other end of the spectrum is a confluent pattern that may affect the interventricular junction or be multifocal. The presence of fibrosis is an important marker of risk. Those patients with greater number of risk factors for SCD typically have more fibrosis, which is consistent with postmortem data (see **Fig. 3**).[21–25] The presence of fibrosis contributes to the disruption of the electrical synchrony that exists between myocytes and hence increases arrhythmia potential.[26–31] Several recent studies have demonstrated risk of ventricular tachyarrhythmias to be associated with LGE.[32–34] It also

promotes increased myocardial stiffness with LV adverse remodeling leading to cavity dilatation and eventually systolic dysfunction, and is detected in 85% of patients with end-stage dilated HCM.[35] The main mechanism driving the formation of fibrosis is thought to be myocardial ischemia due to abnormal microvasculature or a mismatch between the greatly increased LV mass and coronary flow.[36–38] Abnormal perfusion in HCM patients, despite normal coronary angiography, has been linked to SCD. Abnormal perfusion in HCM patients despite normal coronary angiography has been linked to SCD and has been traditionally difficult to assess in HCM patients being principally performed using PET, which to date remains the gold standard tool to evaluate myocardial ischemia. However, PET remains primarily a research tool, delivers significant radiation doses, and is expensive. These limitations have thus restricted the use of PET for HCM patients. CMR stress perfusion, which now can be performed in the same setting as the LGE study and with the same contrast bolus, has been validated against PET perfusion studies (**Fig. 4**).[39–41] A recent paper by Petersen and colleagues[42] demonstrated that severity of myocardial perfusion defects correlate with areas of maximal wall thickness and the presence of fibrosis in patients with HCM. A further hypothesis is that microvascular abnormalities may precede and predispose to the development of myocardial fibrosis and, if present, may represent an earlier risk marker and possible therapeutic target.[43]

A complete CMR examination of a HCM patient can now be performed in 45 minutes and can provide detailed information on volumes, function, peak wall thickness, LV outflow tract obstruction, and systolic anterior motion; quantification of mitral regurgitation; assessment of microvascular perfusion; and measurements of fibrosis. No one doubts that much information is gained in a single comprehensive study. Even so, larger trials are required to determine if the use of CMR to detect and quantify myocardial fibrosis and perfusion abnormalities represent a novel independent risk marker for SCD. Such trials would also help determine whether measurements of fibrosis/perfusion can help in deciding about ICD implantation. Accurate and reproducible serial follow-up of wall thickness, systolic function, perfusion defects, and fibrosis are all possible with CMR and may help identify important changes before symptoms of sudden cardiac events occur. Further work is being carried out to use CMR to detect interstitial fibrosis and myofibrillar disarray. Such work may add to our understanding of this challenging condition and improve related risk assessment.[44]

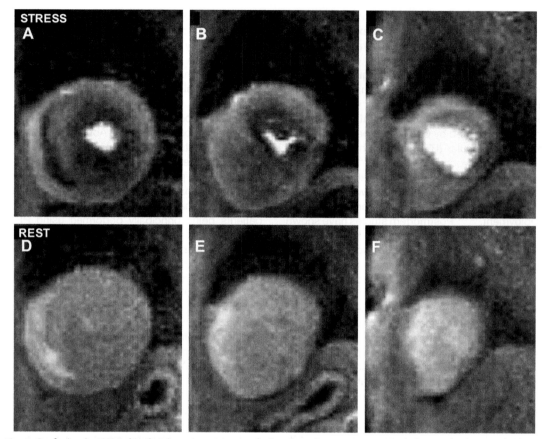

Fig. 4. Perfusion in HCM. (*A–C*) Adenosine stress perfusion from base to apex. Note the marked circumferential perfusion abnormality, best seen at basal and midventricular levels. The abnormality normalizes during the rest perfusion study. (*D–F*) Indications of marked microvascular dysfunction.

IRON-OVERLOAD CARDIOMYOPATHY

For patients with transfusion-dependent anemias, an important consequence is myocardial iron infiltration and subsequent development of cardiomyopathy. The commonest cause worldwide of transfusion dependent anaemia is thalassemia major and unfortunately heart failure due to iron overload is the principle cause of death accounting for up to 71% of all deaths, with 50% of these patients dying before the age of 35, despite iron-chelating therapy.[45–47] This form of cardiomyopathy is reversible but intensive iron chelation is necessary to remove myocardial iron.[48] When a patient develops heart failure, the prognosis is poor. Hence, early detection of myocardial iron overload is required. In the past, total body iron stores and approximation of myocardial iron loading were assessed by serum ferritin levels and liver biopsy. Serum ferritin is also used to monitor success or failure of chelation therapy. Unfortunately, iron deposition is not uniform in the heart and liver. This means significant cardiac iron loading can be present before

the ejection fraction is significantly reduced. Hence, early detection of cardiac iron and indeed monitoring of response to therapeutic interventions can be challenging using conventional techniques.[49] A CMR technique available since 2000 addresses this problem. T2* is a component of the T2 relaxation parameter assessed by CMR arising principally from local magnetic field inhomogeneities that increase in proportion to iron deposition. This simple scan can be performed in a single breath-hold and is validated against both biopsy samples and other markers of myocardial dysfunction, such as LV ejection fraction. This parameter is highly reproducible and correlates with liver and myocardial iron stores. It can be easily imaged and quantified in the heart and the liver using gradient echo techniques (**Fig. 5**). There is no better method to quantify myocardial iron content than with this technique.

Since the implementation of the T2* technique, it has been shown that there is no clinically useful correlation between myocardial iron and liver iron or ferritin levels.[50] In a cross-sectional study,

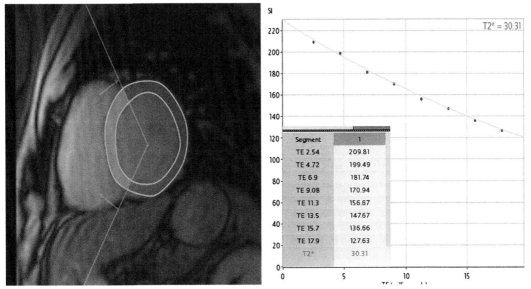

Segment	1
TE 2.54	209.81
TE 4.72	199.49
TE 6.9	181.74
TE 9.08	170.94
TE 11.3	156.67
TE 13.5	147.67
TE 15.7	136.66
TE 17.9	127.63
T2*	30.31

$T2^* = 30.31$

Fig. 5. Myocardial T2* analysis using Thalassemia-Tools (plug-in of CMRtools). The gradient echo images are loaded and the interventricular septum is defined. The software generates the signal against echo-time points and best fits the decay curve to estimate the T2*.

89% of thalassemia patients with new-onset cardiac failure had a T2* less than 10 ms. Therefore the threshold of less than 10 ms for myocardial T2* is now taken as indicating severe iron loading. Mild to moderate iron loading is indicated by a myocardial T2* of 10 to 20 ms, and greater than 20 ms is normal (the median for the normal population is approximately 40 ms). In a prospective follow-up study, the incidence of development of heart failure in those with a T2* less than 6 ms is very high, whereas it is uncommon in patients with a T2* greater than 10 ms. Given the excellent inter-study reproducibility of the technique ($\sim$5%), the efficacy of chelation therapies can be assessed, especially novel therapies with better cardiac iron chelation properties.[51–55]

Since the introduction of the T2* technique to the management of thalassemia patients, with particular emphasis on intensification or alteration of chelation therapies, United Kingdom mortality rates in this condition have been reduced by approximately 70%.[56] This pattern has also been documented in Italy and Cyprus.[57]

Hemochromatosis, a genetically determined disorder of iron metabolism and deposition, is due most commonly to mutations of the HFE gene and rarely the transferrin receptor gene. It most commonly affects the liver, pancreas, and heart, although seldom the heart in isolation. The most common cardiovascular complication is dilated cardiomyopathy. Cardiac hemochromatosis is not strictly an infiltrative disorder since iron is localized to the sarcoplasm and not the interstitium. Myocardial fibrosis is rare and hence LGE is not a common finding, but CMR is ideal for the evaluation and monitoring response to treatment using the T2* technique. Early diagnosis and treatment is essential since the relationship between cardiac iron load and function declines with more severe disease.[58]

SARCOIDOSIS

Sarcoidosis, a multisystem granulomatous disease of unknown etiology, can affect any organ in the body. It typically affects the lungs but can affect the heart in 5% to 7% of cases. In those with cardiac involvement, sarcoidosis accounts for over half of sudden deaths. It is accepted that the prognosis for patients with clinical cardiac sarcoidosis is poor.[59] The prevalence of cardiac involvement may in fact be considerably higher and, in numerous postmortem studies, cardiac involvement has been documented in 30% to 50% of cases.[60] The prognosis for sarcoidosis without cardiac involvement is favorable with the majority achieving remission within a few years. Myocardial involvement, however, is associated with a worse outcome and ventricular tachyarrhythmia is presumed to be the leading cause of death due to reentrant circuits caused by focal granulomatous infiltrates and replacement myocardial fibrosis.[61] Unfortunately in those with considerable cardiac involvement noted at postmortem, ECGs have been shown to be normal in 25% of cases during life. Furthermore, echocardiography imaging focused on regional wall thickening due to edema and granulomata infiltration or to thinning from fibrosis is likely to miss subtle changes. Nuclear T1 imaging can be performed to look for a phenomenon known as reverse distribution, although the spatial resolution is poor. Unfortunately, however, a normal T1 scan does not exclude the presence of cardiac sarcoid and an abnormal result provides no prognostic information.[62-65] In a recent study, half of the cases of confirmed cardiac sarcoid were not detected by single photon emission CT, but were all picked up by CMR.[66] CMR allows for detailed imaging of cardiac structure and function to accurately assess for regional wall thickening or wall motion abnormalities. The wide field of view means that mediastinal lymph nodes can be looked for and, if present, can assist in strengthening the diagnosis. Cardiac sarcoidosis has three successive histological stages: edema, noncaseating granulomatous infiltration, and patchy myocardial fibrosis. Each of these can be imaged successfully using specific CMR sequences. Granulomatous infiltrates are imaged using T2-weighted short tau inversion recovery imaging since such infiltrates tend to produce high signals because of their high water content resulting from myocardial edema.[67] Following intravenous gadolinium, these regions enhance further and both the pattern and location of LGE assist in strengthening the diagnosis and indeed may help guide clinicians in determining where to perform an endomyocardial biopsy, especially since the diagnostic accuracy of "blind" nontargeted biopsy is low (<20%) owing to the patchy nature of the disease.[68] While almost any pattern of LGE is seen in cardiac sarcoidosis, typical findings are patchy midwall and epicardial enhancement affecting the basal lateral walls (**Fig. 6**). CMR is able to demonstrate early signs of myocardial infiltration before more routine imaging modalities, such as scintigraphy or echocardiography, detect these changes. Spotting these early signs is important because early initiation of steroid therapy in this group can prevent ventricular remodeling and reduce the risk of ventricular tachyarrhythmias.[69,70] Smedema and colleagues[71] evaluated the incremental value of CMR to currently employed techniques to detect cardiac sarcoid involvement. Fifty-five patients with known pulmonary sarcoid were screened for cardiac involvement either routinely or because of cardiac symptoms. Twenty-three percent of the group were diagnosed with cardiac involvement using conventional tools, such as ECG, echocardiography, thallium scintigraphy, and Holter monitoring. LGE CMR, however, detected a further 11% of patients with cardiac involvement who were missed using conventional criteria, and the localization of myocardial inflammation and scar correlated well with regions identified at postmortem. Because CMR involves no ionizing radiation, serial studies to monitor results of therapeutic interventions are possible.[72]

AMYLOIDOSIS

Amyloidosis causes the deposition of fibrils composed of low–molecular-weight proteins in extracellular tissue. Perivascular and valvular tissues may also be involved. Deposition of these fibrils in the body is not uniform and depends on the fibril composition. The commonest amyloid subtype is primary amyloid (AL) and, although rare (<10 per million), cardiac involvement is common and can be severe.[73] Other forms of amyloid that involve the heart are rarer and include hereditary amyloid (*TTR* mutation) and senile systemic amyloid. Secondary amyloid almost never involves cardiac tissue.[74,75] Amyloid deposition can involve both the atrial and ventricular myocardium, leading to biatrial enlargement and typically a restrictive cardiomyopathy. Pericardial involvement is not uncommon in cardiac amyloid cases and can lead to pericardial effusion or tamponade. SCD is common in cardiac amyloid cases and thought principally to be secondary to complex ventricular arrhythmias. Studies have shown that these arrhythmias are seen in greater than 50% of cardiac amyloid cases and are associated with a worse prognosis.[76,77] The median survival of untreated amyloidosis with heart failure is less than 6 months. Chemotherapy with autologous stem cell replacement is associated with significant reversal of the clinical manifestations of AL amyloidosis but many do not survive the procedure and, for those patients with heart failure due to amyloid infiltration, the chances of surviving the procedure is even lower. Hence, many are deemed unsuitable. Thus, early detection of cardiac involvement is critical and may significantly improve clinical outcome. As highlighted earlier, amyloid infiltration in the heart typically leads to LV hypertrophy and may form part of a differential in the evaluation of a patient with suspected HCM, hypertensive heart disease, or diastolic heart failure with LV hypertrophy. The gold standard diagnostic tool for cardiac amyloidosis is endomyocardial biopsy, which is invasive, limited to more experienced centers, and not widely available. In the absence of other systemic features of amyloid, or when amyloid only forms part of the differential of a patient with LV hypertrophy, echocardiography is often used, but is limited in its ability to differentiate cardiac amyloidosis from other causes of restrictive

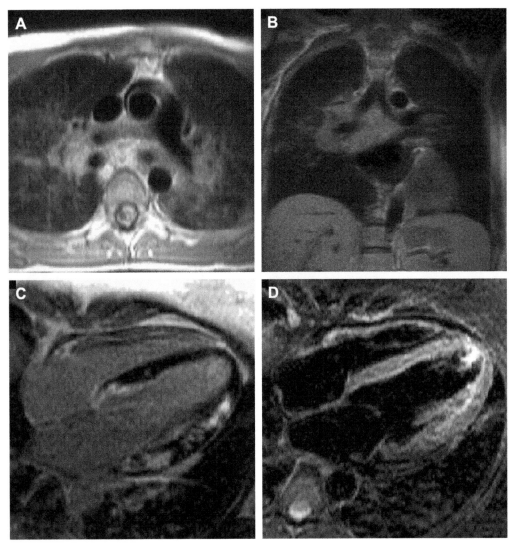

Fig. 6. Cardiac sarcoidosis. (*A* and *B*) Transaxial and coronal half-Fourier single-shot turbo spin-echo (HASTE) images demonstrating striking mediastinal lymphadenopathy. In the four-chamber images (*C* and *D*), patchy mid-wall LGE patterns are seen affecting the inferolateral wall at the base and apex (*C*). These regions correspond to areas of high short tau inversion recovery signal (STIR) (*D*), indicative of myocardial inflammation.

cardiomyopathy. The wide field of view that CMR provides allows imaging of the heart, lungs, pericardium, and extracardiac tissues in a single setting. The finding of a thick heart that thickens poorly in systole, along with pericardial and pleural effusions, often raises suspicions of the diagnosis early in the scan. In contrast to cardiac amyloidosis, where the ventricular contraction normal or reduced, in HCM the ventricular contraction is normal or reduced, in HCM the ventricular contraction is hyperdynamic, which is a useful feature in differentiation. Disease-specific patterns of LGE are seen. Amyloid fibrils preferentially deposit in the subendocardium and affect wash-in and wash-out gadolinium kinetics, which makes

setting the inversion time challenging. A dark blood pool, bright LV and RV subendocardium, and dark midmyocardium are typical findings, and have been described as the "zebra" pattern of enhancement (**Fig. 7**).[78] Other features characteristic of cardiac amyloidosis include a thickened interatrial septum and right atrial free wall hypertrophy. The LGE in amyloidosis is not representative of fibrosis but instead represents interstitial expansion by amyloid fibrils (protein). The localization of enhancement by CMR has also been shown useful in guiding endomyocardial biopsies.[79] These typical patterns of enhancement are not described in any other cardiomyopathic process and can be considered pathognomonic for cardiac

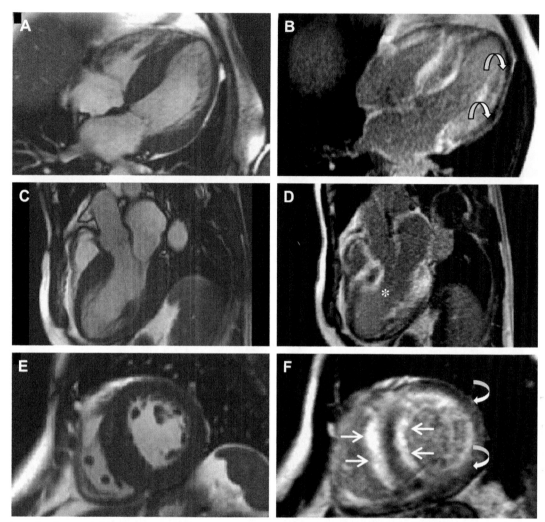

Fig. 7. Cardiac amyloidosis. Long- and short-axis cine images (*A*, *C*, and *E*) demonstrating asymmetrical wall thickening but poor systolic thickening. Following intravenous gadolinium, late imaging demonstrates characteristic low-intensity blood pool (*D, asterisk*) (LGE usually has high signal in the blood pool), and diffuse subendocardial enhancement in both LV and RV (*F, straight arrows*) with sparing of the epicardium and midwall (*zebra pattern indicated by curved arrows*).

amyloidosis. This typical pattern of LGE seen in amyloid is likely to reduce the need for endomyocardial biopsy because the subtype of amyloidosis can be determined by biopsy of extracardiac tissue. Atypical LGE patterns, although rare, are described in confirmed cardiac amyloid cases. LGE quantification in amyloid may also prove useful in the staging of disease and potentially for monitoring response to therapies over time, but further studies are required.

ENDOMYOCARDIAL FIBROSIS

Endomyocardial fibrosis can be classified as tropical, hypereosinophilia associated, or iatrogenic in origin. Tropical endomyocardial fibrosis is commonly seen in sub-Saharan African countries, India, and Brazil. It is the commonest restrictive cardiomyopathy worldwide and accounts for 20% of heart failure deaths in these regions. It was first described in 1948 in Uganda and may potentially cause as many heart failure deaths as those due to Chagas cardiomyopathy.[80] Typically, the heart is small with prominent fibrous thickening of both ventricles. Fibrotic plaques often involve the papillary muscles and apices, leading to apical thrombi, obliteration, and mitral and tricuspid valve regurgitation. Diagnosis with noninvasive imaging techniques is frequently challenging and RV biopsies are often required. CMR is a powerful and unrivaled tool for defining and localizing endomyocardial disease affecting the ventricular apices.

Early imaging following gadolinium administration is a highly accurate method of visualizing thrombus formation and late imaging detects regions of endomyocardial fibrosis and inflammation with proven histopathological correlation (**Fig. 8**).[81]

EOSINOPHILIA-ASSOCIATED CARDIOMYOPATHIES

A number of diseases are characterized by eosinophilia. These include the hypereosinophilic syndrome, Churg-Strauss syndrome (CSS), and the eosinophilic leukemias. They can manifest with a number of cardiac sequelae, which can often be difficult to differentiate using standard imaging modalities. Cardiac involvement occurs in more than 75% of patients with hypereosinophilic conditions, and the endocardium seems to be the region most at risk. The individual eosinophilic conditions shall be described individually.

Hypereosinophilic Syndrome

Idiopathic hypereosinophilic syndrome is a rare disorder characterized by persistent eosinophilia of more than 1.5×10^9/L for longer than 6 months with evidence of multiorgan dysfunction, including that of the heart.[82] Long-term hypereosinophilia not uncommonly leads to eosinophilic infiltration of the myocardium, typically at the apices, which can lead to acute necrosis, thrombus formation, and consequently diffuse apical fibrous thickening. This leads to a restrictive cardiomyopathy, and consequently atrial fibrillation, mural thrombi,

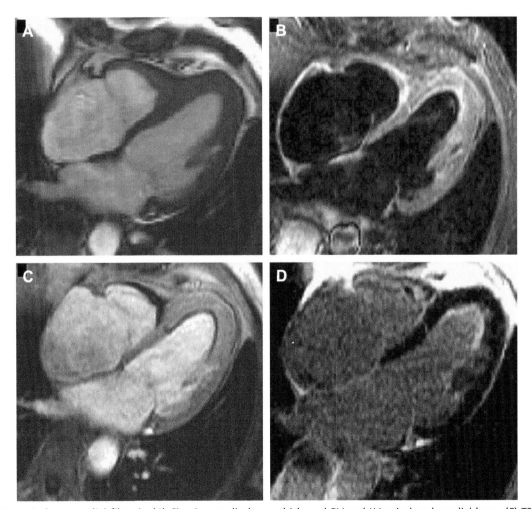

Fig. 8. Endomyocardial fibrosis. (*A*) Cine image displays a thickened RV and LV apical endocardial layer. (*B*) T2-weighted images demonstrate diffuse circumferential subendocardial layer of inflammation. (*C*) Early imaging following intravenous gadolinium demonstrates nonenhancing laminar thrombus. (*D*) Endocardial apical fibrosis seen on later imaging (LGE).

and death. Echocardiography is limited in its ability to visualize the LV and RV apices and fibrous thickening in these regions can often be missed, often necessitating the need for an endomyocardial RV biopsy. CMR is well suited for evaluating suspected hypereosinophilic syndrome because the apices are easily imaged for structure, wall thickness, and function. Early imaging following intravenous gadolinium is an extremely reliable and sensitive imaging tool for the presence or absence of atrial or ventricular thrombi. LGE images typically show diffuse endocardial enhancement of the apices leading to reduced ventricular chamber dimensions (see **Fig. 8**).

Churg-Strauss Syndrome

CSS is a rare systemic disorder characterized by asthma, transient pulmonary infiltrates, hypereosinophilia, and systemic vasculitis. It was first described in 1951 and its prevalence is estimated at 1 to 1.7 per 130,000, with an annual incidence of approximately 2.4 per million.[83] Although CSS has long been considered a rare disease, it is much more frequent in asthmatic patients (around 1:15,000), and may be associated with certain asthmatic medication used. Leukotriene receptor antagonists have recently been associated with the onset of CSS, but a causative role in the induction of the disease has not yet been demonstrated.[84,85] Onset usually occurs between 15 and 70 years of age and there are three distinct phases to the condition described. The first or prodromal phase is characterized by asthma with or without allergic rhinitis. Peripheral eosinophilia (typically >10%) then follows with eosinophilic tissue infiltration. The third, vasculitic phase may involve multiple organs, especially the skin, lungs, kidneys, and nervous system. Cardiac involvement in CSS is not infrequent (17%–92%) and is associated with a worse prognosis, accounting for approximately 50% of deaths.[86–92] Recognized manifestations include eosinophilic vasculitis, pericarditis, myocarditis, myocardial infarction, dilated cardiomyopathy, tamponade, mitral regurgitation, and SCD. CMR is well placed to clinically evaluate these potential cardiac consequences. Pericardial effusions, thickening, and inflammation are well visualized using standard cine imaging, T1- and T2-weighted turbo spin-echo images, and short tau inversion recovery imaging. LGE imaging also can help differentiate CSS and hypereosinophilic syndrome from other cardiomyopathies given the characteristic findings of diffuse enhancement of the subendocardium. CMR is well suited to identify less marked subendocardial thickening, which echocardiography is likely to miss. The noninvasive nature of CMR allows for accurate and reproducible follow-up of LV and RV volumes and function over time and to assess response to immunosuppressive therapies on cardiac function.[93]

CHAGAS DISEASE

Chagas disease is an inflammatory disease caused by the protozoan parasite *Trypanosoma cruzi*. It is the commonest cause of death in many Latin American countries, and over 200,000 new cases are reported each year.[94] An initial self-limiting illness occurs following infection, which lasts for 4 to 8 weeks. Through the development of immunity, the majority of cases are controlled. Persistent parasitemia can occur during latent infection and can lead to direct invasion of myocardial fibers during a latent phase, which can last for 10 to 20 years. Over this period, the inflammatory process may become progressive, resulting in a chronic disease characterized by prominent fibrosis, cardiac dysfunction, and a dilated cardiomyopathy. This progression can develop in up to 30% of individuals, and carries a 50% 5-year mortality. The LV wall typically thins, leading to apical aneurysm formation, which is a distinctive feature of the disease and is easily imaged with CMR. Rochitte and colleagues[95] imaged 51 patients with Chagas disease, and found that over two thirds of patients overall demonstrated LGE, typically in a distribution similar to that in viral myocarditis, involving the epicardial portion of the lateral LV wall (**Fig. 9**). The frequency that LGE was seen increased as the clinical cardiac spectrum of disease worsened, and was seen in all patients with Chagas heart disease and ventricular tachycardia. The pattern of LGE is in keeping with known histopathology that demonstrates inflammatory myocardial infiltrate in the absence of demonstrable parasites in the myocardium. Due to the scarcity of parasites in the myocardium, an autoimmune process is thought to be key in the development of Chagas heart disease.[96] An important predictor of survival in Chagas heart disease is RV function. CMR is the gold standard imaging modality for the LV apex and the RV. Thus, along with LGE imaging, CMR is ideal in the evaluation of these patients.[97]

GLYCOGEN STORAGE DISEASES

Glycogen storage disease is a group of inherited metabolic disorders characterized by abnormalities in the enzymes that regulate the synthesis or degradation of glycogen. Depending on the affected enzyme, 11 different types have been described so far. Among these, subtypes II, III,

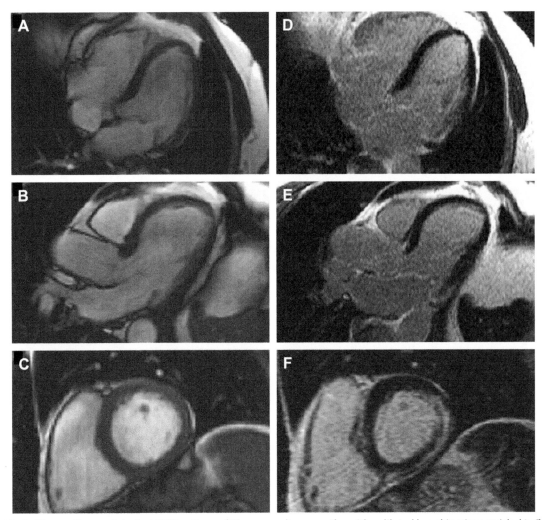

Fig. 9. Chagas disease. A typical CMR pattern of Chagas cardiomyopathy with a dilated hypokinetic ventricle (A–C) and epicardial LGE pattern on inferolateral walls (D–F) quite similar to the pattern seen in viral myocarditis.

and IV are known to affect the heart. Cardiac manifestations include severe LV hypertrophy, which may mimic HCM, and restrictive cardiomyopathy. In advanced stages, cavity dilatation occurs and dilated cardiomyopathy ensues. Though few reports in the literature describe the use of CMR in the assessment of glycogen storage disorders, CMR may aid in determining the etiology, especially in patients labeled as HCM.[98] In one study by Arad and colleagues,[99] the investigators identified glycogen storage disorders caused by *LAMP2* or *PRKAG2* mutations in 3 of 75 patients with HCM diagnosed by echocardiography. The onset of disease during adolescence is followed by a rapid progression toward end-stage heart failure early in adulthood, often resulting in death. Symptomatic treatment is required for the cardiac manifestations and patients may require a heart transplant. Patients are at risk of sudden death

due to arrhythmia during early adulthood. In patients with unexplained LV hypertrophy and ventricular preexcitation, glycogen storage cardiomyopathies due to *PRKAG2* or *LAMP2* mutations should be considered.[99–101]

FABRY DISEASE

Fabry disease is an X-linked inborn error of glycosphingolipid metabolism due to a deficient activity of alpha-galactosidase A, a lysosomal homodimeric enzyme. This leads to progressive intracellular accumulation of neutral glycosphingolipids, mainly globotriaosylceramide in hemizygous male and heterozygous female carriers. The major clinical manifestations in affected hemizygous males, with no detectable alpha-galactosidase A activity, are primarily due to a progressive small vessels disease pathology with angiokeratoma,

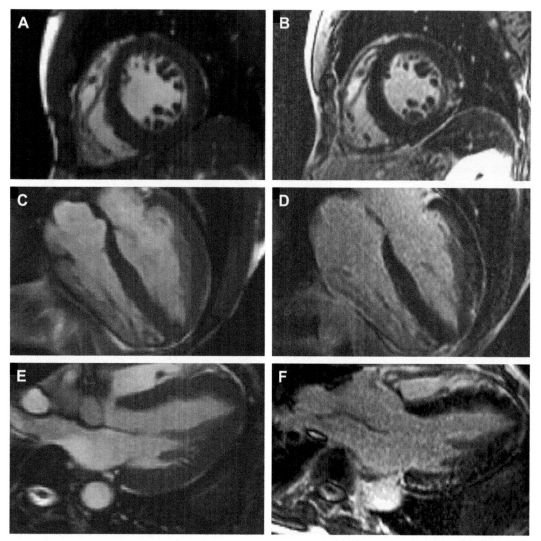

Fig. 10. Fabry disease. (*A, C,* and *E*) Marked increase in LV wall thickness, which can often be mistaken for HCM. (*B, D,* and *F*) LGE images demonstrate typical midwall fibrosis sparing the subendocardium in the basal inferolateral wall.

autonomic dysfunction, and lifelong pain. Renal failure and vasculopathy of the heart and brain are the primary causes of death, typically in early adulthood. Fabry disease may occasionally present with cardiac involvement as the primary feature, typically in individuals with partial enzyme activity. It is increasingly recognized as a cause of LV hypertrophy in middle-aged men, and can account for 6% of late-onset HCM.[102,103] CMR LGE has been shown to be a useful imaging modality in the evaluation of Fabry patients and, in over 50% of cases, LGE can be visualized in the basal inferolateral segments (**Fig. 10**). The pattern of LGE is different from that seen in HCM or hypertension and thus is a useful discriminating factor. LGE in these cases is thought to represent both sphingolipid accumulation and interstitial expansion due to myocardial fibrosis.[104,105] The presence of LGE may be an important marker of risk in these patients and also an important predictor of response to enzyme replacement therapy.[106,107] In a study by Beer and colleagues,[108] LGE was an important marker of impaired regional function that did not improve after 12 months of enzyme replacement therapy, whereas patients without LGE showed an improvement in regional function and a regression of LV hypertrophy with enzyme replacement.

SUMMARY

The evaluation of nonischemic cardiomyopathies is greatly improved with the use of CMR. More accurate identification of etiology, better monitoring of response to treatments, and improved risk stratification are all now possible in a single-scan setting without the need for ionizing radiation. Contrast agents used have an excellent safety profile and hence CMR is an ideal imaging modality to carry out follow-up imaging over time. Tissue characterization with gadolinium has expanded our understanding of these conditions and is likely to expand our understanding of genotype–phenotype correlations.

REFERENCES

1. Maron BJ. Hypertrophic cardiomyopathy: a systematic review. JAMA 2002;287:1308–20.
2. Marian AJ, Roberts R. Recent advances in the molecular genetics of hypertrophic cardiomyopathy. Circulation 1995;92:1336–47.
3. Roberts R, Sigwart U. New concepts in hypertrophic cardiomyopathy, part I. Circulation 2001;104:2113–6.
4. Maron BJ, McKenna WJ, Danielson GK, et al. ACC/ESC clinical expert consensus document on hypertrophic cardiomyopathy: a report of the American College of Cardiology Task Force on Clinical Expert Consensus Documents and the European Society of Cardiology Committee for Practice Guidelines (Committee to Develop an Expert Consensus Document on Hypertrophic Cardiomyopathy). J Am Coll Cardiol 2003;42:1687–713.
5. Seidman JG, Seidman CE. The genetic basis for cardiomyopathy: from mutation identification to mechanistic paradigms. Cell 2001;104:557–67.
6. Watkins H, McKenna WJ, Thierfelder L, et al. Mutations in the genes for cardiac troponin T and alpha-tropomyosin in hypertrophic cardiomyopathy. N Engl J Med 1995;332:1058–64.
7. Klues HG, Schiffers A, Maron BJ. Phenotypic spectrum and patterns of left ventricular hypertrophy in hypertrophic cardiomyopathy: morphologic observations and significance as assessed by two-dimensional echocardiography in 600 patients. J Am Coll Cardiol 1995;26:1699–708.
8. Rickers C, Wilke NM, Jerosch-Herold M, et al. Utility of cardiac magnetic resonance imaging in the diagnosis of hypertrophic cardiomyopathy. Circulation 2005;112:855–61.
9. Moon JCC, Fisher NG, McKenna WJ, et al. Detection of apical hypertrophic cardiomyopathy by cardiovascular magnetic resonance in patients with nondiagnostic echocardiography. Heart 2004;90:645–9.
10. Pennell DJ, Sechtem UP, Higgins CB, et al. Society for Cardiovascular Magnetic Resonance; Working Group on Cardiovascular Magnetic Resonance of the European Society of Cardiology. Clinical indications for cardiovascular magnetic resonance (CMR): Consensus Panel report. Eur Heart J 2004;25:1940–65.
11. Schulz-Menger J, Abdel-Aty H, Busjahn A, et al. Left ventricular outflow tract planimetry by cardiovascular magnetic resonance differentiates obstructive from non-obstructive hypertrophic cardiomyopathy. J Cardiovasc Magn Reson 2006;8:741–6.
12. Olivotto I, Maron MS, Autore C, et al. Assessment and significance of left ventricular mass by cardiovascular magnetic resonance in hypertrophic cardiomyopathy. J Am Coll Cardiol 2008;52:559–66.
13. Maron MS, Hauser TH, Dubrow E, et al. Right ventricular involvement in hypertrophic cardiomyopathy. Am J Cardiol 2007;100:1293–8.
14. Abdel-Aty H, Cocker M, Strohm O, et al. Abnormalities in T2-weighted cardiovascular magnetic resonance images of hypertrophic cardiomyopathy: regional distribution and relation to late gadolinium enhancement and severity of hypertrophy. J Magn Reson Imaging 2008;28:242–5.
15. Maron BJ, Shen WK, Link MS, et al. Efficacy of implantable cardioverter-defibrillators for the prevention of sudden death in patients with hypertrophic cardiomyopathy. N Engl J Med 2000;342:365–73.
16. Vassalli G, Seiler C, Hess OM. Risk stratification in hypertrophic cardiomyopathy. Curr Opin Cardiol 1994;9:330–6.
17. Spirito P, Bellone P, Harris KM, et al. Magnitude of left ventricular hypertrophy predicts the risk of sudden death in hypertrophic cardiomyopathy. N Engl J Med 2000;342:1778–85.
18. Elliott PM, Poloniecki J, Dickie S, et al. Sudden death in hypertrophic cardiomyopathy: identification of high risk patients. J Am Coll Cardiol 2000;36:2212–8.
19. Reynolds MR, Cohen DJ, Kugelmass AD, et al. The frequency and incremental cost of major complications among Medicare beneficiaries receiving implantable cardioverter-defibrillators. J Am Coll Cardiol 2006;47:2493–7.
20. Maron BJ, Spirito P, Shen W-K, et al. Implantable cardioverter-defibrillators and prevention of sudden cardiac death in hypertrophic cardiomyopathy. JAMA 2007;298:405–12.
21. Moon JC, McKenna WJ, McCrohan JA, et al. Toward clinical risk assessment in hypertrophic cardiomyopathy with gadolinium cardiovascular magnetic resonance. J Am Coll Cardiol 2003;41:1561–7.
22. Shirani J, Pick R, Roberts WC, et al. Morphology and significance of the left ventricular collagen network in young patients with hypertrophic cardiomyopathy and sudden cardiac death. J Am Coll Cardiol 2000;35:36–44.
23. Basso C, Thiene G, Corrado D, et al. Hypertrophic cardiomyopathy and sudden death in the young.

Pathologic evidence of myocardial ischemia. Hum Pathol 2000;31:988–98.

24. Varnava AM, Elliott PM, Sharma S, et al. Hypertrophic cardiomyopathy: the interrelation of disarray, fibrosis, and small vessel disease. Heart 2000;84: 476–82.

25. Choudhury L, Mahrholdt H, Wagner A, et al. Myocardial scarring in asymptomatic or mildly symptomatic patients with hypertrophic cardiomyopathy. J Am Coll Cardiol 2002;40:2156–64.

26. Kuribayashi T, Roberts WC. Myocardial disarray at junction of ventricular septum and left and right ventricular free walls in hypertrophic cardiomyopathy. Am J Cardiol 1992;70:1333–40.

27. Ursell PC, Gardner PI, Albala A, et al. Structural and electrophysiological changes in the epicardial border zone of canine myocardial infarcts during infarct healing. Circ Res 1985;56:436–51.

28. de Bakker JM, van Capelle FJ, Janse MJ, et al. Slow conduction in the infarcted human heart: "zigzag" course of activation. Circulation 1993;88: 915–26.

29. Kawara T, Derksen R, de Groot JR, et al. Activation delay after premature stimulation in chronically diseased human myocardium relates to the architecture of interstitial fibrosis. Circulation 2001;104: 3069–75.

30. Anyukhovsky EP, Sosunov EA, Plotnikov A, et al. Cellular electrophysiologic properties of old canine atria provide a substrate for arrhythmogenesis. Cardiovasc Res 2002;54:462–9.

31. St John Sutton MG, Lie JT, Anderson KR, et al. Histopathological specificity of hypertrophic obstructive cardiomyopathy. Myocardial fibre disarray and myocardial fibrosis. Br Heart J 1980; 44:433–43.

32. Adabag AS, Maron BJ, Applebaum E, et al. Occurence and frequency of arrhythmias in hypertrophic cardiomyopathy in relation to delayed enhancement on cardiovascular magnetic resonance. J Am Coll Cardiol 2008;51:1369–74.

33. Dimitrow PP, Klimeczek P, Vliegenthart R, et al. Late hyperenhancement in gadolinium-enhanced magnetic resonance imaging: comparison of hypertrophic cardiomyopathy with and without sustained ventricular tachycardia. Int J Cardiovasc Imaging 2008;24:77–83.

34. Kwon DH, Setser R, Popovic ZB, et al. Association of myocardial fibrosis, electrocardiography and ventricular tachyarrhythmia in hypertrophic cardiomyopathy: a delayed contrast enhanced MRI study. Int J Cardiovasc Imaging 2008;24: 617–25.

35. Harris KM, Spirito P, Maron MS, et al. Prevalence, clinical profile, and significance of left ventricular remodeling in the end-stage phase of hypertrophic cardiomyopathy. Circulation 2006;114:216–25.

36. Cecchi F, Olivotto I, Gistri R, et al. Coronary microvascular dysfunction and prognosis in hypertrophic cardiomyopathy. N Engl J Med 2003;349:1027–35.

37. Olivotto I, Cecci F, Gistri R, et al. Relevance of coronary microvascular flow impairment to long-term remodelling and systolic dysfunction in hypertrophic cardiomyopathy. J Am Coll Cardiol 2006;47: 1043–8.

38. Maron BJ, Wolfson JK, Epstein SE, et al. Intramural ("small vessel") coronary artery disease in hypertrophic cardiomyopathy. J Am Coll Cardiol 1986; 8:545–57.

39. Sipola P, Lauerma K, Husso-Saastamoinen M, et al. First-pass MR imaging in the assessment of perfusion impairment in patients with hypertrophic cardiomyopathy and the Asp175Asn mutation of the alpha-tropomyosin gene. Radiology 2002;226: 129–37.

40. Matsunaka T, Hamada M, Matsumoto Y, et al. First-pass myocardial perfusion and delayed contrast enhancement in hypertrophic cardiomyopathy assessed with MRI. Magn Reson Med Sci 2003;2: 61–9.

41. Knaapen P, van Dockum WG, Gotte MJW, et al. Regional heterogeneity of resting perfusion in hypertrophic cardiomyopathy is related to delayed contrast enhancement but not to systolic function: a PET and MRI study. J Nucl Cardiol 2006;13:660–7.

42. Petersen SE, Jerosch-Herold M, Hudsmith L, et al. Evidence for microvascular dysfunction in hypertrophic cardiomyopathy: new insights from multiparametric magnetic resonance imaging. Circulation 2007;115:2418–25.

43. Sotgia B, Sciagra R, Olivotto I, et al. Spatial relationship between coronary microvascular dysfunction and delayed contrast enhancement in patients with hypertrophic cardiomyopathy. J Nucl Med 2008;49:1090–6.

44. Tseng WI, Dou J, Reese TG, et al. Imaging myocardial fiber disarray and intramural strain hypokinesis in hypertrophic cardiomyopathy with MRI. J Magn Reson Imaging 2006;23:1–8.

45. Olivieri NF, Nathan DG, MacMillan JH, et al. Survival in medically treated patients with homozygous beta-thalassemia. N Engl J Med 1994;331: 574–8.

46. Borgna-Pignatti C, Rugolotto S, De Stefano P, et al. Survival and complications in patients with thalassemia major treated with transfusion and deferoxamine. Haematologica 2004;89:1187–93.

47. Modell B, Khan M, Darlison M. Survival in beta thalassaemia major in the UK: data from the UK Thalassaemia Register. Lancet 2000;355:2051–2.

48. Wacker PHD, Balmer-Ruedin D, Oberhansli I, et al. Regression of cardiac insufficiency after ambulatory intravenous deferoxamine in thalassaemia major. Chest 1993;103:1276–8.

49. Anderson LJ, Holden S, Davis B, et al. Cardiovascular T2-star (*) magnetic resonance for the early diagnosis of myocardial iron overload. Eur Heart J 2001;21:2171–9.

50. Tanner MA, Galanello R, Dessi C, et al. Myocardial iron loading in patients with thalassemia major on deferoxamine chelation. J Cardiovasc Magn Reson 2006;8:543–7.

51. Anderson LJ, Westwood MA, Holden S, et al. Myocardial iron clearance during reversal of siderotic cardiomyopathy with intravenous desferrioxamine: a prospective study using T2* cardiovascular magnetic resonance. Br J Haematol 2004;127:348–55.

52. Anderson LJ, Wonke B, Prescott E, et al. Comparison of effects of oral deferiprone and subcutaneous desferrioxamine on myocardial iron concentrations and ventricular function in beta-thalassemia. Lancet 2002;360:516–20.

53. Pennell DJ, Berdoukas V, Karagiorga M, et al. Randomised controlled trial of deferiprone or deferoxamine in beta-thalassemia major in patients with asymptomatic myocardial siderosis. Blood 2006; 107:3738–44.

54. Tanner MA, Galanello R, Dessi C, et al. A randomized, placebo-controlled, double-blind trial of the effect of combined therapy with deferoxamine and deferiprone on myocardial iron in thalassemia major using cardiovascular magnetic resonance. Circulation 2007;115:1876–84.

55. Tanner MA, Galanello R, Dess I, et al. Combined chelation therapy in thalassemia major for the treatment of severe myocardial siderosis with severe left ventricular dysfunction. J Cardiovasc Magn Reson 2008;10(1):12.

56. Modell B, Khan M, Darlison M, et al. Falling mortality and changing causes of death in thalassaemia major: data from the UK Thalassaemia Register and possible contribution from T2* cardiovascular magnetic resonance. J Cardiovasc Magn Reson 2008;10(1):42.

57. Telfer P, Coen PG, Christou S, et al. Survival of medically treated thalassemia patients in Cyprus. Trends and risk factors over the period 1980–2004. Haematologica 2006;91:1187–92.

58. Westra WH, Hruban RH, Baughman KL, et al. Progressive hemochromatosis cardiomyopathy despite reversal of iron deposition after liver transplantation. Am J Clin Pathol 1993;99: 39–44.

59. Roberts W, McAllister H, Ferrans V. Sarcoidosis of the heart: a clinicopathologic study of 35 necropsy patients (group 1) and review of 78 previously described necropsy patients (group II). Am J Med 1977;63:86–108.

60. Silverman K, Hutchins G, Bulkley B. Cardiac sarcoidosis: a clinico-pathological study of 84 in selected patients with systemic sarcoidosis. Circulation 1978;58:1204–11.

61. Ardehali H, Howard DL, Hariri A, et al. A positive endomyocardial biopsy result for sarcoid is associated with poor prognosis in patients with initially unexplained cardiomyopathy. Am Heart J 2005; 150:459–63.

62. Mana J. Nuclear imaging: 67 Gallium, 201 thallium, 18 F labeled fluoro-2 deoxy-D glucose position emission tomography. Clin Chest Med 1997;18: 799–811.

63. Kinney E, Caldwell J. Do thallium myocardial perfusion scan abnormalities predict survival in sarcoid patients without cardiac symptoms? Angiology 1990;41:573–6.

64. Hirose Y, Ishida Y, Hayashida K. Myocardial involvement in patients with sarcoidosis: an analysis of 75 patients. Clin Nucl Med 1994;19:522–6.

65. Bulkley BH, Rouleau JR, Whitaker JQ, et al. The use of 201thallium for myocardial perfusion imaging in sarcoid heart disease. Chest 1977;72:27–32.

66. Tadamura E, Yamamuro M, Kubo S, et al. Effectiveness of delayed enhanced MRI for identification of cardiac sarcoidosis: comparison with radionucleotide imaging. AJR Am J Roentgenol 2005;185:110–5.

67. Matsuki M, Matsuo M. MR findings of myocardial sarcoidosis. Clin Radiol 2000;55:323–5.

68. Iannuzzi MC, Rybicki BA, Teirstein AS. Sarcoidosis. N Engl J Med 2007;357:153–65.

69. Bargout R, Kelly RF. Sarcoid heart disease: clinical course and treatment. Int J Cardiol 2004;97: 173–82.

70. Vignaux O, Dhote R, Duboc D, et al. Clinical significance of myocardial magnetic resonance abnormalities in patients with sarcoidosis: a 1-year follow-up study. Chest 2002;122:1895–901.

71. Smedema JP, Snoep G, van Kroonenburgh. The additional value of gadolinium-enhanced MRI to standard assessment for cardiac involvement in patients with pulmonary sarcoidosis. Chest 2005; 128:1629–37.

72. Doherty MJ, Kishor Kumar S, Nicholson AA, et al. Cardiac sarcoidosis: the value of magnetic resonance imaging in diagnosis and assessment of response to treatment. Respir Med 1998;92: 697–9.

73. Shah KB, Inoue Y, Mehra MR. Amyloidosis and the heart: a comprehensive review. Arch Intern Med 2006;166:1805–13.

74. Dubrey SW, Cha K, Simms RW, et al. Electrocardiography and Doppler echocardiography in secondary (AA) amyloidosis. Am J Cardiol 1996; 77:313–5.

75. Falk RH. Diagnosis and management of the cardiac amyloidoses. Circulation 2005;112:2047–60.

76. Falk RH, Rubinow A, Cohen AS. Cardiac arrhythmias in systemic amyloidosis: correlation with

echocardiographic abnormalities. J Am Coll Cardiol 1984;3:107–13.

77. Palladini G, Malamani G, Co F, et al. Holter monitoring in AL amyloidosis: prognostic implications. Pacing Clin Electrophysiol 2001;24:1228–33.

78. Maceira AM, Joshi J, Prasad SK, et al. Cardiovascular magnetic resonance in cardiac amyloidosis. Circulation 2005;111:186–93.

79. Vogelsberg H, Mahrholdt H, Deluigi CC, et al. Cardiovascular magnetic resonance in clinically suspected cardiac amyloidosis: noninvasive imaging compared to endomyocardial biopsy. J Am Coll Cardiol 2008;51:1022–30.

80. Davies JNP. Endomyocardial fibrosis in Uganda. East Afr Med J 1948;25:10–6.

81. Cury RC, Abbara S, Sandoval LJ, et al. Visualisation of endomyocardial fibrosis by delayed enhancement magnetic resonance imaging. Circulation 2005;111:e115–7.

82. Katz HT, Haque SJ, Hsieh FH. Pediatric hypereosinophilic syndrome (HES) differs from adult HES. J Pediatr 2005;46:134–6.

83. Churg J, Strauss L. Allergic granulomatosis, allergic angiitis, and periarteritis nodosa. Am J Pathol 1951;27:277–94.

84. Tuggey JM, Hosker HS. Churg-Strauss syndrome associated with montelukast therapy. Thorax 2000;55:805–6.

85. Martin RM, Wilton LV, Mann RD. Prevalence of Churg-Strauss syndrome, vasculitis, eosinophilia, and associated conditions: retrospective analysis of 58 prescription-event monitoring cohort studies. Pharmacoepidemiol Drug Saf 1999;8: 179–89.

86. Val-Bernal JF, Mayorga M, Garcia-Alberdi E, et al. Churg-Strauss syndrome and sudden cardiac death. Cardiovasc Pathol 2003;12:94–7.

87. Hellemans S, Dens J, Knockaert D. Coronary involvement in the Churg-Strauss syndrome. Heart 1997;77:576–8.

88. Abu-Shakra M, Smythe H, Lewtas J, et al. Outcome of polyarteritis nodosa and Churg-Strauss syndrome. An analysis of twenty-five patients. Arthritis Rheum 1994;37:1798–803.

89. Guillevin L, Cohen P, Gayraud M, et al. Churg-Strauss syndrome. Clinical study and long term follow-up of 96 patients. Medicine 1999;78: 26–37.

90. Lanham JG, Elkon KB, Pusey CD, et al. Systemic vasculitis with asthma and eosinophilia: a clinical approach to the Churg-Strauss syndrome. Medicine 1984;63:65–81.

91. Guillevin L, Pagnoux C, Mouthon L. Churg-Strauss syndrome. Semin Respir Crit Care Med 2004;25: 535–45.

92. Pela G, Tirabassi G, Pattoneri P, et al. Cardiac involvement in the Churg-Strauss syndrome. Am J Cardiol 2006;97:1519–24.

93. Rosenberg M, Lorenz HM, Gassler N, et al. Rapid progressive eosinophilic cardiomyopathy in a patient with Churg-Strauss syndrome (CSS). Clin Res Cardiol 2006;95:289–94.

94. World Health Organization. Control of Chagas disease. World Health Organ Tech Rep Ser 1991;81: 27–31.

95. Rochitte CE, Oliviera PF, Andrade JM. Myocardial delayed enhancement by magnetic resonance imaging in patients with Chagas' disease: a marker of disease severity. J Am Coll Cardiol 2005;46(1): 553–8.

96. Marin-Neto JA, Cunha-Neto E, Maciel BC, et al. Pathogenesis of chronic Chagas heart disease. Circulation 2007;115:1109–23.

97. Nunes MP, Rocha MOC, Ribeiro ALP, et al. Right ventricular dysfunction is an independent predictor of survival in patients with dilated chronic Chagas' cardiomyopathy. Int J Cardiol 2008;127:372–9.

98. Moon JC, Mundy HR, Lee PJ, et al. Myocardial fibrosis in glycogen storage disease type III. Circulation 2003;107:e47.

99. Arad M, Woodrow Benson D, Perez-Atayade AR, et al. Constitutively active AMP-kinase mutations cause glycogen storage disease mimicking hypertrophic cardiomyopathy. J Clin Invest 2002;109: 357–62.

100. Arad M, Maron BJ, Gorham JM, et al. Glycogen storage diseases presenting as hypertrophic cardiomyopathy. N Engl J Med 2005;352:362–72.

101. Laforet P, Richard P, Said MA, et al. A new mutation in PRKAG2 gene causing hypertrophic cardiomyopathy with conduction system disease and muscular glycogenosis. Neuromuscul Disord 2006;16:178–82.

102. Nakao S, Takenaka T, Maeda M, et al. An atypical variant of Fabry's disease in men with left ventricular hypertrophy. N Engl J Med 1995;333:288–93.

103. Sachdev B, Takenaka T, Teraguchi H. Prevalence of Anderson-Fabry disease in male patients with late onset hypertrophic cardiomyopathy. Circulation 2002;105:1407–11.

104. Moon JC, Sachdev B, Elkington AG, et al. Gadolinium enhanced cardiovascular magnetic resonance in Anderson-Fabry disease. Evidence for a disease specific abnormality of the myocardial interstitium. Eur Heart J 2003;23:2151–5.

105. Takenaka T, Teraguchi H, Yoshida A, et al. Terminal stage cardiac findings in patients with cardiac Fabry disease: an electrocardiographic, echocardiographic, and autopsy study. J Cardiol 2008;51: 50–9.

106. Teraguchi H, Takenaka T, Yoshida A, et al. End-stage cardiac manifestations and autopsy findings in patients with cardiac Fabry disease. J Cardiol 2004;43:98–9.

107. Hughes DA, Elliott PM, Shah J, et al. Effects of enzyme replacement therapy on the cardiomyopathy of Anderson-Fabry disease: a randomised, double blind, placebo-controlled clinical trial of agalsidase alfa. Heart 2008;94:153–8.

108. Beer M, Weidemann F, Breunig F, et al. Impact of enzyme replacement therapy on cardiac morphology and function and late enhancement in Fabry's cardiomyopathy. Am J Cardiol 2006;97:1515–8.

Valvular and Hemodynamic Assessment with CMR

Saul G. Myerson, MD, MRCP*

KEYWORDS

- Cardiovascular magnetic resonance
- Valve disease • Hemodynamic assessment
- Flow quantification • Cardiac anatomy

The unique capabilities of CMR are well suited to the assessment of valvular function and hemodynamics of the heart. In particular, the combination of several techniques (anatomic and functional imaging, flow quantification, and angiography) allows a full assessment that would not be possible with only one or two components of the study. The ability to image all areas of the heart and surrounding vessels allows the identification of narrow pathways, conduits, and shunts that can be difficult or impossible to visualize by other means, and their hemodynamic impact on the heart can be assessed. Clear views of outflow tracts can be obtained, even in complex congenital conditions, along with valvular anatomy (including orifice area by direct planimetry rather than calculation) and assessment of anomalous vessel positions that may be important (eg, drainage of the pulmonary veins in cases of suspected sinus venosus atrial septal defects).

The section on hemodynamic assessment includes flow and its relationship to function but excludes left and right ventricular contractility and diastolic function assessment because they are dealt with in the article by Grothues and colleagues, elsewhere in this issue.

ADVANTAGES OF CARDIOVASCULAR MAGNETIC RESONANCE
Accurate and Reproducible Volumes, Function, and Mass

Precise measurements of left ventricular (LV) and right ventricular (RV) volumes, function, and mass are vital for assessing the impact of valvular and hemodynamic lesions on both ventricles, which can ultimately lead to ventricular failure if the impact is great. Cardiovascular magnetic resonance (CMR) is the most accurate and reproducible technique for assessing ventricular volumes and mass,[1–3] and RV volumes are difficult to achieve by other methods. Additional insights into the effect of valve disease on the myocardium may also be gained, for example, by accurately measuring LV mass in patients with aortic stenosis, rather than relying on wall thickness. Reproducibility is important for serial assessment, because valvular and other hemodynamic lesions are often present for many years or even decades before cardiac deterioration or symptoms are present, and long-term follow up is important. By its very nature as a three-dimensional technique, CMR is more sensitive to changes in volume or mass than a unidimensional technique (eg, left ventricular diameter). The latter is also more prone to measurement error because the exact position for measurement has the potential to vary, despite guidelines which aim to standardize the measurement.[4] Precise measurements of LV or RV function are also required for the quantification of certain valve lesions (eg, mitral or tricuspid regurgitation), in conjunction with flow measurement (see later discussion). Accurate stroke volumes also can be used to quantify isolated valve regurgitation without flow data.[5]

Flow Quantification

The ability to measure flow through an image slice[6] is a major advantage of CMR and a crucial

University of Oxford, Oxford, UK
* Department of Cardiovascular Medicine, University of Oxford, John Radcliffe Hospital, Headley Way, Oxford OX3 9DU.
E-mail address: saul.myerson@cardiov.ox.ac.uk

Heart Failure Clin 5 (2009) 389–400
doi:10.1016/j.hfc.2009.02.004

aspect of hemodynamic assessment. Whether quantifying the degree of valve regurgitation or the pulmonary/systemic shunt ratio or determining relative flow in vessels, the facility to actually measure flow rather than calculate it from complex equations is a feature unique to CMR.

The measurement of flow is based on a phenomenon of MR. Standard MRI uses the hydrogen nuclei in water molecules, which are placed in a higher energy state than at baseline by the delivery of energy in the form of radiowaves. As they return to their baseline (lower) energy state, they emit a radiofrequency signal that is picked up and turned into an image. This signal, in common with all radiofrequency waves, has a phase and amplitude. If the water molecules are moving through a magnetic field gradient (eg, blood flowing along a vessel inside an MR scanner), the phase of the emitted signal changes. The faster the water is moving, the greater the change in phase (phase shift) of the signal, and this relationship is linear. By measuring the phase shift, the velocity of flowing blood in the selected imaging plane can be measured. The velocity of blood can be measured in line with the image plane (in-plane velocity measurement) or in blood flowing through the plane (through-plane velocity measurement). Flow can be derived from through-plane velocity mapping by measuring the velocity in each voxel in a selected area (eg, the ascending aorta) and integrating these over a time period (eg, one cardiac cycle) to obtain flow.[7] The measurement of flow is normally synchronized to the electrocardiogram, and the formulas for calculating flow are usually built into the cardiac software distributed with each scanner.

The accuracy of flow measurement is excellent for in vitro studies and it correlates well with invasive in vivo measurements.[8–11] In vivo studies are hampered, however, by the lack of a true gold standard technique for comparison; invasive measures of flow rely on complex calculations and assumptions that may not hold true in all cases. Temporal resolution is typically 25 to 45 msec, which is lower than for continuous wave Doppler velocity measurements in echocardiography but is good enough for most flow and velocity measurements. The measurement of peak velocity in a stenotic lesion may be slightly underestimated, however, because of the lower temporal resolution. Flow quantification relies on a homogenous magnetic field and laminar flow in a vessel. Complex (non-laminar) flow patterns, such as turbulent or high-velocity jets distal to a stenosis, can give rise to additional phase shifts that reduce the accuracy

of the measurement.[12] These errors are only significant however above velocities of 3.5 to 4 m/s.[11,13] Using sequences with a short echo-time (approximately 2 msec) can reduce these errors[13] and future applications may use these ultra-short echo time sequences. To achieve the most homogenous magnetic field, the image slice should be at the center of the magnet, and some modern scanners automatically position the patient for flow sequences to achieve this. Errors in velocity (and flow) measurement also can occur because of partial volume effects, in which several velocities occur within a single voxel and an averaged phase shift is measured.[12] In practice, through-plane flow mapping typically has an in-plane resolution of approximately 1 mm, and with thin imaging slices (typically 5–7 mm), partial volume errors are only really a problem for narrow flow jets (eg, tight aortic stenosis).

Advanced in-plane flow sequences can measure velocity in three dimensions, with all three directions measured simultaneously.[14,15] This allows complex flow patterns to be assessed, and future work may examine the use of this technique for clinical work.

Noninvasive Technique Without Ionizing Radiation

The need for multiple serial measurements in valve disease and other conditions that require hemodynamic assessment heightens the need for a safe, noninvasive technique. CMR has both of these features in addition to accurate and reproducible measurements and is well placed for the serial assessment of patients. There are also no reported adverse effects of CMR during pregnancy, either for the mother or fetus, although data in this area are scarce. Young women can have important valve disease diagnosed for the first time when pregnant, and increasing numbers of women with congenital heart disease survive to child-bearing age. When important hemodynamic information is required during pregnancy (eg, severity of a valve lesion or coarctation, RV function), CMR is able to provide it, although echocardiography remains the first-line investigation.

DIFFICULT AREAS
Arrhythmias

The main problematic area with CMR assessment of valve disease and hemodynamics is irregular cardiac rhythms. Cine image quality can be reduced, affecting the assessment of ventricular function, although the effect on this is usually small. The accuracy of flow measurement also can be reduced because flow sequences are acquired over several cardiac cycles (typically 10–12), with data acquired in a complex manner and reconstructed based on the assumption of a regular rhythm. In patients with an irregular rhythm, the complexity of the data acquisition means that although acquired over several cardiac cycles, the flow is not averaged over these, as might be expected.

Where the beat-to-beat variability is small (eg, atrial fibrillation with a controlled rate), these errors are usually not clinically significant. Irregular rhythms (uncontrolled atrial fibrillation, multiple ventricular ectopics) can present a challenge, particularly to acquiring accurate flow data. Intelligent planning of the timing of data acquisition to the electrocardiogram can offset some of the problems, but some patients still present a challenge and caution should be exercised in interpreting the flow data in these. Cine imaging is more reliable because it is more amenable to intelligent electrocardiogram gating and is less affected by arrhythmias, particularly during systole. Newer electrocardiogram gating techniques are specifically designed to cope with arrhythmias for cine sequences but have yet to be developed for flow imaging. Ventricular volumes vary with differing heart rates because of differential filling; these physiologic changes do still occur and result in slight blurring of the myocardial borders. The result is an approximate averaging of the volumes over the several cardiac cycles of image acquisition, which is usually acceptable.

Younger Children

Smaller children present particular challenges for hemodynamic assessment with CMR. First, the MR environment can be frightening, and general anesthesia may be required to facilitate a scan, which is a significant undertaking for the patient and medical staff. In practice, older children (from approximately the age of 6 to 8 years) often can be imaged successfully without anesthesia or sedation if appropriate communication and reassurance are provided, sometimes with the help of the parents. The second challenge is the small size of the patient; imaging small structures can be difficult, and increasing the image resolution results in a decrease in MR signal from the smaller voxels, with reduced image quality. This is further compounded by the limited ability to breath-hold and the lower reproducibility of the breath-holding position in conscious subjects. Ultra-fast sequences using the latest parallel acquisition techniques are often used, and flow can be quantified using non–breath-holding

techniques. Image slice thickness is reduced, but only to 4 to 5 mm to balance the reduced signal to noise ratio that results from this.

INDIVIDUAL VALVE LESIONS
Aortic Stenosis

CMR aids the assessment of aortic stenosis through accurate assessment of the anatomy of the valve and aortic root, measurement of the velocity of the stenotic jet, and quantification of LV mass and function to indicate the precise effect on the LV. The aortic root is often angulated, which can make assessment with echocardiography difficult. In particular, aligning a continuous wave Doppler beam with the direction of the stenotic jet may prove impossible to achieve. With the free choice of imaging planes available in CMR, visualizing the valve and root and measuring the velocity are straightforward. Good visualization of the anatomy is complemented by accurate quantitation of the severity of aortic stenosis.[16]

First, direct planimetry of the aortic valve orifice is feasible by placing the imaging plane through the valve tips in systole (Fig. 1). This technique agrees well with aortic valve area measured directly by transoesophageal echocardiography[17,18] and with estimated valve area from the continuity equation.[17,18] Second, peak transvalvar velocity can be measured by the velocity mapping technique described earlier.[19,20] The optimal assessment involves initially the in-plane flow in the outflow tract to identify the location of maximal velocity (usually just distal to the valve tips), followed by through-plane flow in a plane perpendicular to the direction of flow and positioned at the identified location of maximal velocity (see Fig. 1). This minimizes the partial volume effects while ensuring that peak velocity is measured, and mean velocity can be assessed from the through-plane flow measurements. Ensuring the correct slice position for flow measurement is important for accuracy; although this image appears similar to the one through the valve tips, the position of maximal velocity (the vena contracta) may lie a few millimeters distal to the valve tips, so the images may not be in identical locations.

CMR has a lower temporal resolution than echocardiography, however (typically 20–25 msec versus approximately 2 msec for continuous wave Doppler), which can result in a slight underestimation of the peak velocity if the true peak is missed. The complex flow patterns and small jet width of high-velocity jets also can reduce the accuracy of velocity mapping (as described previously). For these reasons, direct planimetry of the

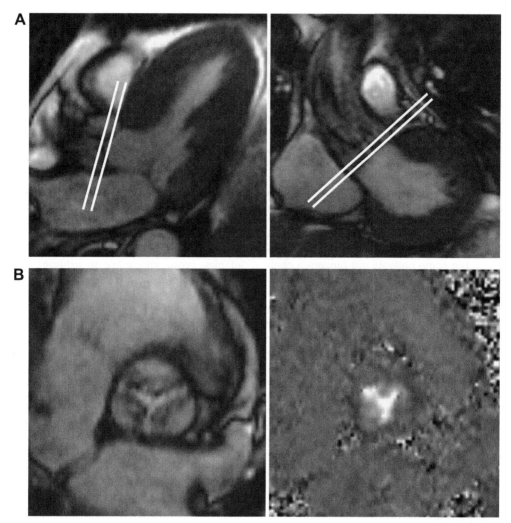

Fig. 1. (*A*) Aortic stenosis. Positioning of image slice through the valve tips in systole to obtain en-face view of aortic valve. (*Left*) Standard left ventricular outflow tract view. (*Right*) Coronal LV outflow tract view (perpendicular to the first view); parallel lines indicate the position of the image slice. Images are still frames from a steady-state free precession cine sequence. (*B*) Resulting view of aortic valve (*left*) demonstrating severe aortic stenosis, and corresponding through-plane flow image (*right*) demonstrating high velocity flow toward the aorta (in *white*). Mid-gray areas on the flow image represent tissue with little or no motion; the black/white speckled areas represent background noise from the lung fields caused by negligible signal from this tissue.

valve orifice area may be a more reliable assessment of aortic stenosis with CMR.

Other advantages in aortic stenosis include the ability to differentiate subvalvar from supravalvar stenosis, which are easily visualized on CMR, and the site of velocity acceleration can be accurately located with in-plane velocity mapping. The ascending aorta may be dilated, particularly with bicuspid aortic valves, and CMR can accurately assess the diameter of any dilation. Finally, highly accurate LV mass measurement provides a more precise and sensitive measure of the effect

of the stenosis on the LV than measuring myocardial wall thickness.

Aortic Regurgitation

Aortic regurgitation is difficult to quantify with echocardiography, which mostly relies on qualitative and semi-quantitative measures of severity. CMR can accurately quantify the amount of regurgitation using flow mapping, and derived values such as regurgitant fraction (regurgitant volume/ forward volume × 100%) can be obtained. This is achieved by placing an imaging slice for flow mapping in the aorta, just above the aortic valve, and measuring both the forward and regurgitant flow per cardiac cycle.[10,21,22] Positioning the imaging slice as close to the valve as possible is important (**Fig. 2**), despite the higher and more turbulent velocities encountered here, because underestimation of the regurgitation can occur otherwise.[8] Underestimation is caused by several factors, including the apical movement of the valve during systole, which allows blood to flow into the gap between the imaging plane and the valve, which may then return to the ventricle during diastole and not flow through the imaging plane. Aortic distension during systole exacerbates this, and coronary flow can reduce the accuracy of measurement if the imaging plane is above the coronary ostia. An ideal flow sequence would incorporate slice tracking to minimize these errors, which tracks the aortic valve and moves the imaging slice accordingly, but this procedure involves complex software programming and has only been developed at a single center so far.[23]

The accuracy of aortic regurgitation quantification by CMR is excellent when compared with in vitro studies[24] or in vivo volumetric CMR measurement,[10] and it correlates well with angiographic or echocardiographic grades of severity.[8,10,22] Because it remains the only technique capable of true in vivo quantification of aortic regurgitation, there is no other technique to compare it to for in vivo accuracy. Reproducibility is also good for interstudy and intra- and interobserver comparisons.[21,22]

Further studies are required to determine which quantitative thresholds are clinically meaningful, but one echocardiographic study of aortic regurgitation quantification (using a highly derived and less accurate measure) showed aortic regurgitation quantification provided good prediction of clinical outcomes.[25] Accurate LV volumes with CMR can also aid clinical assessment of the impact of the regurgitation, and a detailed assessment of aortic root anatomy can assist in identifying the cause of the regurgitation and whether the root needs replacing at the time of valve replacement surgery.

Mitral Regurgitation

CMR can quantify mitral regurgitation, although direct measurement using flow mapping at the mitral annulus is difficult because of the highly mobile valve and the high frequency of atrial fibrillation affecting flow accuracy. Consequently, quantification is usually performed indirectly either by measuring the difference in ventricular stroke volumes (which assumes a single valve lesion) or by subtracting aortic systolic flow (measured by aortic flow mapping) from LV stroke volume.[16] This latter technique is not affected by right-sided valve lesions but is still subject to inaccuracies in flow if atrial fibrillation is present. The quantification of mitral regurgitation correlates well with echocardiographic and angiographic assessment and has good reproducibility.[26–28] Studies are required to determine the clinical use of mitral regurgitation quantification with CMR, but one echocardiographic study using the proximal isovolumetric surface area technique for estimating mitral regurgitant orifice area showed good correlation with clinical outcome.[29]

CMR also can assess leaflet morphology and function of the individual scallops and identify the site of localized prolapse/regurgitation.[30] Multiple contiguous cine images perpendicular to the mitral valve plane provide the anatomic detail, and this technique has good agreement with transesophageal echocardiography for assessing mitral valves for repair.[30] Although transesophageal echocardiography is likely to remain first line for leaflet assessment, CMR could be used if the transesophageal echocardiography was not possible. Direct measurement of the regurgitant orifice area is also possible using this technique, although it is perhaps less useful than accurate quantification of the regurgitation.

Mitral Stenosis

Echocardiography, particularly transesophageal echocardiography, remains the first-line technique for assessing mitral stenosis because of its excellent visualization of the mitral leaflets. CMR can be

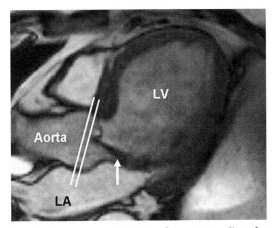

Fig. 2. Aortic regurgitation. The image slice for through-plane flow measurement is positioned just above the aortic valve (*parallel lines*) to measure flow in the regurgitant jet (*arrow*). LA, left atrium; LV, left ventricle.

helpful in selected cases, however, with good visualization of the restricted mitral leaflets and direct measurement of the orifice area in much the same way as for aortic stenosis, by placing an imaging plane at the mitral valve tips during systole (**Fig. 3**). Care needs to be taken to position the plane at the tips to obtain an accurate valve area, as is required for echocardiographic assessment. Diastolic flow and velocity can be measured, although the frequency of atrial fibrillation in severe cases reduces the accuracy.

Pulmonary Stenosis

CMR provides excellent visualization of the RV outflow tract and can identify the site and severity of pulmonary stenosis (**Fig. 4**). Assessment is similar to aortic stenosis, with direct planimetry of the valve orifice and measurement of peak velocity, with through-plane velocity mapping preferred for velocity measurements. Identifying subvalvar and supravalvar stenosis is also straightforward, and RV mass and function can be assessed to determine the effect on the RV.

Pulmonary Regurgitation

Pulmonary regurgitation is an increasingly recognized cause of long-term RV dysfunction.[31,32] Particular patients at risk are individuals with repaired tetralogy of Fallot, who commonly have a significant degree of pulmonary regurgitation,[32–34] and patients who have undergone valvuloplasty for congenital pulmonary stenosis. Identifying patients at risk for heart failure has been problematic in the past, but the accurate assessment of quantity of regurgitation and RV volumes/function with CMR has revolutionized this area.[35]

In a similar way to aortic regurgitation, pulmonary regurgitation can be quantified accurately rather than graded from mild to severe. The superb visualization of the RV outflow tract allows accurate placement of an image slice for through-plane flow mapping. This method of quantification compares well to assessment by comparison of ventricular stroke volumes[34] and correlates with echocardiographic parameters.[36] Accurate measurement of RV volumes and function with CMR are as important as assessment of the valve dysfunction and can guide the timing of valve replacement,[32,37] although the optimal thresholds for recommending valve replacement have yet to be determined. With the emergence of CMR, studies to assess the clinical use of these measurements and the optimal thresholds for intervention are ongoing.

Using CMR, the improvements in valvular function and RV volumes and function after valve replacement have been documented.[35] Percutaneous stent valves for pulmonary valve replacement have increased the number of patients likely to benefit, and the use of CMR is likely to increase as a result. Despite the metal content of the stents, follow-up flow imaging can still occur above and below the stent, and some newer nitinol stents can allow flow assessment within the stent.[38]

Percutaneous Pulmonary Valve Replacement

Percutaneous pulmonary valve replacement using a stent valve is increasing in popularity, and accurate sizing and anatomy of the pulmonary outflow tract are important to facilitate this.[39,40] CMR provides the required detail and accurate

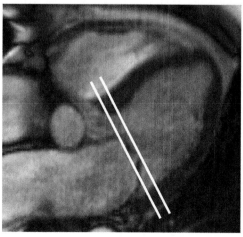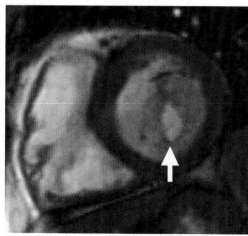

Fig. 3. Mitral stenosis. Positioning of the image slice at the mitral tips in systole (*left*) and resultant view of the mitral orifice (*right, arrow*).

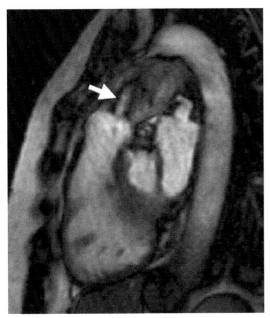

Fig. 4. Pulmonary stenosis. Right ventricular outflow tract view shows the high velocity jet of pulmonary stenosis (*arrow*).

assessment of the valve lesion itself and is invaluable in the assessment of patients for this procedure.[39] It is likely to become the dominant form of pulmonary valve replacement in the future, particularly for patients with multiple previous cardiac operations.

Tricuspid Regurgitation

Severe tricuspid regurgitation can result in significant symptoms of right heart failure. Quantifying RV volumes and function, and the tricuspid regurgitation itself, can be valuable in patient assessment and are feasible with CMR.[41] Pulmonary flow measurement (as used for pulmonary regurgitation) can be combined with RV stroke volume to calculate the quantity of tricuspid regurgitation (RV stroke volume – pulmonary forward flow) and the regurgitant fraction (TR/RV stroke volume × 100%), in much the same way as for mitral regurgitation. The same limitations apply, with the importance of locating the flow imaging slice close to the magnet isocenter and the reduced accuracy of irregular rhythms. It also can be assessed by the difference in ventricular stroke volumes if only a single valve leak is present.[42]

Patients with abnormal placement of the tricuspid valve (eg, Ebstein's anomaly) often present a challenge for assessing true RV volumes and function and the extent of tricuspid regurgitation. Combined with good processing software

that allows identification of the valve position in calculating RV volumes, however, CMR can produce accurate assessments and aid management.[43,44]

Tricuspid Stenosis

Although rare and not routinely assessed with CMR, this valve lesion can be examined when required. Valve area can be measured by placement of an image slice through the valve tips in diastole, as for mitral stenosis, and forward velocity through the valve can be measured, although this parameter is perhaps less useful.

Multiple Valve Lesions

The CMR techniques can be used to assess patients with multiple valve lesions and obtain a detailed assessment of the severity of each component. Assessing the degree of stenosis or quantifying regurgitation can be undertaken, whether they occur in the same valve (ie, mixed valve disease) or in different valves. For example, a patient with mixed aortic and mixed mitral valve disease can have the area of each valve measured with cine imaging at the appropriate time in the cardiac cycle to assess stenosis, the aortic regurgitation quantified from the diastolic (regurgitant) flow above the aortic valve, and the mitral regurgitation quantified by subtracting the systolic (forward) flow above the aortic valve from the LV stroke volume. In this way, a comprehensive assessment can be undertaken.

Prosthetic Valves

Despite perceptions to the contrary, most metallic prosthetic heart valves are safe in the MR scanner at 1.5 and 3 T.[45,46] The forces exerted on the valves by the scanner are negligible when compared with those that occur with each heartbeat. More than merely safe, prosthetic heart valves can be assessed using CMR, including flow patterns and local anatomy.[47,48] The artifact produced is small, and as long as this is avoided when placing an imaging plane for through-plane flow imaging, satisfactory results can be obtained (**Fig. 5**). Newer valve types, such as the bileaflet tilting disc, have a smaller artifact area than older ball-and-cage valves, although some bioprosthetic valves have significant amounts of metal in the frame, which can have a larger artifact. All are suitable for CMR assessment.

HEMODYNAMIC ASSESSMENT

The key aspects of CMR that enable the evaluation of valvular disease—free choice of imaging planes,

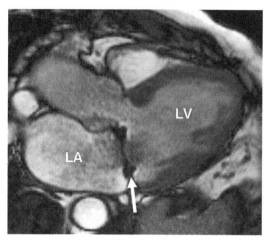

Fig. 5. Prosthetic mitral valve (bileaflet tilting disc type) demonstrates the small artifact area. LA, left atrium; LV, left ventricle.

accurate ventricular volumes (including stroke volume), and quantification of flow through a vessel—are also crucial to other areas of hemo-dynamic assessment. The ability to measure the output from each ventricle and quantify flow in selected vessels allows a full assessment of the problem in individual patients. This is particularly useful in patients who have congenital heart disease, in whom abnormal anatomy and connec-tions are often further complicated by multiple cardiac operations. Each case is different, and individual assessments are required.

PARTICULAR AREAS IN WHICH CARDIOVASCULAR MAGNETIC RESONANCE AIDS HEMODYNAMIC ASSESSMENT
Shunts

Atrial and ventricular septal defects can be visualized accurately and the quantity of shunt measured. The defect is often seen on a four-chamber (horizontal long-axis) view (**Fig. 6**A) but can be identified with short-axis views perpendic-ular to the septum, either targeted or using an entire stack of short-axis images through the rele-vant chambers. The ability to image in any plane allows all borders of the defect to be identified, which is particularly important for atrial septal defects, in which there may not be a rim of tissue (see **Fig. 6**B), or the defect may be a sinus venosus defect, which also may involve anomalous pulmo-nary venous drainage. Targeted imaging can illustrate the anatomy, even imaging the defect en-face and measuring flow through this.[49] Finally, measuring left and right ventricular volumes and quantifying aortic and pulmonary flow to measure the left-to-right shunt ratio are important for

determining the hemodynamic consequences of the lesion and the response to treatment.[50] Increasingly, percutaneous closure of these defects is undertaken, but it requires accurate assessment of the size of the defect, detailed knowledge of the surrounding anatomy, and quan-tification of the hemodynamic effects, all of which CMR provides. This can alter the clinical manage-ment in a significant proportion of cases.[49]

Extracardiac shunts also can be identified and the shunt quantified, but it depends on the size and nature of the shunt. A patent ductus arteriosus is usually straightforward to identify—often from an oblique sagittal view in line with the aortic arch. The size, location, and quantity of flow through the shunt can then be obtained. Major aortopulmonary collateral arteries may be identified, but it depends on their number, size, and location; small and tortuous vessels are difficult to identify. One of the more useful techniques is MR angiography, in which a bolus of contrast is imaged as it passes through a chosen area, and three-dimensional reconstruction of the bolus distribution can be undertaken using appropriate software. If imaging is timed to take place as the contrast passes through the aortic arch, it may be possible to iden-tify any major aortopulmonary collateral arteries. The degree of shunting can be measured from the difference between aortic and pulmonary flows.

Surgical Conduits

Surgical conduits, mostly used for the alleviation of congenital heart disease, can become blocked or relatively stenosed (as a patient grows). Assessing the patency of the conduit is usually possible with CMR cine imaging, and velocity or flow through the conduit can be quantified. The location for imaging depends on the circumstances of each individual, and a good knowledge of the known anatomy and nature of previous operations is help-ful before CMR assessment. Examples of surgical conduits include Glenn and Waterston shunts and RV to pulmonary artery conduits.

Other Flow Assessments

The versatility of CMR allows the assessment of flow in any large vessel, which can be tailored to individual circumstances. An example of this would be measurement of the relative flow in the left and right pulmonary arteries to assess the importance of unilateral pulmonary arterial disease or anomalous connections.

Venous Assessment

Venous anatomy, connections, and flow also can be assessed. The systemic vena cavae are well

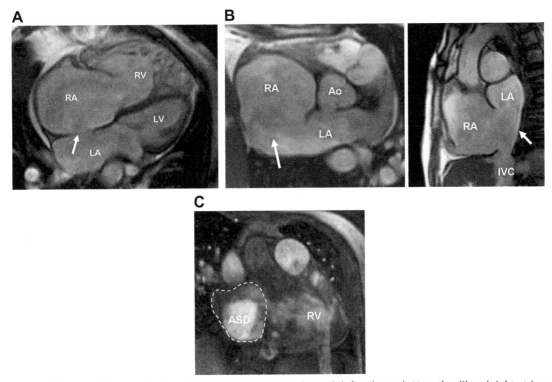

Fig. 6. (*A*) Horizontal long-axis view of a patient with an atrial septal defect (*arrow*). Note the dilated right atrium and ventricle. LA, left atrium; LV, left ventricle; RA, right atrium; RV, right ventricle. (*B*) The same patient shown in part A. Modified oblique transverse view (*left*) and modified atrial short axis view (*right*) demonstrates the lack of an inferoposterior rim of the ASD (*arrows*). (*C*) En-face view of the same ASD shown in part B shows the view from the right atrium, with the atrial septum outlined (*dashed line*) and the defect visible inferoposteriorly within it. RV, right ventricle.

visualized entering the right atrium (in normally connected hearts) and often can be visualized in a modified sagittal plane planned to include the insertion of the veins into the atrium. Flow in the veins can be measured if required, although a low-velocity window (<1 m/s) is usually indicated. Significant stenoses, thrombi, and other masses can be identified in the larger veins.

The insertion of the pulmonary veins into the left atrium often can be identified from cine imaging (a stack of contiguous transverse planes can be helpful), but MR angiography is rapid and particularly applicable to imaging the pulmonary veins. Imaging should coincide with the contrast bolus passing through the pulmonary veins and left atrium, and the precise location of each vein can be identified.[51] Anomalous pulmonary veins usually can be identified in this way, and CMR agrees well with surgical findings.[52] Left atrial circumferential ablation for atrial fibrillation is significantly aided by pulmonary venous imaging, because the left atrium is a complex three-dimensional shape and the location of the venous insertions is variable.[51] Although visualization of the left

atrium and pulmonary veins is helpful, the latest equipment and software in the cardiac catheterization laboratory can merge image data with electrophysiologic mapping of the left atrium and with the real-time position of the ablation catheter,[53] which significantly improves the speed and accuracy of the procedure.

Limitations of Hemodynamic Assessment

One important aspect of hemodynamic measurement that CMR is unable to measure directly is pressure inside a vessel or cardiac chamber. As with echocardiography, CMR can measure velocity across a stenosis and derive a pressure drop from this, but absolute pressure quantification remains elusive. One recent paper identified how CMR may indirectly indicate pressure by examining the complex flow patterns in the pulmonary artery using a new three-dimensional flow assessment technique.[54] This article suggested that pulmonary pressure (measured invasively) was strongly linked with the type of flow pattern in the main pulmonary artery. The data require further validation but indicate the novel approaches to assessment that CMR may bring in the future.

SUMMARY

CMR is able to provide a comprehensive assessment of valvular and hemodynamic function, including quantification of valve regurgitation and other flows, and accurate cardiac volumes and mass for assessing the effect on both ventricles. Combined with the ability to image all areas of the heart (including difficult areas such as the right ventricle and pulmonary veins), it is an ideal technique for investigating patients who have heart failure in whom these areas need to be examined.

REFERENCES

1. Bellenger NG, Burgess MI, Ray SG, et al. Comparison of left ventricular ejection fraction and volumes in heart failure by echocardiography, radionuclide ventriculography and cardiovascular magnetic resonance: are they interchangeable? Eur Heart J 2000; 21:1387–96.

2. Myerson SG, Bellenger NG, Pennell DJ. Assessment of left ventricular mass by cardiovascular magnetic resonance. Hypertension 2002;39:750–5.

3. Koch JA, Poll LW, Godehardt E, et al. Right and left ventricular volume measurements in an animal heart model in vitro: first experiences with cardiac MRI at 1.0 T. Eur Radiol 2000;10:455–8.

4. Cheitlin MD, Armstrong WF, Aurigemma GP, et al. ACC/AHA/ASE 2003 guideline update for the clinical application of echocardiography: summary article. A report of the American College of Cardiology/ American Heart Association Task Force on Practice Guidelines (ACC/AHA/ASE Committee to Update the 1997 Guidelines for the Clinical Application of Echocardiography). J Am Soc Echocardiogr 2003; 16:1091–110.

5. Globits S, Frank H, Mayr H, et al. Quantitative assessment of aortic regurgitation by magnetic resonance imaging. Eur Heart J 1992;13:78–83.

6. Gatehouse PD, Keegan J, Crowe LA, et al. Applications of phase-contrast flow and velocity imaging in cardiovascular MRI. Eur Radiol 2005;15:2172–84.

7. Nayler GL, Firmin DN, Longmore DB. Blood flow imaging by cine magnetic resonance. J Comput Assist Tomogr 1986;10:715–22.

8. Chatzimavroudis GP, Oshinski JN, Franch RH, et al. Quantification of the aortic regurgitant volume with magnetic resonance phase velocity mapping: a clinical investigation of the importance of imaging slice location. J Heart Valve Dis 1998;7:94–101.

9. Hundley WG, Li HF, Hillis LD, et al. Quantitation of cardiac output with velocity-encoded, phase-difference magnetic resonance imaging. Am J Cardiol 1995;75:1250–5.

10. Sondergaard L, Lindvig K, Hildebrandt P, et al. Quantification of aortic regurgitation by magnetic resonance velocity mapping. Am Heart J 1993; 125:1081–90.

11. Sondergaard L, Thomsen C, Stahlberg F, et al. Mitral and aortic valvular flow: quantification with MR phase mapping. J Magn Reson Imaging 1992;2:295–302.

12. Firmin DN, Nayler GL, Kilner PJ, et al. The application of phase shifts in NMR for flow measurement. Magn Reson Med 1990;14:230–41.

13. O'Brien KR, Cowan BR, Jain M, et al. MRI phase contrast velocity and flow errors in turbulent stenotic jets. J Magn Reson Imaging 2008;28:210–8.

14. Canstein C, Cachot P, Faust A, et al. 3D MR flow analysis in realistic rapid-prototyping model systems of the thoracic aorta: comparison with in vivo data and computational fluid dynamics in identical vessel geometries. Magn Reson Med 2008;59:535–46.

15. Hope TA, Markl M, Wigstrom L, et al. Comparison of flow patterns in ascending aortic aneurysms and volunteers using four-dimensional magnetic resonance velocity mapping. J Magn Reson Imaging 2007;26:1471–9.

16. Kramer CM, Barkhausen J, Flamm SD, et al. Standardized cardiovascular magnetic resonance imaging (CMR) protocols, society for cardiovascular magnetic resonance: board of trustees task force on standardized protocols. J Cardiovasc Magn Reson 2008;10:35–40.

17. John AS, Dill T, Brandt RR, et al. Magnetic resonance to assess the aortic valve area in aortic stenosis: how does it compare to current diagnostic standards? J Am Coll Cardiol 2003;42:519–26.

18. Tanaka K, Makaryus AN, Wolff SD. Correlation of aortic valve area obtained by the velocity-encoded phase contrast continuity method to direct planimetry using cardiovascular magnetic resonance. J Cardiovasc Magn Reson 2007;9:799–805.

19. Kilner PJ, Manzara CC, Mohiaddin RH, et al. Magnetic resonance jet velocity mapping in mitral and aortic valve stenosis. Circulation 1993;87: 1239–48.

20. Sondergaard L, Hildebrandt P, Lindvig K, et al. Valve area and cardiac output in aortic stenosis: quantification by magnetic resonance velocity mapping. Am Heart J 1993;126:1156–64.

21. Dulce MC, Mostbeck GH, O'Sullivan M, et al. Severity of aortic regurgitation: interstudy reproducibility of measurements with velocity-encoded cine MR imaging. Radiology 1992;185:235–40.

22. Honda N, Machida K, Hashimoto M, et al. Aortic regurgitation: quantitation with MR imaging velocity mapping. Radiology 1993;186:189–94.

23. Kozerke S, Scheidegger MB, Pedersen EM, et al. Heart motion adapted cine phase-contrast flow

measurements through the aortic valve. Magn Reson Med 1999;42:970–8.

24. Chatzimavroudis GP, Oshinski JN, Franch RH, et al. Evaluation of the precision of magnetic resonance phase velocity mapping for blood flow measurements. J Cardiovasc Magn Reson 2001; 3:11–9.

25. Detaint D, Messika-Zeitoun D, Maalouf J, et al. Quantitative echocardiographic determinants of clinical outcome in asymptomatic patients with aortic regurgitation. J Am Coll Cardiol Img 2008;1: 1–11.

26. Fujita N, Chazouilleres AF, Hartiala JJ, et al. Quantification of mitral regurgitation by velocity-encoded cine nuclear magnetic resonance imaging. J Am Coll Cardiol 1994;23:951–8.

27. Gelfand EV, Hughes S, Hauser TH, et al. Severity of mitral and aortic regurgitation as assessed by cardiovascular magnetic resonance: optimizing correlation with Doppler echocardiography. J Cardiovasc Magn Reson 2006;8:503–7.

28. Kon MW, Myerson SG, Moat NE, et al. Quantification of regurgitant fraction in mitral regurgitation by cardiovascular magnetic resonance: comparison of techniques. J Heart Valve Dis 2004;13:600–7.

29. Enriquez-Sarano M, Avierinos JF, Messika-Zeitoun D, et al. Quantitative determinants of the outcome of asymptomatic mitral regurgitation. N Engl J Med 2005;352:875–83.

30. Buchner S, Debl K, Poschenrieder F, et al. Cardiovascular magnetic resonance for direct assessment of anatomic regurgitant orifice in mitral regurgitation. Circ Cardiovasc Imaging 2008;1:148–55.

31. Frigiola A, Redington AN, Cullen S, et al. Pulmonary regurgitation is an important determinant of right ventricular contractile dysfunction in patients with surgically repaired tetralogy of Fallot. Circulation 2004;110:II153–7.

32. Geva T. Indications and timing of pulmonary valve replacement after tetralogy of Fallot repair. Semin Thorac Cardiovasc Surg Pediatr Card Surg Annu 2006;11–22.

33. Karamlou T, McCrindle BW, Williams WG. Surgery insight: late complications following repair of tetralogy of Fallot and related surgical strategies for management. Nat Clin Pract Cardiovasc Med 2006;3:611–22.

34. Rebergen SA, Chin JG, Ottenkamp J, et al. Pulmonary regurgitation in the late postoperative follow-up of tetralogy of Fallot: volumetric quantitation by nuclear magnetic resonance velocity mapping. Circulation 1993;88:2257–66.

35. Vliegen HW, van Straten A, de Roos A, et al. Magnetic resonance imaging to assess the hemodynamic effects of pulmonary valve replacement in adults late after repair of tetralogy of Fallot. Circulation 2002;106:1703–7.

36. Li W, Davlouros PA, Kilner PJ, et al. Doppler-echocardiographic assessment of pulmonary regurgitation in adults with repaired tetralogy of Fallot: comparison with cardiovascular magnetic resonance imaging. Am Heart J 2004;147:165–72.

37. Ammash NM, Dearani JA, Burkhart HM, et al. Pulmonary regurgitation after tetralogy of Fallot repair: clinical features, sequelae, and timing of pulmonary valve replacement. Congenit Heart Dis 2007;2:386–403.

38. Kuehne T, Saeed M, Reddy G, et al. Sequential magnetic resonance monitoring of pulmonary flow with endovascular stents placed across the pulmonary valve in growing swine. Circulation 2001;104: 2363–8.

39. Lurz P, Coats L, Khambadkone S, et al. Percutaneous pulmonary valve implantation: impact of evolving technology and learning curve on clinical outcome. Circulation 2008;117:1964–72.

40. Schievano S, Coats L, Migliavacca F, et al. Variations in right ventricular outflow tract morphology following repair of congenital heart disease: implications for percutaneous pulmonary valve implantation. J Cardiovasc Magn Reson 2007;9:687–95.

41. Mahle WT, Parks WJ, Fyfe DA, et al. Tricuspid regurgitation in patients with repaired tetralogy of Fallot and its relation to right ventricular dilatation. Am J Cardiol 2003;92:643–5.

42. Rees S, Somerville J, Warnes C, et al. Comparison of magnetic resonance imaging with echocardiography and radionuclide angiography in assessing cardiac function and anatomy following Mustard's operation for transposition of the great arteries. Am J Cardiol 1988;61:1316–22.

43. Choi YH, Park JH, Choe YH, et al. MR imaging of Ebstein's anomaly of the tricuspid valve. AJR Am J Roentgenol 1994;163:539–43.

44. Eustace S, Kruskal JB, Hartnell GG. Ebstein's anomaly presenting in adulthood: the role of cine magnetic resonance imaging in diagnosis. Clin Radiol 1994;49:690–2.

45. Shellock FG. MR imaging of metallic implants and materials: a compilation of the literature. AJR Am J Roentgenol 1988;151:811–4.

46. Shellock F. Reference manual for magnetic resonance safety, implants and devices. 2008 edition. Los Angeles (CA): Biomedical Research Publishing Group; 2008.

47. Botnar R, Nagel E, Scheidegger MB, et al. Assessment of prosthetic aortic valve performance by magnetic resonance velocity imaging. MAGMA 2000;10:18–26.

48. Hasenkam JM, Ringgaard S, Houlind K, et al. Prosthetic heart valve evaluation by magnetic resonance imaging. Eur J Cardiothorac Surg 1999;16:300–5.

49. Thomson L, Crowley A, Heitner J, et al. Direct en face imaging of secundum atrial septal defects by velocity-encoded cardiovascular magnetic

resonance in patients evaluated for possible trans-catheter closure. Circ Cardiovasc Imaging 2008;1: 31–40.

50. Webb G, Gatzoulis MA. Atrial septal defects in the adult: recent progress and overview. Circulation 2006;114:1645–53.

51. Mansour M, Holmvang G, Sosnovik D, et al. Assessment of pulmonary vein anatomic variability by magnetic resonance imaging: implications for catheter ablation techniques for atrial fibrillation. J Cardiovasc Electrophysiol 2004;15: 387–93.

52. Festa P, Ait-Ali L, Cerillo AG, et al. Magnetic resonance imaging is the diagnostic tool of choice in the preoperative evaluation of patients with partial anomalous pulmonary venous return. Int J Cardiovasc Imaging 2006;22:685–93.

53. Dong J, Dickfeld T, Dalal D, et al. Initial experience in the use of integrated electroanatomic mapping with three-dimensional MR/CT images to guide catheter ablation of atrial fibrillation. J Cardiovasc Electrophysiol 2006;17:459–66.

54. Reiter G, Reiter U, Kovacs G, et al. Magnetic resonance–derived 3-dimensional blood flow patterns in the main pulmonary artery as a marker of pulmonary hypertension and a measure of elevated mean pulmonary arterial pressure. Circ Cardiovasc Imaging 2008;1:23–30.

Magnetic Resonance Imaging of Pericardial Disease and Intracardiac Thrombus

John D. Grizzard, MD*

KEYWORDS

- Magnetic resonance • Pericardial disease
- Intracardiac thrombus • Constructive pericarditis
- Pericardial effusion

Multiple imaging modalities are currently available for the comprehensive evaluation of pericardial disease and the detection of intracardiac thrombus. Echocardiography is currently the mainstay of noninvasive cardiac imaging, and CT excels in the evaluation of pericardial calcification. MRI has several advantages over echocardiography and the competing modality of CT (**Table 1**).

Echocardiography is inexpensive, rapidly performed, and portable. It is also ubiquitous, being readily available in virtually all hospital settings. It is often the first modality used in the evaluation of suspected pericardial disease or cardiac masses. It has limitations; specifically, in many patients the acoustic windows are limited, allowing only partial visualization of the global cardiac structure and the adjacent mediastinal contents. Many patients have a large body habitus that also significantly degrades image quality. Pericardial thickening also can be difficult to detect with echocardiography, as can calcification. Finally, echocardiography is limited in its ability to provide tissue characterization.[1]

CT has emerged as a vigorous competitor to MR and echocardiographic imaging. Like MR, CT is capable of high-resolution thin section imaging and can be gated to the cardiac cycle, allowing cinematic displays of cardiac motion, although with a lower temporal resolution than MR. It is more sensitive than MRI for the detection of calcification, which represents an often cited advantage relative to MRI. Current multislice CT

scanners allow multiplanar reconstructions using isotropic voxels, resulting in high-resolution imaging in virtually any plane. The resultant improvement in multiplanar imaging with current generation CT scanner technology has lessened to some extent the prior advantage of multiplanar MR imaging. CT requires the use of ionizing radiation, and gated CT examinations can result in a radiation dose that exceeds that of cardiac catheterization.[2] It usually requires the administration of iodinated contrast, with the attendant risks of nephrotoxicity and potential allergic reactions. Its efficacy in tissue characterization is inferior to MRI.

For various reasons, MRI remains the gold standard for comprehensive imaging of pericardial disease. MRI provides direct multiplanar imaging without the need for reconstructions and in any freely selectable imaging plane. There are no limitations regarding acoustic windows. No radiation is required, and no nephrotoxic contrast media are administered. Gadolinium is frequently administered but is widely regarded as significantly safer than iodinated contrast material.

Most importantly, MR provides superior tissue characterization relative to CT and echocardiography. Various imaging sequences, including fast spin-echo (T1-weighted and T2-weighted), cine, and delayed enhancement cardiovascular MR (DE-CMR) techniques, provide a broad palette from which the examiner can choose to localize and characterize various pericardial and cardiac disorders.[3,4] Perfusion imaging can be performed

Virginia Commonwealth University Medical Center, Richmond, VA, USA
* Non-invasive Cardiovascular Imaging, Department of Radiology, Virginia Commonwealth University Medical Center, 1250 E. Marshall Street, P.O. Box 980615, Richmond, VA 23298-0615.
E-mail address: jdgrizzard@vcu.edu

Heart Failure Clin 5 (2009) 401–419
doi:10.1016/j.hfc.2009.02.006
1551-7136/09/$ – see front matter © 2009 Elsevier Inc. All rights reserved.

Table 1
Comparsion of cross-sectional imaging modalities

Modality	Multiplanar Capability	Soft-Tissue Contrast	Temporal Resolution	Windows
ECHO	+++	+	++++	Limited
CT	++	++	+	Unlimited
MR	++++	++++	+++	Unlimited

for evaluation of lesion vascularity. Finally, MRI using real-time sequences can provide depiction of dynamic processes, thereby furnishing hemodynamic and structural information. The multisequence, multiplanar capability of MRI makes it the ideal method for the evaluation of pericardial diseases and detection of intracardiac thrombus.

Although pericardial disease and cardiac thrombi are clearly separate and discrete entities, there are significant similarities in the use of MRI for their diagnosis and overlap in the MR techniques used. These disorders are considered together in this article.

MAGNETIC RESONANCE IMAGING TECHNIQUES

In early implementations, cardiac MRI for the evaluation of pericardial disease was performed with gated spin-echo examinations without breath holding. Typically, two signal acquisitions were averaged to diminish breathing-induced motion artifacts, and a study yielding five dual-echo slices required 45 minutes to obtain. Subsequently, fast spin-echo sequences were developed that allow image acquisition in a single breath-hold. A single image using this technique requires between 10 and 15 heartbeats, and a comprehensive examination of the entire chest requires 5 to 10 minutes for one sequence type. Pre- and postcontrast T1-weighted imaging and comprehensive T2-weighted imaging of the entire chest using this type of sequence is a time-consuming exercise. This sequence often results in suboptimal T1 weighting because of the long TR used. Finally, breathing artifact often diminishes the image quality.

In the last several years, however, significant technical improvements have been made to MR scanner hardware, such as powerful gradients capable of more rapid imaging and coils that facilitate parallel imaging. Software improvements in the form of new and robust sequences also have been developed that provide unique information not previously available with the former imaging sequences.[5,6] These changes have resulted in a significant improvement in image quality

and decreases in scan time. For example, comprehensive multislice dark-blood morphologic imaging of the entire chest can be performed with double-inversion recovery fast spin-echo (HASTE) imaging in approximately 1 minute. Similarly, cine imaging is performed with the balanced steady-state free precession (b-SSFP) sequence, resulting in improved image quality and diminished scan time. Certain compromises have been made, as will be described, and in selected instances conventional fast spin-echo T1- or T2-weighted sequences may be appropriate. The more modern techniques usually demonstrate superior image quality with less respiratory artifact and superior image information.[7]

Standard Cardiac Magnetic Resonance Examination

A cardiac examination designed for evaluation of suspected thrombus or pericardial disease should begin with the standard sequences used in essentially all cardiac MRI: initial static morphologic images and high-resolution cine images of the heart. These sequences are supplemented by delayed enhancement and perfusion imaging for tissue characterization. The examination also should be tailored to the specific clinical circumstance, and various other sequences can be added as necessary (**Table 2**).

Previously, dark-blood morphologic sequences were most often performed with fast spin-echo imaging, which as described previously could be time consuming. Recently, the HASTE (half-Fourier acquisition turbo spin-echo) sequence has largely replaced the older fast spin-echo technique because it allows dark-blood imaging with a greatly reduced acquisition time, with one entire image acquisition occurring in a single-shot fashion at every other heartbeat (**Fig. 1**A, B). This represents a tremendous acceleration relative to the former technique. There is slightly increased blurring with this technique, however, relative to the standard gated spin-echo techniques. The resistance of the single-shot sequence to respiratory motion artifact, which frequently degrades spin-echo image

Table 2
Suggested imaging protocol

Sequence	Planes	Coverage
Core examination		
Localizer	Axial, coronal, sagittal	Entire chest
HASTE	Axial, sagittal, or coronal	Entire chest
b-SSFP cines	Short- and long-axis views	Heart from base to apex
Single-shot b-SSFP delayed-enhancement images with inversion time set to null normal myocardium	Short- and long-axis views	Copy the cines
Single-shot b-SSFP delayed-enhancement images with inversion time of 600 msec (for thrombus detection)	Short- and long-axis views	Copy the cines
Optional for pericardium		
Real-time SSFP cine images	Short-axis and four-chamber views during deep inspiration	To evaluate septal motion

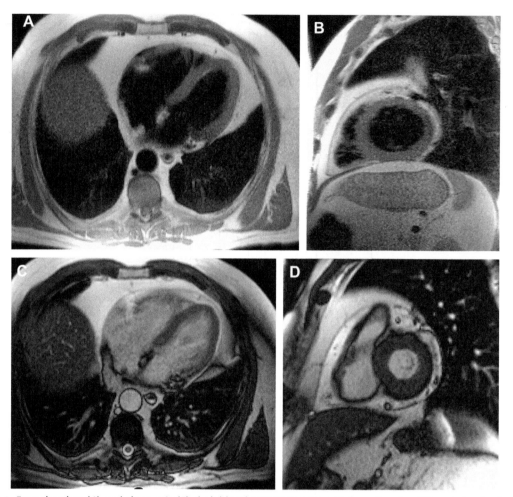

Fig. 1. Four-chamber (*A*) and short-axis (*B*) dark-blood HASTE images and four-chamber (*C*) and short-axis (*D*) bright-blood b-SSFP images show normal pericardium.

quality, usually offsets this minimal disadvantage. Standard dark-blood T1- and T2-weighted fast spin-echo gated acquisitions can be obtained as needed for further evaluation of selected findings.

Cine imaging through the entire myocardium in the short- and long-axis planes as routinely performed for cardiac evaluation is appropriate for the imaging of suspected pericardial disease and the detection of thrombus. b-SSFP sequences are the standard for cine imaging because they demonstrate improved image quality in comparison with segmented gradient-echo imaging techniques.[5] The signal intensity in the b-SSFP technique depends on the T2/T1 ratio. Structures with a high T2/T1 ratio, such as fat, fluid, and intracavitary blood, demonstrate similar high signal despite their significantly different T1 and T2 properties. The myocardium is relatively low in signal intensity on precontrast images, which provides excellent contrast between the blood pool and the

endocardium and is often helpful in the delineation of intracavitary lesions. The pericardium usually can be depicted with great clarity, and the normal gliding movement of the visceral pericardium attached to the heart relative to the parietal pericardium can be easily assessed (see **Fig. 1**C, D).

Newer scanners are also often able to perform real-time cine image acquisitions, which allow images to be performed without breath holding, and without segmentation.[8] These nongated b-SSFP images are acquired in the cine mode in real-time and can be used for the evaluation of dynamic processes.

Uncommonly, sequences using tagging to evaluate for pericardial/myocardial adhesions also can be performed.[9] In this sequence, a grid of saturation bands is placed over the heart, and their deformation can provide information about regional wall motion. This sequence also has been used to depict abnormal adherence of the visceral pericardium to the parietal pericardium or of the pericardium to the chest wall. (The grid lines remain unbroken as opposed to demonstrating the normal disruption caused by cardiac motion.) Given the high-resolution imaging possible at the current time with SSFP cine sequences, these are usually not necessary. Perfusion sequences are used to evaluate the vascularity of a lesion and can be obtained in multiple imaging planes with one injection. These are heavily T1-weighted imaging sequences that can provide information regarding tumor vascularity and are helpful in the evaluation of masses and thrombi.

The same delayed enhancement sequences that are used for the detection of myocardial infarction are also used for the evaluation of masses and thrombus. The standard delayed enhancement (DE-CMR) sequence is a segmented T1-weighted inversion recovery gradient-echo sequence with an inversion time chosen that provides nulling of the signal of normal myocardium, accentuating the contrast differences between normal myocardium and areas of infarction.[6] The same sequence can be used for the characterization of masses, which typically demonstrate hyperenhancement. Single-shot delayed enhancement images using an inversion recovery b-SSFP sequence can provide similar information in a fraction of the imaging time.[10,11] The same sequences also can be performed with a long inversion time (> 600 msec), which is often helpful in the detection of thrombus, as described later.[12]

PERICARDIAL DISEASE

The pericardium is a mesothelial-lined serous sac into which the heart has been invaginated, much like placing one's hand into a balloon and then deflating it. The visceral pericardium is composed of a thin layer of mesothelial cells overlying the epicardial surface of the heart. The parietal pericardium is a somewhat thicker and more collagenous layer. The normal thickness of the pericardium is less than 2 mm on MRI, and even this measurement actually represents a summation of both pericardial layers and a small amount of intervening fluid usually present, along with chemical shift artifact.[13] The actual pericardial thickness is probably less than 1.5 mm. Normally, between 25 and 50 mL of clear serous fluid is present in the pericardial sac, providing lubrication. The normal pericardium is readily depicted on MRI as a thin low-signal intensity line on static morphologic or cine images.[13] It is usually most easily seen overlying the right ventricular free wall and at the left ventricular apex (see **Fig. 1**).

The pericardium normally provides a barrier to the spread of infection and limits the degree to which the myocardium can be acutely distended. A certain amount of physiologic ventricular coupling is facilitated by the presence of the intact pericardium. It is infrequently the subject of consideration, except in instances of a significant alteration of sensation or function. These disorders fall into only a few clinical syndromes: acute pericarditis, pericardial effusion (with or without tamponade), and constrictive pericarditis. In the setting of heart failure, evaluation of the pericardium with MRI is most often performed to aid in the differentiation between constrictive pericarditis and restrictive cardiomyopathy.

Acute Pericarditis

Acute pericarditis is usually a clinical diagnosis and infrequently requires imaging. It is likely that 90% or more of isolated cases of acute pericarditis are either idiopathic or viral in origin, but various causes, including uremia, acute myocardial infarction, and neoplasm, can result in the clinical pattern of acute pericarditis (**Box 1**).

On imaging, one may observe a small amount of pericardial effusion, and minimal pericardial thickening may be seen. Significant pericardial thickening usually implies chronicity, however, and would be uncommon in acute pericarditis.[14] Occasionally, pericardial enhancement may be seen.[15] Most cases respond readily to symptomatic therapy and treatment with nonsteroidal anti-inflammatory agents.

Pericardial Effusion

Any of the disorders that can cause acute pericarditis also may result in pericardial effusion (see **Box 1**). Although echocardiography is the usual initial imaging modality chosen to detect and

Box 1
Causes of acute pericarditis/pericardial effusion
Idiopathic
Infection: viral, bacterial, fungal/tuberculosis
Injury: radiation, surgery, trauma, myocardial infarction
Postinjury: postmyocardial infarction, postpericardiotomy
Connective tissue disease: rheumatoid arthritis, systemic lupus
Malignancies: breast, lung, lymphoma
Metabolic: uremia

characterize pericardial effusions, MRI is helpful in various circumstances. It is more sensitive than echocardiography for the detection of small effusions and is superior to echocardiography in the detection of loculated effusions or effusions complicated by pericardial thickening.[16–18]

Magnetic Resonance Findings

Uncomplicated effusions are usually low in signal on T1-weighted images and high in signal intensity on T2-weighted images. Cine gradient echo images performed with SSFP often demonstrate pericardial effusions as having uniformly high signal intensity. This high signal intensity on cine and T2-weighted images allows clear

differentiation from the fibrous pericardium, which is low in signal on these sequences (**Fig. 2**).

Complicating hemorrhage can be suspected when high signal intensity is seen within the pericardial sac on T1-weighted images. Hemorrhage or infection should be suspected on cine imaging when the effusion fluid is clearly complex and inhomogeneous, containing regions of different signal intensity (**Fig. 3**).[19–22] Delayed enhancement imaging can demonstrate abnormal pericardial enhancement, indicative of inflammation or infection. Imaging with a delayed enhancement sequence using a long inversion time can demonstrate intrapericardial thrombus as a region of low signal intensity (**Fig. 4**). Most importantly, MRI can depict the effect of the effusion on the myocardium.

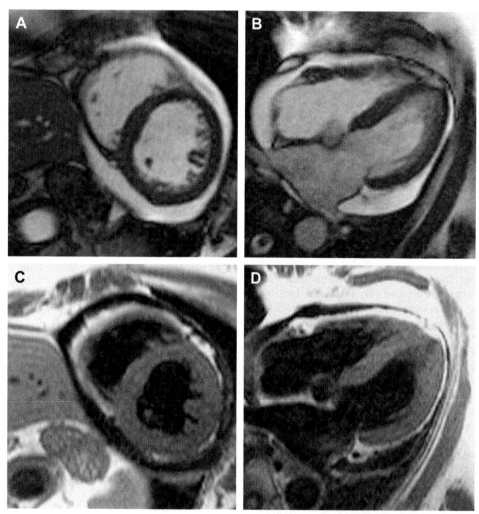

Fig. 2. Moderate-sized simple pericardial effusion on short-axis (*A*) and four-chamber (*B*) b-SSFP images and corresponding T1-weighted short-axis (*C*) and four-chamber (*D*) views. Note the uniform high signal on b-SSFP images and the low signal on T1-weighted images.

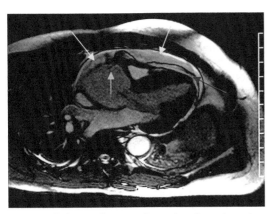

Fig. 3. Still frame from a three-chamber cine view demonstrates complex pericardial fluid (*yellow arrows*), which represents intrapericardial hemorrhage caused by an aortic dissection (*blue arrow* denotes the dissection flap). The red arrow points to an epicardial fat pad. Note also the small jet of aortic insufficiency.

CARDIAC TAMPONADE

The pericardium normally demonstrates a steep pressure/volume curve, such that even small increases in volume beyond a certain point result in a significant rise in intrapericardial pressure.[23–25] This is particularly true in the acute setting, in which the rapid accumulation of a pericardial effusion may result in cardiac tamponade that would not develop if the effusion developed more slowly. Specifically, the slow, progressive development of pericardial effusion (or progressive cardiomegaly) results in a shift of the pressure/volume relationship to the right and produces flattening of the slope of the curve such that greater volumes of intrapericardial fluid are tolerated before a significant rise in pressure occurs. The rate at which a small volume increase results in a pressure increase is also diminished. As little as 200 to 250 mL of pericardial fluid can result in tamponade if it develops rapidly, whereas a significantly larger effusion may be well tolerated if it develops slowly.

Clinically, patients with large pericardial effusions that produce hemodynamic compromise often demonstrate venous distention and peripheral edema. The lungs may be relatively clear, although patients frequently complain of dyspnea.[26] In patients with cardiac tamponade, the stroke volume cannot be increased because of the impairment of ventricular filling, and tachycardia is often seen as a physiologic response to maintain cardiac output. In many cases, the chest radiograph alone may be diagnostic, with echocardiography obtained for confirmation. Significant diagnostic difficulty can arise occasionally, and MRI can be helpful. This is particularly true in patients with uremia, in whom pericardial effusions are frequent. In this population, it may be difficult to distinguish the hemodynamic effects of the pericardial effusion from symptoms of right heart failure caused by inadequate dialysis.

Magnetic Resonance Findings

A large circumferential pericardial effusion is usually evident, although a focal loculated effusion that significantly impairs right ventricular filling may produce significant hemodynamic impairment. The character of the effusion may be inferred, as described previously. Large effusions may be

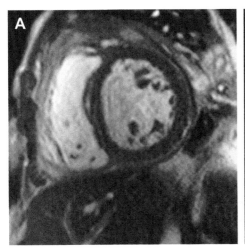
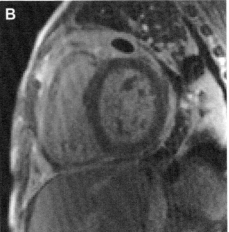

Fig. 4. (*A*) Postcontrast cine image shows a complex effusion in a patient with uremic pericarditis. Note the small oval mass superior to the left ventricle. (*B*) Delayed enhancement imaging with a long-inversion time (600 msec) shows the mass has low signal intensity consistent with thrombus.

present without producing tamponade, however. A finding indicative of the likely presence of significant hemodynamic compromise is the observation of right atrial and ventricular collapse in diastole.[27–29] This finding is best observed on cine imaging (**Fig. 5**A). Real-time cine imaging has some theoretical advantages over breath-hold cine imaging given that the degree of atrial or ventricular collapse may be variable in certain phases of the respiratory cycle, being more prominent after the first two or three heartbeats following the initiation of breath holding (see **Fig. 5**B).[30]

Real-time imaging that demonstrates abnormal septal movement indicative of abnormal ventricular interdependence is also helpful in confirming the hemodynamic significance of a large pericardial effusion.[31] Specifically, images acquired in the short-axis plane while the patient takes a deep inspiration can be observed for septal flattening or inversion. This is usually observed on the first two heartbeats after a deep inspiration, after which the septal flattening reverses. This sequence allows visual representation of the hemodynamic significance of the pathologic anatomy. Septal flattening or inversion in this circumstance indicates that the distensibility of the pericardial sac has reached its limit, such that any augmentation of right ventricular filling as results from a deep inspiration results in diminished left ventricular filling and displacement of the septum to the left (see **Fig. 5**C). Conversely, a lack of septal flattening or inversion despite the

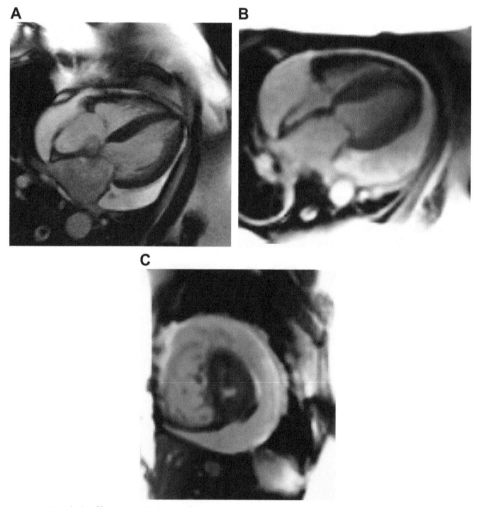

Fig. 5. Large pericardial effusion with hemodynamic compromise. Diastolic atrial collapse noted on standard segmented cine image (*A*) is better seen on real-time cine image (*B*). Real-time cine imaging during a deep inspiration (*C*) demonstrates marked septal flattening.

presence of significant effusion would imply that residual distensibility of the pericardium persists despite the volume of pericardial fluid present.

CONSTRICTIVE PERICARDITIS

Constrictive pericarditis usually results from abnormal thickening of the pericardium, which subsequently limits distention of the heart and results in impairment of diastolic ventricular filling. It was formerly most often caused by tuberculosis, but this is currently an uncommon cause. Currently, the most common identifiable causes include prior surgery and prior irradiation, but many cases are idiopathic in origin.[32-37] Many of the previously listed causes of acute pericarditis also can result in chronic constrictive pericarditis.

Histologically, constrictive pericarditis results from fibrosis of the pericardium, which results in encasement of the heart in a noncompliant, rigid structure. In the recent literature, global pericardial thickening still predominates, but a significant percentage of cases may be caused by only focal thickening, often overlying the right ventricle. In less than 5% of cases, gross pericardial thickening is not evident, although usually areas of adhesion between the visceral and parietal pericardium are seen on microscopic examination.[37,38]

The clinical differentiation between constrictive pericarditis and restrictive cardiomyopathy can be difficult because both lead to impairment of diastolic filling, which can result in venous distention, peripheral edema, passive hepatic congestion, and ascites. The distinction is of critical importance, however, because pericardiectomy can be curative for the appropriate patient with constriction. Although a variety of imaging techniques, including echocardiography and CT, can be helpful in making this determination, MRI is the preferred technique.[39,40] Echocardiography is limited in its ability to detect pericardial thickening, and because the thickening may be focal and not global, this is an important limitation. Doppler flow analyses are sometimes helpful but are not as high in sensitivity and specificity as MRI techniques.[41] CT is superior to MRI in the detection of calcification, but because constriction can occur without calcification and calcification can occur without constriction, this advantage is of limited clinical importance.[34] Although the excellent spatial resolution of CT provides superb definition of static processes, the significantly lower temporal resolution limits its use for the detection of hemodynamic processes that can be readily depicted with MRI. MR is also superior to CT in differentiating pericardial thickening from small effusions.[20] Regardless of the imaging technique

used, however, it is important to remember that the diagnosis of constriction is ultimately that of a hemodynamic derangement, not simply a morphologic abnormality.

Magnetic Resonance Findings

MRI provides excellent differentiation between high signal epicardial fat and pericardial fluid and the low signal of fibrous pericardium and allows clear detection of pericardial thickening. Thickening of the pericardium is diagnosed when its width exceeds 4 mm (**Fig. 6**A, B).[14] Although usually evident on standard cine and single-shot dark-blood static images, gated fast spin-echo T1 images may be helpful in equivocal cases. Small focal areas of thickening should be sought in the appropriate clinical circumstance, because constriction may result from localized thickening. Cine imaging is often helpful in the detection of small foci of localized pericardial adhesions.

Ancillary findings, such as atrial dilatation, distention of the inferior vena cava, hepatomegaly, and ascites, may be seen with restrictive cardiomyopathy and constrictive pericarditis (see **Fig. 6**C). Morphologic images showing pericardial thickening and a normal appearing myocardium are highly predictive of the presence of constriction in the appropriate clinical setting, however. These findings of abnormal pathologic anatomy are helpful in making the diagnosis; however, because ultimately the diagnosis of constriction is one of altered physiology, direct or indirect demonstration of the abnormal hemodynamics is desirable. Cine images that demonstrate altered hemodynamics are a more direct means of confirming the diagnosis of constriction.

DYNAMIC IMAGING

Cine imaging in constrictive pericarditis can demonstrate abnormal ventricular interdependence caused by the lack of pericardial distensibility. An abnormal configuration of the ventricular septum is frequently observed in early diastole on cine imaging. This septal "bounce" or shivering septum is a manifestation of the abnormal ventricular filling dynamics. Specifically, it reflects the limitation of right ventricular filling secondary to the rigid pericardium, with resultant shift of the septum to the left during early diastole. This occurrence results in an abnormal septal curvature, which is normally convex to the right; in patients with constrictive pericarditis, reports indicate that loss of this convexity is frequently seen.[42] This sign has excellent sensitivity and specificity for the diagnosis of constrictive pericarditis, being present in

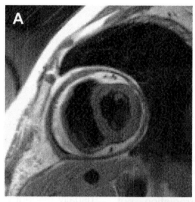

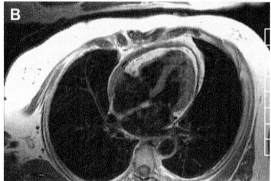

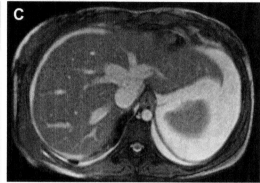

Fig. 6. Short-axis (*A*) and four-chamber views (*B*) demonstrate global pericardial thickening in a patient with constrictive pericarditis. Note the atrial dilatation seen in (*B*). Atrial and caval dilatation (*C*) may be seen in constrictive pericarditis and restrictive cardiomyopathy.

more than 80% of patients on cine MIR and none of the normal controls (**Fig. 7**A, B).

Real-time cine imaging during a deep inspiration also has been reported to be helpful in distinguishing patients with restrictive cardiomyopathy from patients with constrictive pericarditis. In a small series of patients, all cases of constrictive pericarditis were clearly differentiated from cases of restrictive cardiomyopathy on real-time cine imaging performed, with patients taking a deep inspiration. In the patients with constrictive pericarditis, septal flattening or inversion was observed, whereas this finding was absent in patients with restrictive cardiomyopathy.[31] The septal inversion noted in these cases is indicative of the diminished compliance of the pericardium such that any increase in right ventricular filling (such as that caused by a deep inspiration) results in shift of the septum to the left (see **Fig. 7**C). Patients with restrictive cardiomyopathy did not show such septal abnormalities. The use of real-time cine MRI seems to provide direct visualization of the pathologic hemodynamics and abnormal ventricular interdependence characteristic of constrictive pericarditis.

EFFUSIVE/CONSTRICTIVE PERICARDITIS

This disorder represents a combination of a significant pericardial effusion producing increased intrapericardial pressure along with pericardial thickening; the diagnosis is based on the persistence of abnormal pericardial dynamics even after the raised intrapericardial pressure secondary to the effusion has been relieved.[43,44] It is most often seen after radiation therapy. It is diagnosed at cardiac catheterization, in which pressure measurements before and after pericardiocentesis confirm the hemodynamic alterations. Some authors feel that this may represent an intermediate phase in the transition from acute effusive pericarditis to the development of chronic fibrous pericarditis.

OTHER PERICARDIAL DISORDERS
Congenital Absence of the Pericardium

This is a rare developmental abnormality in which the pericardium may be partially or completely absent. Most cases are comprised of partial agenesis of the pericardium, usually involving the left side. It may be associated with underlying

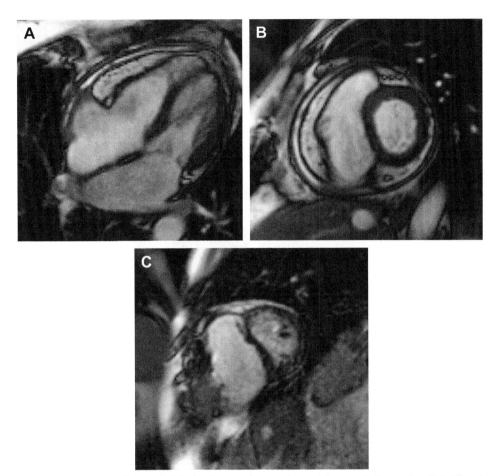

Fig. 7. Four-chamber (A) and short-axis (B) cine images in a patient with constrictive pericarditis. The abnormal septal curvature seen on standard cine images obtained in diastole (A, B) is indicative of impaired RV diastolic filling. Real-time cine imaging (C) shows septal inversion apparent during a deep-inspiration, consistent with abnormal ventricular interdependence.

congenital heart disease, including atrial septal defects, patent ductus arteriosus, and other disorders. It is most often recognized on chest radiography, which demonstrates the characteristic abnormal rotation of the heart into the left side of the chest in the usual case of left-sided partial agenesis. The left atrial appendage is often abnormally prominent, and rare cases of herniation of the left atrial appendage through the defect with resultant strangulation have been reported.[20,45,46] This abnormality is recognized on MRI when lung tissue is seen interposed between the aorta and pulmonary artery, an appearance not possible with intact pericardium. Also, occasionally lung tissue can be observed inferior to the heart and interposed between the heart and diaphragm.

Pericardial Masses

Primary pericardial masses are most commonly caused by pericardial cysts. These benign lesions

are believed to originate from portions of the pericardium being pinched off from the remainder of the pericardium during embryologic development. They most commonly occur along the right (70%) cardiophrenic angle and are less commonly left-sided. They can occur anywhere along the margin of the pericardium, however.

Magnetic Resonance Findings

Pericardial cysts are low in signal intensity on T1 images and high in signal intensity on T2 images, which is consistent with their fluid character. They do not enhance and usually are unilocular (**Fig.** 8A–D).[47,48]

OTHER PERICARDIAL TUMORS

Other benign pericardial tumors are rare and include teratomas, solitary benign fibrous tumors of the pericardium, and hemangiomas.[49] Primary

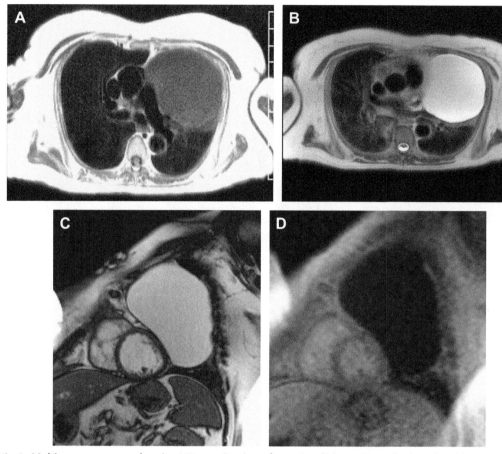

Fig. 8. Multisequence comprehensive MR examination of a pericardial cyst. Note the low signal intensity on the T1-weighted image (*A*), the high signal on the T2-weighted and cine images (*B, C*), and the lack of enhancement on the perfusion image (*D*). Note how the comprehensive nature of the MR examination allows one to visualize the relationship of the lesion to the myocardium and characterize this lesion as a simple, nonenhancing cyst lacking solid elements.

malignant tumors of the pericardium are also rare, and metastatic disease is significantly more common. Mesothelioma is the most common primary malignant tumor, although sarcomas occasionally may be seen. Mesothelioma may present with multiple confluent soft-tissue masses that engulf the heart. MRI findings include the presence of pericardial effusion along with a nodular appearance of the pericardium.[49]

Intracardiac Thrombus

Evaluation of a suspected or known cardiac mass or thrombus is a frequent source of referrals for cardiac MRI, and MRI is often requested for further evaluation of a mass or thrombus suspected but incompletely characterized on echocardiography.[50] Another frequent source of referrals is for evaluation of a possible pseudomass, with clarification desired as to the significance of this finding in question. Increasingly, however, CMR imaging incidentally detects intracardiac thrombus in patients scanned for other indications, such as the evaluation of myocardial function and viability in the setting of heart failure. In all of these instances, the superior tissue characterization and high-resolution imaging capable with MR usually provide a definitive evaluation.

Pseudomasses

Any discussion of cardiac masses or thrombus should first begin with a discussion of lesions that can mimic a significant cardiac mass. The most common of these entities is the right atrial pseudotumor produced by a prominent crista terminalis (**Fig. 9**A), which can be mistaken for a right atrial mass or thrombus on echocardiography. A prominent Chiari network also can be mistaken for a right atrial mass, as can a prominent

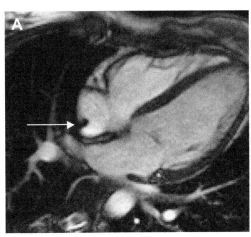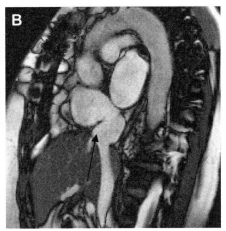

Fig. 9. (*A*) Still-frame cine image demonstrates a prominent crista terminalis (*arrow*) producing a right atrial pseudomass. (*B*) Arrow denotes the Eustachian valve in another patient on a short-axis view at the level of the interatrial septum.

Eustachian valve (see **Fig. 9**B). All of these normal structures can be well visualized on MR and a true mass excluded.[51] Of note, these pseudomasses obviously do not show abnormal enhancement on delayed enhancement MR.

Intracardiac Thrombus

Although not a neoplasm, thrombus is actually the most common cardiac "mass." Thrombi occur in a wide variety of clinical circumstances, but there is usually an underlying disorder or circumstance that predisposes a patient to its formation. For example, atrial fibrillation predisposes the patient to the formation of left atrial thrombi, particularly involving the left atrial appendage, whereas central venous catheters are associated with the development of right atrial thrombi.[52] Patients who have heart failure are known to be at increased risk for the development of ventricular thrombi, with a recent study indicating a prevalence of 7% in an unselected population of 784 patients with reduced systolic function (left ventricular ejection fraction < 50%).[12] That study also indicated that patients with ischemic cardiomyopathy were at an approximately fourfold greater risk of developing thrombi than patients with similar levels of systolic dysfunction because of nonischemic cardiomyopathy. Importantly, the authors noted that the presence of areas demonstrating more than 50% transmural infarction on delayed enhancement imaging was also an independent risk factor for thrombus development, information only available with DE-CMR. Clinically, it is frequently noted that ventricular thrombi are found adherent to sites of prior infarction, where wall motion abnormalities and denudation of the endothelium produced by prior infarction result in a nidus for thrombus formation (**Fig. 10**A, B). In particular, thrombi are often noted along the endocavitary aspect of ventricular aneurysms (see **Fig. 10**C, D).

Imaging Evaluation

Currently, echocardiography is often chosen as the initial imaging modality for the detection of intracardiac thrombus. Echocardiography has been shown to be significantly less sensitive than cardiac MRI for the detection of ventricular thrombus, however. Several studies have demonstrated an approximately twofold increase in sensitivity for the detection of ventricular thrombus when comparison is made with echocardiography.[53–55] For example, in the study by Srichai and colleagues,[54] the sensitivity and specificity of CMR for the diagnosis of ventricular thrombus was compared with transthoracic echocardiography and transesophageal echocardiography (TEE) in 361 patients with ischemic heart disease scheduled for ventricular reconstructive surgery. Of these, 160 patients underwent all three studies within 30 days of surgical/pathologic confirmation. The authors found that CMR (including cine and DE-CMR) was significantly more sensitive and specific (88% and 99%, respectively) than transthoracic echocardiography (23% and 96%, respectively) or TEE (40% and 96%, respectively).

Other authors have noted that the sensitivity of MRI for the detection of ventricular thrombus is significantly improved by the administration of intravenous contrast material (see **Fig. 10**C, D). For example, in the study by Weinsaft and colleagues[12] the authors noted that noncontrast cine MR

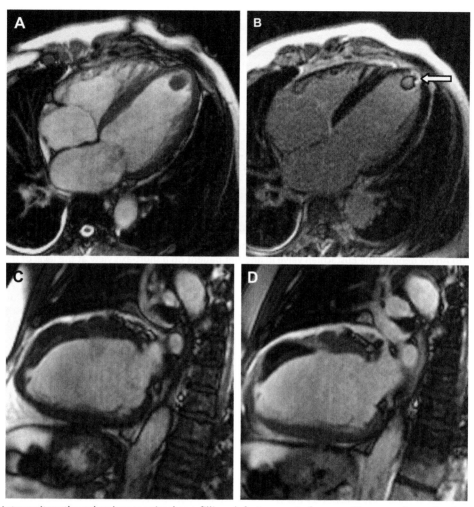

Fig. 10. Intracavitary thrombus is recognized as a filling defect separate from papillary muscles and trabeculae on the four-chamber cine view (*A*) and is noted on the delayed enhancement image (*B*) to be adherent to a site of previous apical infarction (*arrow*). Note that mural thrombus can be difficult to detect in the absence of contrast, as in this two-chamber cine view (*C*). After the administration of contrast, the anterior mural thrombus is readily detected (*D*).

detected only 40% of intraventricular thrombi that were subsequently detected with DE-CMR. Mollet and colleagues[53] also noted that precontrast cine imaging often failed to detect ventricular thrombi that were clearly seen as low-signal intensity foci after the administration of contrast. Weinsaft and colleagues[12] also noted that postcontrast delayed enhancement inversion recovery images with a long inversion time (600 msec) were often helpful in the characterization and delineation of thrombi. In this instance, the long inversion time allows recovery of signal by virtually all tissues except thrombus, which remains low in signal intensity and dark on imaging (**Fig. 11**A, B).

Only two small studies have evaluated the use of CMR for the detection of left atrial appendage thrombus—and with conflicting results. In the study

by Ohyama and colleagues,[56] double and triple inversion-recovery noncontrast sequences were used, and the results were compared with TEE. All cases of left atrial appendage thrombi by TEE were detected with CMR. There was one false-positive result on MR. Mohrs and colleagues,[57] however, found that CMR using a contrast-enhanced two-dimensional perfusion sequence, a contrast-enhanced three-dimensional gradient echo inversion recovery sequence, or the combination of both sequences failed to detect more than half of the left atrial appendage thrombi detected with TEE. Currently, the literature does not allow a definite determination of the relative merits of CMR compared with the standard of TEE for the detection of left atrial appendage thrombus. No studies have evaluated the improved sensitivity of

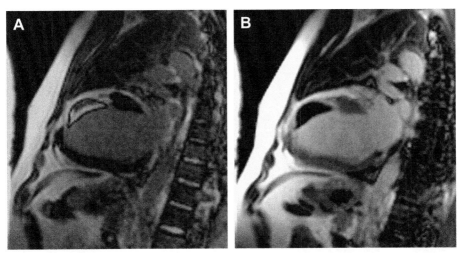

Fig. 11. Two-chamber single-shot delayed enhancement images with inversion times of 300 msec (*A*) and 600 msec (*B*) demonstrate a mural thrombus adherent to an anterior wall infarct. Note that on (*A*), where the inversion time was chosen to null the signal from myocardium, the thrombus has a dark rim surrounding a bright center, whereas on (*B*) the thrombus is uniformly dark. See the accompanying text for explanation of this finding.

the delayed enhancement technique for the detection of left atrial thrombi. One could reasonably speculate that a comprehensive combination of dark-blood double inversion recovery (HASTE) sequences, two-dimensional perfusion sequences during the administration of contrast, postcontrast echocardiographic-triggered angiographic datasets, and DE-CMR using a standard (250–350 msec) and long (600 msec) inversion time might have a sensitivity and specificity rivaling that of transesophageal echo (**Fig. 12**A–D).

Magnetic Resonance Findings

Cine MR images demonstrate ventricular thrombus as having a low signal on b-SSFP cine images, similar to normal myocardium. Thrombus is then recognized when it presents as an intracavitary filling defect that is discernible from adjacent trabeculations and papillary muscles (see **Fig. 10**A, B). Recognition of mural thrombus, however, can be difficult on noncontrast cine images and likely accounts for the lower sensitivity of cine CMR relative to contrast-enhanced CMR (see **Fig. 10**C, D). There are currently no reports of the sensitivity of postcontrast cine imaging for thrombus detection.

Dark-blood static morphologic sequences, such as the double-inversion HASTE sequence, may show thrombus as a focal high-signal intracavitary lesion but are relatively insensitive, with a sensitivity of 46%, as reported by Barkhausen and colleagues.[55] Because they are avascular, thrombi do not show contrast uptake on perfusion

sequences and usually appear as dark foci bordering the endocardium.

The delayed enhancement (DE-CMR) sequence is the most sensitive sequence for the depiction of thrombus. Thrombus usually appears as a dark intracavitary or mural filling defect, often attached to foci of hyperenhanced, infarcted myocardium (see **Fig. 10**B). The segmented inversion-recovery delayed enhancement sequence is the imaging standard and has a typical spatial resolution of 1.3 mm × 1.6 mm × 6 mm. In patients with arrhythmia or limited ability to cooperate with breath holding, a newer single-shot b-SSFP inversion recovery sequence is available from some vendors and is resistant to degradation from arrhythmia or breathing artifact. Although of slightly lower spatial resolution, this sequence allows rapid coverage in multiple planes, even in the most uncooperative patients or patients who have arrythmia.

Although thrombi usually are low in signal intensity on DE-CMR obtained with an inversion time chosen to null normal myocardium, not infrequently they may show a black border with central higher signal, which results in an "etched" appearance. This appearance may lead to some confusion. It is likely caused by the fact that thrombus has no contrast uptake and has a long T1 value such that following an inversion pulse it remains far below the zero-crossing line at the time point where normal myocardium is at the zero-crossing point (see **Fig. 11**A). Because the standard inversion recovery sequence is sensitive only to magnitude and not to phase, it seems to have "positive"

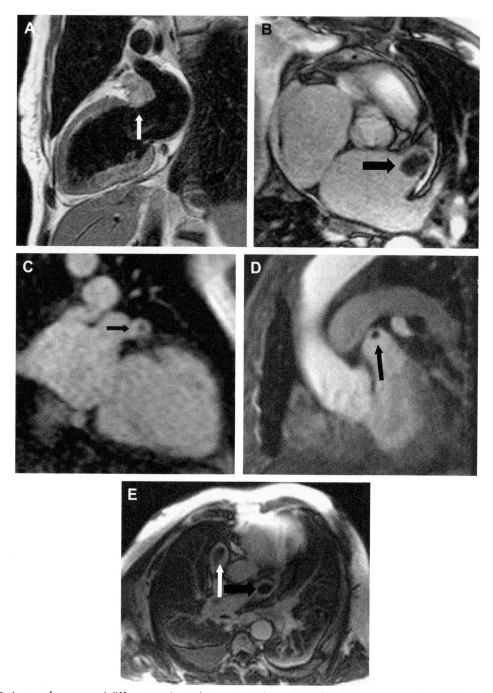

Fig. 12. Images from several different patients demonstrate the variety of techniques currently available with MR for the detection of left atrial appendage thrombus (*arrows*). T2-weighted spin-echo two-chamber view (*A*), cine b-SSFP image in the aortic valve plane (*B*), two-chamber perfusion image (*C*), sagittal MR angiographic image (*D*), and axial single-shot delayed enhancement image (*E*) demonstrate thrombi in the left atrial appendage. Right atrial appendage thrombus also is noted in (*E*) (*white arrow*).

or bright signal. Acquiring the image at a later time point, such as an inversion time of 600 msec, allows the thrombus to recover longitudinal magnetization and arrive at or approach the zero-crossing point, whereas normal myocardium and infarct have recovered above the zero-crossing and are light gray in signal intensity (see **Fig. 11**B). If there is any confusion regarding the signal characteristics of a suspected thrombus, repeating the inversion recovery

DE-CMR sequence with a long inversion time (600 msec) is suggested. This same long-inversion recovery variation of DE-CMR can be acquired using a single-shot b-SSFP sequence in multiple planes to rapidly screen for thrombus, even in the most uncooperative patients or patients who have arrhythmia.

Differential Diagnosis

The differential diagnosis of thrombus includes other intracavitary lesions, primarily myxomas. Although they occasionally can present a diagnostic dilemma, usually characteristic imaging findings provide accurate differentiation. For instance, myxomas are located in the left atrium in approximately 75% of cases and are usually attached to the fossa ovalis. Approximately 15 to 20% of myxomas arise in the right atrium, with a small percentage extending across the fossa ovalis to involve both atria. They are rare in the ventricles (< 2% of cases). Importantly, the signal characteristics are usually different from thrombus. Specifically, on b-SSFP cine imaging, myxomas often demonstrate high signal intensity because of their gelatinous composition (**Fig. 13**A). In contrast, thrombus is dark on b-SSFP cine imaging, with signal intensity similar to normal myocardium (see **Fig. 13**B). Myxomas usually demonstrate heterogenous enhancement on DE-CMR rather than the low signal seen with thrombus. DE-CMR and perfusion imaging of myxomas may demonstrate an enhancing stalk, a finding not seen with thrombus.[58]

KEY POINTS

- MRI is superior to echocardiography and CT in the comprehensive evaluation of pericardial disease and intracardiac thrombus.
- In the modern MR examination, the older spin-echo morphologic sequences have been replaced by single-shot double inversion recovery sequences (eg, HASTE) for dark-blood imaging, and SSFP cine imaging has replaced gradient-echo techniques.
- Improved tissue characterization is provided by the combination of perfusion and delayed enhancement imaging.
- Pericardial effusions and thickening, whether global or localized, can be well depicted with MR.
- In addition to imaging the anatomic abnormality present in constrictive pericarditis, MR with real-time cine imaging can demonstrate the pathologic hemodynamics.
- Thrombus is the most common cardiac "mass," and MR detects twice as many as echocardiography.
- Single-shot delayed enhancement images with a long inversion time (600 msec) can be used even in uncooperative patients to screen rapidly for thrombus.

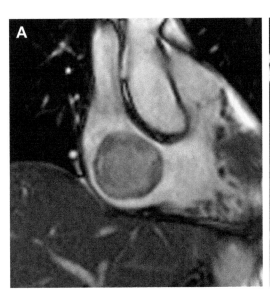
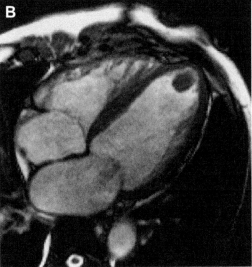

Fig. 13. Still-frame b-SSFP cine images of a two-chamber right ventricular view of a right atrial myxoma (*A*) and a four-chamber view of a left ventricular thrombus (*B*). Note the relatively high signal intensity of the myxoma on b-SSFP cine imaging indicative of its gelatinous composition, whereas the thrombus is isointense to myocardium.

ACKNOWLEDGMENTS

The author wishes to thank Ms. Fi Fi LeBlanc for her invaluable secretarial assistance and Dr. Sarah Joyner for her helpful suggestions.

REFERENCES

1. Gulati G, Sharma S, Kothari SS, et al. Comparison of echo and MRI in the imaging evaluation of intracardiac masses. Cardiovasc Intervent Radiol 2004; 27(5):459–69.
2. Shuman WP, Branch KR, May JM, et al. Prospective versus retrospective ECG gating for 64-detector CT of the coronary arteries: comparison of image quality and patient radiation dose. Radiology 2008;248(2): 431–7.
3. Semelka RC, Shoenut JP, Wilson ME, et al. Cardiac masses: signal intensity features on spin-echo, gradient-echo, gadolinium-enhanced spin-echo, and TurboFLASH images. J Magn Reson Imaging 1992;2(4):415–20.
4. Hoffmann U, Globits S, Schima W, et al. Usefulness of magnetic resonance imaging of cardiac and paracardiac masses. Am J Cardiol 2003;92(7):890–5.
5. Pereles FS, Kapoor V, Carr JC, et al. Usefulness of segmented trueFISP cardiac pulse sequence in evaluation of congenital and acquired adult cardiac abnormalities. AJR Am J Roentgenol 2001;177(5): 1155–60.
6. Simonetti OP, Kim RJ, Fieno DS, et al. An improved MR imaging technique for the visualization of myocardial infarction. Radiology 2001;218(1):215–23.
7. Fuster V, Kim RJ. Frontiers in cardiovascular magnetic resonance. Circulation 2005;112(1): 135–44.
8. Kuhl HP, Spuentrup E, Wall A, et al. Assessment of myocardial function with interactive non-breath-hold real-time MR imaging: comparison with echocardiography and breath-hold Cine MR imaging. Radiology 2004;231(1):198–207.
9. Reichek N. MRI myocardial tagging. J Magn Reson Imaging 1999;10(5):609–16.
10. Sievers B, Elliott MD, Hurwitz LM, et al. Rapid detection of myocardial infarction by subsecond, free-breathing delayed contrast-enhancement cardiovascular magnetic resonance. Circulation 2007;115(2):236–44.
11. Huber A, Schoenberg SO, Spannagl B, et al. Single-shot inversion recovery TrueFISP for assessment of myocardial infarction. AJR Am J Roentgenol 2006; 186(3):627–33.
12. Weinsaft JW, Kim HW, Shah DJ, et al. Detection of left ventricular thrombus by delayed-enhancement cardiovascular magnetic resonance prevalence and markers in patients with systolic dysfunction. J Am Coll Cardiol 2008;52(2):148–57.
13. Sechtem U, Tscholakoff D, Higgins CB. MRI of the normal pericardium. Part I. AJR Am J Roentgenol 1986;147(2):239–44.
14. Sechtem U, Tscholakoff D, Higgins CB. MRI of the abnormal pericardium. Part II. AJR Am J Roentgenol 1986;147(2):245–52.
15. Teraoka K, Hirano M, Yannbe M, et al. Delayed contrast enhancement in a patient with perimyocarditis on contrast-enhanced cardiac MRI: case report. Int J Cardiovasc Imaging 2005;21(2–3): 325–9.
16. Rienmuller R, Groll R, Lipton MJ. CT and MR imaging of pericardial disease. Radiol Clin North Am 2004; 42(3):587–601, vi.
17. Breen JF. Imaging of the pericardium. J Thorac Imaging 2001;16(1):47–54.
18. White CS. MR evaluation of the pericardium. Top Magn Reson Imaging 1995;7(4):258–66.
19. Kastler B, Germain P, Dietemann JL, et al. Spin echo MRI in the evaluation of pericardial disease. Comput Med Imaging Graph 1990;14(4):241–7.
20. Wang ZJ, Reddy GP, Gotway MB, et al. CT and MR imaging of pericardial disease. Spec No. Radiographics 2003;23:S167–80.
21. Glockner JF. Imaging of pericardial disease. Magn Reson Imaging Clin N Am 2003;11(1):149–62, vii.
22. Frank H, Globits S. Magnetic resonance imaging evaluation of myocardial and pericardial disease. J Magn Reson Imaging 1999;10(5):617–26.
23. Refsum H, Junemann M, Lipton MJ, et al. Ventricular diastolic pressure-volume relations and the pericardium: effects of changes in blood volume and pericardial effusion in dogs. Circulation 1981;64(5): 997–1004.
24. Freeman GL, LeWinter MM. Pericardial adaptations during chronic cardiac dilation in dogs. Circ Res 1984;54(3):294–300.
25. Freeman GL, LeWinter MM. Determinants of intrapericardial pressure in dogs. J Appl Phys 1986; 60(3):758–64.
26. Little WC, Freeman GL. Pericardial disease. Circulation 2006;113(12):1622–32.
27. Tsang TS, Oh JK, Seward JB. Diagnosis and management of cardiac tamponade in the era of echocardiography. Clin Cardiol 1999;22(7):446–52.
28. Tsang TS, Barnes ME, Hayes SN, et al. Clinical and echocardiographic characteristics of significant pericardial effusions following cardiothoracic surgery and outcomes of echo-guided pericardiocentesis for management: Mayo Clinic experience, 1979–1998. Chest 1999;116(2):322–31.
29. Singh S, Wann LS, Schuchard GH, et al. Right ventricular and right atrial collapse in patients with cardiac tamponade: a combined echocardiographic and hemodynamic study. Circulation 1984;70(6):966–71.
30. Appleton CP, Hatle LK, Popp RL. Cardiac tamponade and pericardial effusion: respiratory variation

in transvalvular flow velocities studied by Doppler echocardiography. J Am Coll Cardiol 1988;11(5): 1020–30.

31. Francone M, Dymarkowski S, Kalantzi M, et al. Real-time cine MRI of ventricular septal motion: a novel approach to assess ventricular coupling. J Magn Reson Imaging 2005;21(3):305–9.

32. Myers RB, Spodick DH. Constrictive pericarditis: clinical and pathophysiologic characteristics. Am Heart J 1999;138(2 Pt 1):219–32.

33. Ling LH, Oh JK, Schaff HV, et al. Constrictive pericarditis in the modern era: evolving clinical spectrum and impact on outcome after pericardiectomy. Circulation 1999;100(13):1380–6.

34. Ling LH, Oh JK, Breen JF, et al. Calcific constrictive pericarditis: is it still with us? Ann Intern Med 2000; 132(6):444–50.

35. Nishimura RA. Constrictive pericarditis in the modern era: a diagnostic dilemma. Heart 2001; 86(6):619–23.

36. Nishimura RA, Connolly DC, Parkin TW, et al. Constrictive pericarditis: assessment of current diagnostic procedures. Mayo Clin Proc 1985;60(6):397–401.

37. Oh KY, Shimizu M, Edwards WD, et al. Surgical pathology of the parietal pericardium: a study of 344 cases (1993–1999). Cardiovasc Pathol 2001; 10(4):157–68.

38. Talreja DR, Edwards WD, Danielson GK, et al. Constrictive pericarditis in 26 patients with histologically normal pericardial thickness. Circulation 2003; 108(15):1852–7.

39. Mertens LL, Denef B, De Geest H. The differentiation between restrictive cardiomyopathy and constrictive pericarditis: the impact of the imaging techniques. Echocardiography 1993;10(5):497–508.

40. Masui T, Finck S, Higgins CB. Constrictive pericarditis and restrictive cardiomyopathy: evaluation with MR imaging. Radiology 1992;182(2):369–73.

41. Sengupta PP, Mohan JC, Mehta V, et al. Accuracy and pitfalls of early diastolic motion of the mitral annulus for diagnosing constrictive pericarditis by tissue Doppler imaging. Am J Cardiol 2004;93(7):886–90.

42. Giorgi B, Mollet NR, Dymarkowski S, et al. Clinically suspected constrictive pericarditis: MR imaging assessment of ventricular septal motion and configuration in patients and healthy subjects. Radiology 2003;228(2):417–24.

43. Hancock EW. A clearer view of effusive-constrictive pericarditis. N Engl J Med 2004;350(5):435–7.

44. Hancock EW. Subacute effusive-constrictive pericarditis. Circulation 1971;43(2):183–92.

45. Yamano T, Sawada T, Sakamoto K, et al. Magnetic resonance imaging differentiated partial from complete absence of the left pericardium in a case of leftward displacement of the heart. Circ J 2004; 68(4):385–8.

46. Faridah Y, Julsrud PR. Congenital absence of pericardium revisited. Int J Cardiovasc Imaging 2002; 18(1):67–73.

47. Oyama N, Oyama N, Komuro K, et al. Computed tomography and magnetic resonance imaging of the pericardium: anatomy and pathology. Magn Reson Med Sci 2004;3(3):145–52.

48. Vander Salm TJ. Unusual primary tumors of the heart. Semin Thorac Cardiovasc Surg 2000;12(2): 89–100.

49. Gilkeson RC, Chiles C. MR evaluation of cardiac and pericardial malignancy. Magn Reson Imaging Clin N Am 2003;11(1):173–86, viii.

50. Link KM, Lesko NM. MR evaluation of cardiac/juxta-cardiac masses. Top Magn Reson Imaging 1995; 7(4):232–45.

51. Meier RA, Hartnell GG. MRI of right atrial pseudo-mass: is it really a diagnostic problem? J Comput Assist Tomogr 1994;18(3):398–401.

52. Kingdon EJ, Holt SG, Davar J, et al. Atrial thrombus and central venous dialysis catheters. Am J Kidney Dis 2001;38(3):631–9.

53. Mollet NR, Dymarkowski S, Volders W, et al. Visualization of ventricular thrombi with contrast-enhanced magnetic resonance imaging in patients with ischemic heart disease. Circulation 2002;106(23): 2873–6.

54. Srichai MB, Junor C, Rodriguez LL, et al. Clinical, imaging, and pathological characteristics of left ventricular thrombus: a comparison of contrast-enhanced magnetic resonance imaging, transthoracic echocardiography, and transesophageal echocardiography with surgical or pathological validation. Am Heart J 2006;152(1):75–84.

55. Barkhausen J, Hunold P, Eggebrecht H, et al. Detection and characterization of intracardiac thrombi on MR imaging. AJR Am J Roentgenol 2002;179(6): 1539–44.

56. Ohyama H, Hosomi N, Takahashi T, et al. Comparison of magnetic resonance imaging and transesophageal echocardiography in detection of thrombus in the left atrial appendage. Stroke 2003; 34:2436–9.

57. Mohrs OK, Nowak B, Petersen SE, et al. Thrombus detection in the left atrial appendage using contrast-enhanced MRI: a pilot study. AJR Am J Roentgenol 2006;186(1):198–205.

58. Grizzard JD, Ang GB. Magnetic resonance imaging of pericardial disease and cardiac masses. Cardiol Clin 2007;25(1):111–40, vi.

Expanding Role of Cardiovascular Magnetic Resonance in Left and Right Ventricular Diastolic Function

Vikas K. Rathi, MD, FACC*, Robert W.W. Biederman, MD, FACC

KEYWORDS

- Diastolic function • Left ventricle • Right ventricle
- Congestive heart failure
- Cardiovascular magnetic resonance

One of the most important prognostic variables in clinical cardiology is left ventricular functional status. As dynamic pumping chambers, the left and right ventricles undergo contraction, termed *systole*, and relaxation, termed *diastole*, and their performance is termed *systolic function* and *diastolic function* respectively. Numerous investigators, using tools ranging from microscopes to various invasive and noninvasive methodologies, have advanced our understanding of ventricular function and have established that ventricular systolic and diastolic function are equally important for the heart to work efficiently.[1–3] The earliest accounts of congestive heart failure, which included systolic and diastolic ventricular function, come from Fishberg[4] over 70 years ago. Fishberg described the two forms of heart failure as hypo-diastolic and hyposystolic failure. Since the era of Fishberg, the incidence and prevalence of heart failure have increased exponentially. According to statistics from the American Heart Association, the prevalence in 2005 of congestive heart failure in adults age 20 and older was 5.3 million. Half of those adults had pure diastolic heart failure.[5] The estimated direct and indirect cost of congestive heart failure in the United States for 2008 was $34.8 billion.[5] Despite such vast prevalence and socioeconomic burden of diastolic heart failure, numerous impediments have stood in the way of

appropriate management. These impediments include controversies over the definition of diastolic heart failure and misunderstanding about diastolic dysfunction and diagnosis of diastolic heart failure. Thanks to efforts of some established investigators, a consensus has emerged on the definition of diastolic heart failure. At the same time, we have now come to better understand the mechanisms and diagnosis of the diastolic heart failure, including those mechanisms associated with cell biology and how they relate to the hemodynamics of diastolic heart failure.[6–9]

DEFINITION OF DIASTOLIC HEART FAILURE

Recent literature gives various definitions of diastolic heart failure, but the one most commonly used is that offered in the Consensus Statement on the Diagnosis of Diastolic Heart Failure with Normal Left Ventricular Ejection Function.[10] The three main elements of this definition are (1) presence of signs or symptoms of congestive heart failure, (2) presence of normal or mildly abnormal left ventricular systolic function, and (3) evidence of left ventricular diastolic dysfunction. While the signs and symptoms are clinical markers of the heart failure, the left ventricular diastolic dysfunction is a laboratory marker assessed by various diagnostic modalities.

Allegheny General Hospital, Pittsburgh, PA, USA
* Corresponding author. Center for Cardiovascular MRI, Division of Cardiology, Gerald McGinnis Cardiovascular Institute, Allegheny General Hospital, 320 E North Avenue, Pittsburgh, PA 15237.
E-mail address: vrathi@wpahs.org (V.K. Rathi).

Heart Failure Clin 5 (2009) 421–435
doi:10.1016/j.hfc.2009.02.005

Currently, our understanding of the diastole is incomplete, with explanations that are innumerable and complex. More problematic is the lack of proven therapeutic strategies, further impeding development of advanced diagnostic techniques as the perception exists that "diagnosis without therapy is not warranted." It is understood that normal diastole represents a complex interplay of factors, including left ventricular relaxation, diastolic suction, viscoelastic forces in the myocardium, ventricular interaction, atrial booster contribution, chronotropy, preload, and afterload. Additionally, these factors are themselves affected by additional factors, including the pericardium and intrathoracic pressures. Most of these factors relate to one or both of two biomechanical phenomena: (1) left ventricular relaxation and (2) left ventricular compliance.[6,8,9,11] Therefore, any diagnostic study for diastolic heart failure should incorporate thorough evaluation of parameters as they relate to ventricular relaxation and compliance or stiffness.

For mainstream and routine diagnosis and follow-up of the diastolic heart failure, clinicians need a noninvasive technique for gathering accurate, reproducible, and reliable diastolic function data along with various other functional data, such as systolic function, valvular function, and myopericardial interaction. In the quest to understand the pathophysiology of diastolic heart failure, various investigators have proposed various theories and have published findings regarding ventricular remodeling. Recent studies have shown that patients with isolated diastolic heart failure with preserved systolic function have an increased left ventricular end-diastolic volume, increased left ventricular end-diastolic long-axis dimension, and eccentric geometry.[12,13] These interesting results are contrary to the traditional understanding that in diastolic heart failure left ventricular remodeling is characterized by normal left ventricular end-diastolic volume, increased left ventricular mass, increased relative wall thickness, and concentric geometry.[14,15] However, these recent studies have relied almost exclusively on two-dimensional (2D) echocardiography. The use of comprehensive three-dimensional (3D) imaging techniques is apparently needed. Such techniques can provide accurate and reliable information on diastolic function, including precise volumetric data, to improve our fundamental understanding of the pathophysiology of underlying heart failure.

The increasing acceptance and continued developments in the field of cardiovascular magnetic resonance (CMR) has given us the opportunity to gain all necessary anatomic and physiologic information necessary to establish an accurate diagnosis and gain a solid physiologic understanding of diastolic perturbations. This article specifically focuses on the role of CMR, in contrast to various other diagnostic imaging modalities, in understanding the physiology of diastolic function, and on the future applications of CMR as they relate to diastolic function evaluation.

INVASIVE DIAGNOSIS OF DIASTOLIC DYSFUNCTION

The most rigorous assessment of diastolic function for humans is invasive and uses a high-fidelity micromanometer placed in the left ventricle to measure the isovolumic relaxation time (IVRT) and rate of pressure decay during isovolumic relaxation.[16] The rate of pressure decay is described by the equation: $P(t) = P_0 e - t/T$, where $P(t)$ is the rate of pressure decay, P_0 is the left ventricular pressure at maximum derivative of pressure over time, t is the time after the onset of relaxation, and T is the time constant for the left ventricular pressure to decay to $1/e$ of its initial value.

This rate of pressure decay, referred to as *tau*, is the time it takes the left ventricle pressure to fall to approximately two thirds of its peak value. The left ventricular compliance can be assessed by pressure–volume loop constructs. As the compliance of the chamber decreases, the pressure–volume loop shifts upwards, indicating that for the same volume the diastolic pressure is high. While considered the gold standard for measuring rate of pressure decay, tau is not perfect. Its chief drawback is that it does not take into account the effect of transmyocardial pressure on the chamber, including the effect of transmyocardial pressure related to the pericardium and right ventricle. Also, measurement and interpretation of tau requires talent and expertise not always readily available. Furthermore, because it must be obtained from an invasive test, tau cannot be routinely assessed.

CARDIOVASCULAR MAGNETIC RESONANCE DIAGNOSIS OF DIASTOLIC FUNCTION

Left ventricular filling and compliance can be measured by variety of methods in CMR. The choice of which methods to use depends on whether the clinician is following a basic or complex strategy. The basic strategy, which is analogous to the use of single photon emission CT (SPECT) and echocardiography, calls for obtaining (1) ventricular time–volume curves, (2) mitral inflow velocities, (3) pulmonary vein flow, and (4) tissue Doppler. The complex strategies, which have no echocardiography equivalent, call for obtaining (1) the diastolic untwisting rate or torsion recovery rate and (2) the myocardial diastolic strain rate.

When first used to diagnose diastolic function, CMR was employed to measure change of volume over time. This role for CMR was quickly replaced by mitral and pulmonary vein flow velocity imaging. Parameters that are less load-dependent, such as mitral annular tissue imaging, have gained wide acceptance and considerable data exist regarding their diagnostic and prognostic value. Newer imaging principles, such as myocardial strain and torsion recovery rate, which directly relay information regarding myocardial relaxation, are described below.

Diastolic Time–Volume Relationship

The time–volume curve measures relative left ventricular volume change over time and has been used to measure ventricular filling rates by SPECT imaging. CMR, by gathering data on time-resolved 3D left ventricular volumes, can duplicate the measures of the curve.[17,18] Via CMR, the left ventricular endocardial borders are traced for each cardiac phase. These traces provide temporally resolved left ventricular volumes in systole and diastole.[19,20] These volumes can be plotted against time similar to those described in nuclear SPECT studies (**Fig. 1**). The parameters commonly described are peak filling rate and time to peak filling rate computed by fitting third-order polynomial functions to the systolic ejection and rapid diastolic filling portions of the time–volume curves. This method has two main disadvantages: (1) It does not provide any information regarding left ventricular filling characteristics and (2) it is only partially representative of compliance because it is unable to distinguish between contributions from the right ventricle and contributions from the pericardium. This method is rarely used anymore in the diagnosis of diastolic function.

Magnetic Resonance Velocity Imaging

Similar to color Doppler on echocardiography, phase contrast (PC) imaging enables clinicians to use CMR to obtain mitral valve inflow and pulmonary vein flow velocity profiles. CMR-PC imaging is highly reproducible and accurate, and can be routinely used in clinical CMR imaging. In CMR-PC, the spin phase data are used to measure the velocity of a moving structure. A range of velocities can be encoded on the order of 1 mm/s to 11 m/s. The velocity data can be used to calculate pressure gradients using the modified Bernoulli equation ($4V^2$). PC overcomes the majority of the technical limitations of Doppler, such as beam angle, eccentric flows, and multiple velocity directions. Most importantly, in contradistinction to color Doppler echocardiography, CMR-PC can acquire the three direction velocity profiles across the 2D cross section of the imaging plane, whereas Doppler only provides velocity profile across a single line ("icepick"). The precision of CMR-PC for blood flow and velocity measurements has been evaluated in both in vitro and in vivo studies. Chatzimavroudis and colleagues[21] studied both steady flow and pulsatile flow in vitro in an aortic phantom as well as in vivo in aortic regurgitation patients and normal volunteers. The investigators achieved excellent correlation ($r^2 = 0.99$).

CMR-PC interrogation of mitral and pulmonary vein flow velocity information can be used to classify various grades of diastolic dysfunction similar to that described using color Doppler in echocardiography. The principles of CMR-PC can also be applied for the assessment of myocardial velocities similar to tissue Doppler imaging of the myocardium using color Doppler. Furthermore, myocardial tissue tagging, which is unique to CMR, provides high-resolution 3D assessment of myocardial strain rate and rate of torsion recovery (untwisting), which can be used for gaining incremental information on myocardial compliance.

Mitral and pulmonary vein phase velocity imaging

Employed in a way similar to 2D color Doppler echocardiography, CMR-PC has been used in a limited fashion to survey diastolic mitral and pulmonary venous flows. The initial study, by Mohiaddin and colleagues[22] in 1991 using normal controls and mitral stenosis patients, characterized flow velocities in diastole using CMR-PC. In this study, no direct comparison was made of CMR-PC mitral or pulmonary flow velocity to mitral or pulmonary flow velocity obtained by color Doppler. However, findings correlated with the historical data available from color Doppler of mitral and pulmonary veins. Hartiala and colleagues[23] in 1993 compared 2D color Doppler echocardiography and CMR-PC–derived mitral (early filling [E] and atrial systolic filling [A]) and pulmonary venous (systolic [S] and diastolic [D]) velocities. The mitral E and A velocities by CMR-PC 3D encoding were slightly lower than the Doppler-derived velocities, but linear correlation between the two modalities was excellent. Consequently the E/A and S/D ratios measured by these two methods showed significant linear correlations. These studies suffered from technical

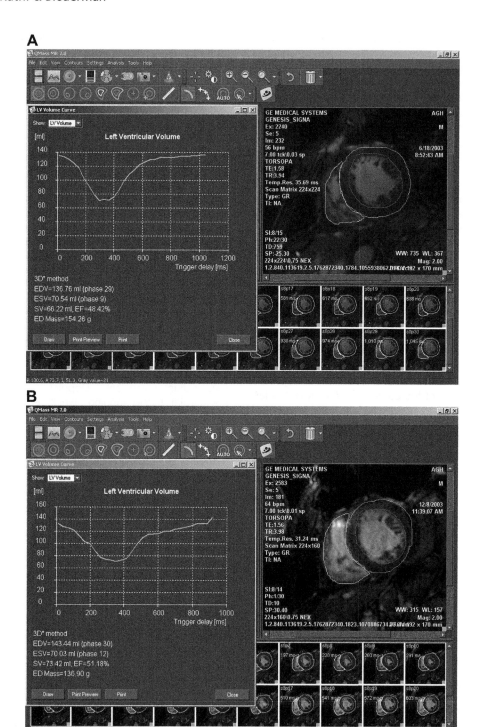

Fig. 1. This figure demonstrates the postprocessing of the 3D volumetric data and analysis of the time–volume relationship (QMass MRI 7.0, Medis, The Netherlands). The CMR left ventricular endocardial borders are traced phase by phase for each slice to achieve time-resolved volumetric data. (*A*) The time–volume relationship pre–aortic valve replacement (AVR) demonstrate that diastolic dysfunction with peak filling rate (PFR) = 321 mL/s, PFR/EDV = 2.3 EDV/s, time to peak filling rate (TPFR) = 143 ms. The pre-AVR left ventricular ejection fraction (LVEF) = 48.42% and the left ventricular mass = 154 g. (*B*) The time–volume relationship 6 months post-AVR shows improvement in the diastolic filling parameters: PFR = 394 mL/s; PFR/EDV = 2.7 EDV/s; and TPFR = 94 ms. The post-AVR LVEF and left ventricular mass had also improved to 52% and 136 g respectively. ESV, end-systolic volume; SV, systolic volume; ED mass, end-diastolic mass.

limitations, such as low field-strength magnets and temporal resolution for CMR-PC of only 16 phases per cardiac cycle. These limitations meant that 256 cycles were required to complete the data set and investigators were unable to assess the E-wave deceleration time and IVRT. Also, each CMR-PC data set took 5 minutes to acquire and images were obtained in vertical or horizontal long-axis modes, which are not optimal for 3D assessment of mitral or pulmonary vein velocities. Similar studies were performed by Karwatowski and colleagues[24] using CMR-PC evaluation of mitral inflow in patients with ischemic heart disease to assess left ventricular diastolic function. The E velocities by CMR-PC (60.1 ± 14.3 cm/s) correlated with the Doppler velocities (59.4 ± 13.7 cm/s; P not significant). However, the A velocities were underestimated by the CMR-PC (51 ± 14.6 cm/s versus 62 ± 17.2 cm/s; P = .002). In this study, the pulmonary vein velocities were not measured.

The recent study by Rathi and colleagues[25] for the first time demonstrates the direct correlation of CMR-PC mitral and pulmonary vein diastolic function parameters with those of color Doppler in a variety of diastolic dysfunction patients. A total of 31 subjects (21 male and 10 female) were studied. These subjects included 21 patients with mean age of 60 years (± 14 years) and 10 controls with mean age of 33 years (± 9 years). The E and A velocities measured by CMR-PC correlated well with Doppler (r = 0.81; $P<.001$), but demonstrated a systematic underestimation by CMR-PC compared with Doppler (slope = 0.77). Bland-Altman analysis of E/A and deceleration time calculated from each modality showed excellent agreement (bias −0.29 and −10.3 ms for E/A and deceleration time, respectively). When assessing morphology using echocardiography, CMR correctly identified all patients as having normal or abnormal inflow conditions. Morphologic identification based on the mitral inflow patterns (normal, impaired relaxation, pseudonormal, and restrictive) attained 100% agreement between CMR and echocardiography (**Fig. 2**). Moreover, this step added an average only of 4 minutes to the total patient imaging time. This cardinal study establishes the present utility and current accuracy for the assessment of diastolic function as a routine practice for CMR similar to the most echocardiographic laboratories across the world.

Research conducted at various centers, including ours, has addressed several limitations associated with conventional CMR-PC techniques available on standard CMR scanners. Newer techniques, such as the block regional interpolation scheme of k-space (BRISK), developed at our center, incorporate rarified sampling of the k-space, thereby decreasing scan time on the order of two- to four-fold, while maintaining signal to noise ratio, spatial resolution and temporal resolution of conventional CMR-PC techniques.[26] The BRISK sequences can be applied to CMR-PC techniques to acquire flow data within a single breath-hold of 15 to 17 seconds. Flow studies comparing conventional CMR-PC techniques with BRISK CMR-PC techniques have been performed at our laboratory on phantom with excellent correlation (r = 0.98–0.99).[27] Moreover these BRISK sequences are easily ported into conventional scanners, requiring no hardware upgrades as they rely only on software modifications.

All experienced centers now routinely acquire basic diastolic function information when necessary by using the CMR-PC technique. The diastolic function assessment can now be routinely used for follow-up evaluation and surveillance (**Fig. 3**). **Box 1** describes a step-by-step approach for acquiring mitral and pulmonary vein flow velocities by CMR.

Myocardial tissue velocity imaging

In an application similar to flow velocity acquisition, CMR-PC can be used to evaluate in vivo myocardial motion velocity. In this role, CMR-PC can perform similar to myocardial tissue Doppler imaging by echocardiography (**Fig. 4**). The inherent advantage of CMR-PC is the ability to acquire images in multiple oblique planes, allowing the operator to choose in-plane or through-plane velocity acquisitions. Karwatowski and colleagues,[28] in their first attempts to obtain myocardial motion velocities, studied the regional myocardial velocities using CMR-PC in three groups of patients: 26 with myocardial infarction, 21 with coronary artery disease but no infarction, and 19 normal subjects. Investigators reported significantly lower maximal early diastolic myocardial velocities in myocardial infarction patients compared with patients with coronary artery disease but without infarction and compared with normal subjects. In another study, Karwatowski and colleagues[29] compared left ventricular diastolic myocardial velocities by CMR-PC with left ventricular filling velocities measured by color Doppler echocardiography and showed that the onset of diastolic long-axis velocity preceded flow across the mitral valve by a mean of 46 ms and the maximal myocardial long-axis velocity correlated with peak early filling velocity (r = 0.56; $P<.01$), early deceleration rate (r = −0.63; $P<.001$) and E/A (r = 0.53, $P<.01$). Similarly the mean myocardial long-axis velocity also correlated with the mitral inflow parameters.

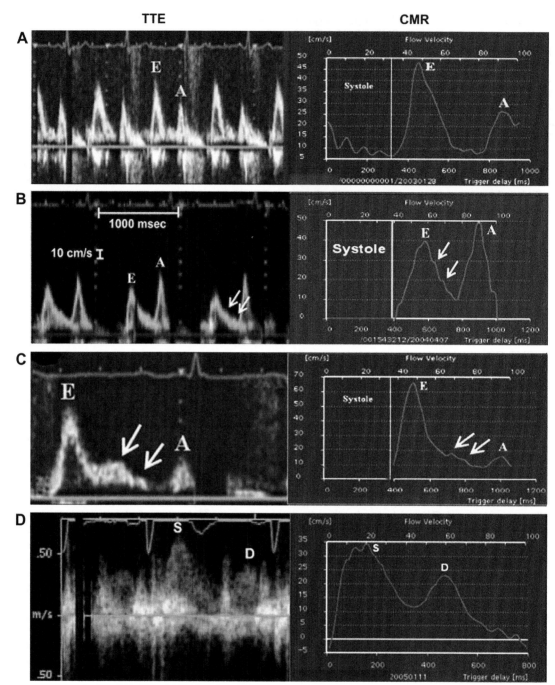

Fig. 2. Morphologic representation of velocities obtained by transthoracic echocardiogram (TTE) and CMR-PC. Note comparability between TTE and CMR-PC representation of E and A waves with respect to their magnitude and temporal presentation in diastole. The x-axis of the TTE panel is labeled on panel B figure and was calibrated to 1000 ms between two vertical dotted lines for all patients. The y-axis is represented by the smaller distance between the dots of the vertical dotted lines and was calibrated to 10 cm/s for all patients. The y-axis calibration for pulmonary vein flow (*D*) was different from the transmitral flow and is shown on the image. However, the x-axis calibration was similar. Panel A demonstrates normal E/A and deceleration time. Panel B shows impaired relaxation with prolonged deceleration time and a high A wave. Panel C demonstrates a restrictive pattern with short deceleration time and an elevated E/A. Note diastasis points (*arrows*) illustrating the similarities in depiction of flow features. In panel D, the flow velocity profile obtained by CMR of the right superior pulmonary vein is similar to that obtained with TTE (S and D are the systolic and diastolic waves of the pulmonary vein). (*From* Rathi VK, Doyle M, Yamrozik J, et al. Routine evaluation of left ventricular diastolic function by cardiovascular magnetic resonance: a practical approach. J Cardiovasc Magn Reson 2008 Jul 8;10(1):36; with permission.)

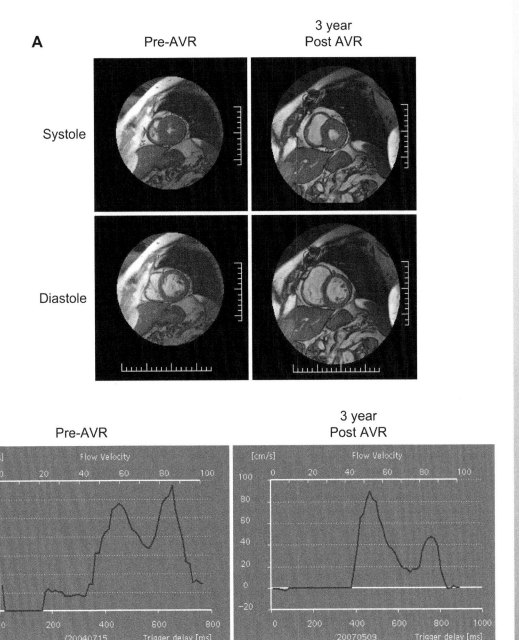

Fig. 3. This figure demonstrates the clinical utility of obtaining diastolic function data by CMR. The left ventricular short-axis images pre-AVR and 3-year post-AVR show regression of left ventricular hypertrophy as shown in diastole of panel A. Panel B shows corresponding improvement in the diastolic function assessed by CMR-PC of the mitral valve inflow. The pre-AVR impaired relaxation with E/A less than 1 has improved at 3-year post-AVR to more normal E/A of greater than 1 corresponding with decline in left ventricular hypertrophy.

In a more recent study, Paelinck and colleagues[30] studied the feasibility of using CMR-PC for estimating pulmonary capillary wedge pressure (PCWP) by normalizing the mitral valve inflow E velocity with the mitral annular septal tissue velocity (E′). Eighteen patients with hypertensive heart disease and absence of valvular regurgitation, and with normal or mildly reduced systolic function referred for cardiac catheterization, underwent consecutive measurement of mitral flow and septal tissue velocities with CMR-PC and Doppler. The data collected was compared with PCWP. There was a strong relation between CMR-PC (11.6 ± 4.3) and Doppler-assessed (12.1 ± 3.5) E/E′ (95% CI of −1.5 to 0.5) (r = 0.89; P<.0001). On CMR-PC, (mean difference = −12.1 ± 25.7 cm/s with a 95% CI of −24.9 to 0.7; P = .063). For both techniques, correlations between invasive PCWP and E/E′ were strong (CMR-PC: r = 0.80; $P<.0001$. Doppler: r = 0.85; $P<.0001$). Furthermore in this study, E/E′ less than 8 had 100% positive predictive value for PCWP less than 15 mm Hg, and E/E′ greater than 15 had a 100% positive predictive value for PCWP greater than 15 mm Hg.

Myocardial Tissue Tagging for Diastolic Function

Ventricular filling, flow velocity, and myocardial velocity reflect diastolic function only indirectly. By comparison direct myocardial diastolic relaxation mechanics, such as left ventricular strain rate recovery and torsion recovery, directly reflect diastolic function. By tagging the myocardial tissue with radiofrequency tissue tags, the ventricular strain rate recovery and torsion recovery can be readily obtained. CMR tissue tagging has been shown to be robust, reproducible, and suitable for research applications when detailed interrogation of myocardial mechanics is necessary. Alternatives methods of obtaining this information are not clinically feasible, and involve myocardial implantation of tantalum markers, piezoelectric crystals, or angiographic tracking of the coronary artery bifurcations.

At ventricular systole, CMR radio-frequency tissue tags are applied in a regular grid to modulate the myocardial signal in a transmural and noninvasive manner (**Fig. 5**). As the heart contracts and relaxes, distortions of the grid permit direct measurements to be made of myocardial deformation.[31–34] These deformations can commonly be described using units of strain (%S) or torsion (degree).

Diastolic torsion recovery rate

The normal left ventricle builds up systolic compressive forces that, upon release, have been shown to enhance diastolic recoil, working through viscoelastic mechanisms in a process that has been termed *diastolic suction*.[35–37] Diastolic suction enhances mitral valve opening. It is suggested that this process relies heavily on release of systolic torsion, which is commonly termed *diastolic recoil* or *untwisting*.[38–40]

Left ventricular torsion is a process of ventricular contraction due to the obliquity of fiber orientation, resulting in a transmural shear force causing angular rotation (twisting) of the myocardium. Systolic torsion promotes a more complete ejection of blood from the left ventricle during systole. Compelling studies from Beyar and colleagues[41] and Rademakers and colleagues[32] suggest that

inferoseptal mitral annular velocities correlated most significantly with the Doppler annular velocities. As seen in prior reports, the mitral A wave velocities by the two techniques were closely related. However, the CMR-PC measurements had a tendency to underestimate A velocity

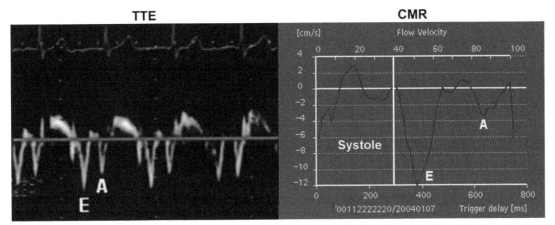

Fig. 4. Myocardial velocities at mitral annulus (septum) by tissue Doppler imaging correlate with those by CMR.

ventricular torsion may permit uniform distribution of systolic stresses across the myocardium, resulting in improved mechanical efficiency and reduced myocardial oxygen uptake. Diastolic recoil or torsion recovery occurs primarily in IVRT and before opening of the mitral valve.[32,35,42] The indices measured in late diastole, including mitral inflow, are subject to pseudonormalization due to left atrial pressure variation, thus confounding the understanding of the physiology and pathophysiology of left ventricular relaxation. The left ventricular recoil, or untwisting rate, being an intrinsic property of the myocardium and occurring primarily during IVRT, has been thought to be independent of such pseudonormalization. In their elegant study in dogs, which correlated the left ventricular untwisting rate with tau, Dong and colleagues[43] demonstrated that diastolic untwisting of normal myocardium begins even before aortic valve closure and is completed before mitral valve opening. The study concluded that the correlation between tau and the untwisting rate was high ($r = -0.86$) and was unaffected by elevated left atrial pressure and that tau was the only independent predictor of untwisting rate. Multiple regression showed that tau, but not left atrial or aortic pressure, was an independent predictor of untwisting rate ($P<.0001$, $P = .99$, and $P = .18$, respectively). Further, they showed that recoil was unrelated to left atrial pressure, aortic pressure, left ventricular pressure, or peak maximum derivative of pressure over time ($+dP/dt$).

Characterization of the diastolic recoil in diastolic dysfunction or diastolic heart failure patients has yet to be systematically explored. Limited studies in aortic stenosis have revealed that the diastolic torsion recovery is prolonged until the end of diastole in pathologic hypertrophy.[44,45] The normal left ventricle performs a systolic wringing motion around the ventricular long axis with clockwise rotation at the base ($-4.4 \pm 1.6°$) and counterclockwise rotation at the apex ($+6.8 \pm 2.5°$) when viewed from the apex. During early diastole, an untwisting motion preceding diastolic filling can be observed. In patients with aortic valve stenosis, systolic

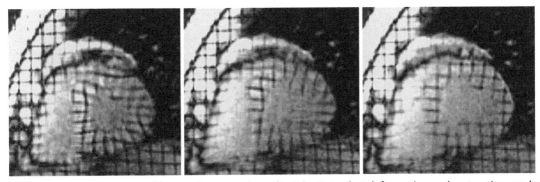

Fig. 5. Common k-space–tagged images from systole to diastole. Note that deformation and restoration can be easily seen and readily quantified.

rotation is reduced at the base ($-2.4 \pm 2.0°$; $P<0.01$) but increased at the apex ($+12.0 \pm 6.0°$; $P<0.05$). Diastolic untwisting is delayed and prolonged with a decrease in normalized rotation velocity (-6.9 ± 1.1 s^{-1}) when compared with controls (-10.7 ± 2.2 s^{-1}; $P<0.001$). Maximal systolic torsion is $8.0 \pm 2.1°$ in controls and $14.1 \pm 6.4°$ ($P<0.01$) in patients with aortic valve stenosis. An elegant study performed by Biederman and colleagues[46] on aortic stenosis patients looked at the change in myocardial strain and torsion pre– and post–aortic valve replacement (AVR) and the influence of coronary artery disease. The torsion data for 1 year post-AVR was available in 17 patients and showed that torsion was elevated pre-AVR and gradually normalized to normal range 1 year post-AVR (**Fig. 6**) in concert with regression of left ventricular mass and an increase in ejection fraction. This suggested that torsion and diastolic untwisting were compensatory properties to augment the fall in classic circumferential and radial myocardial strain, and were tightly governed by the left ventricle, normalizing once the underlying pathologic perturbation (afterload) was removed.

In summary, torsion in normal subjects is usually completed in the first third of diastole (corresponding to tau) but may be significantly delayed in patients with impaired relaxation progressing to restrictive physiology. The left ventricular untwisting rate, being independent of preload, will be prolonged in patients with impaired relaxation and restrictive physiology.

Diastolic strain rate

Deformation patterns based on circumferential or radial strain have not been used to comprehensively evaluate a wide variety of patients with diastolic dysfunction and have never been used to evaluate the right ventricle. To quantify regional strain, the complex 2D motion of the tagged left ventricle tissue is computed using a previously validated tag-detection algorithm that measures the initial position of the tags and their relative displacement as a function of the cardiac cycle. This data can be used to estimate the strain as a measure of underlying myocardial deformation at each point of the left ventricular myocardium. More recently, complex arithmetic and imaging techniques have been developed and validated to speed the acquisition and postprocessing such that a number of approaches can now be efficiently used.[47–50] We currently employ the harmonic phase method (**Fig. 7**) for all our analysis and find it reliable and user-friendly as well as time-sensitive. We formerly used the method of Young and colleagues[49,50] for much of our earlier analytical work. Limitations, however, exist in the current strategies for strain analysis in that typical myocardial tag density drops off exponentially as a function of time (myocardial T1 property) either limiting or negating diastolic assessments unless the sampling is specifically altered to obtain late cardiac cycle data. Currently, alternative strategies either at the vendor or the researcher level are required to completely assess both systole and diastole, limiting acceptance of this important clinical tool.

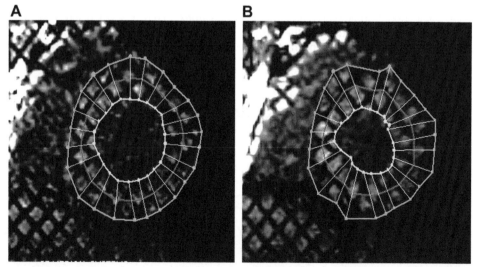

Fig. 6. Harmonic phase left ventricular end-diastolic (*A*) and end-systolic (*B*) images demonstrating tags overlaid by epicardium (*green line*), endocardium (*yellow line*), and midwall (*orange line*) contours (tracing performed semiautomatically). A strain and torsion map is then generated demonstrating intramyocardial deformation.

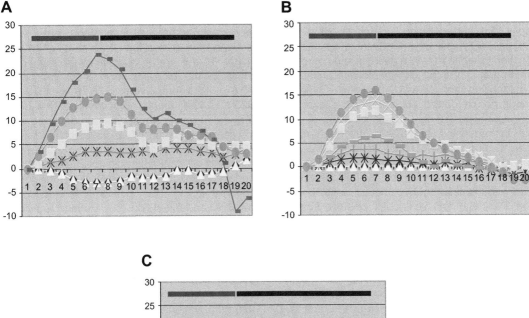

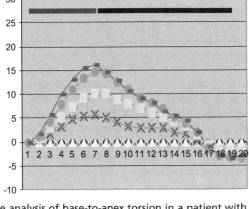

Fig. 7. Harmonic phase off-line analysis of base-to-apex torsion in a patient with aortic stenosis. (*A*) Pre-AVR. (*B*) Post-AVR. (*C*) Fourteen-months post-AVR. The y-axis is torsion (degrees) plotted for all slices. The x-axis is time over the entire cardiac cycle (34-ms phase interval) displaying 12 7-mm contiguous slices starting with end-diastole. Overlap masks display of all slices. Red bar indicates systole. Blue bar indicates diastole. Note the dynamic change in torsion: Apical torsion is maximum pre-AVR, in keeping with supranormal apical function (24°) with basal torsion typically 0° to 4°. Also evident is the failure for diastolic untwisting to rapidly recover during the isovolumic period, revealing severe delay until near atrial-systole. (*From* Biederman RW, Doyle M, Yamrozik J, et al. Physiologic compensation is supranormal in compensated aortic stenosis: Does it return to normal after aortic valve replacement or is it blunted by coexistent coronary artery disease? An intramyocardial magnetic resonance imaging study. Circulation 2005;112(9 Suppl):I429–36; with permission.)

RIGHT VENTRICULAR DIASTOLIC FUNCTION

For the right ventricle, as with the left ventricle, systolic function has gained attention over diastolic function assessment. Thus there is more data available for the value of right ventricular systolic parameters and their prognostic significance. If we enumerate the scheme of things that matter for ventricular function, then the evidence suggests that diastolic function is as important as systolic function and is as important a prognostic indicator as systolic function. This should also be true for the right ventricle. The complexities of diastolic function evaluation and management are further complicated by complex right ventricular geometry, which makes even systolic function difficult to accurately assess. Some recent echocardiographic and CMR studies on right ventricular diastolic function have provided important insights. Using color Doppler of the tricuspid valve, Pye and colleagues[51] found no significant correlation between any tricuspid flow parameters and age. This is in contrast to transmitral flow, on which age has an important effect. In a study on 185 patients by echocardiography, Yu and colleagues[52] for the first time systematically assessed right ventricular diastolic function in left heart failure patients and compared it with that in a group of patients with pulmonary hypertension (and normal left ventricle function) and in normal control subjects. These investigators concluded that right ventricular diastolic function is frequently abnormal in left heart failure patients, and this is not related to elevated pulmonary artery systolic pressure alone, although high pulmonary artery pressure by itself also is associated with impaired right ventricular diastolic function. Recently, right ventricular diastolic function by right ventricular time–volume curve and IVRT measurement on CMR was performed by Gan and colleagues.[53] In this study, 25 patients with pulmonary hypertension underwent cardiac catheterization and CMR. Compared to control subjects, patients with pulmonary hypertension had prolonged mean IVRT, decreased E and E/A, and increased A filling. The IVRT was related to right ventricular mass and pulmonary vascular resistance.

It is unknown if right ventricular diastolic indices mirror those for the left ventricle. In a short study presented as an abstract at the Society of Cardiovascular Magnetic Resonance by our group in 2005,[54] we looked at 14 subjects, of whom four were normal (eight male; six female; mean age 55 years; range 22–79 years). The 10 patients had history of coronary artery disease, hypertensive cardiomyopathy, severe aortic stenosis, and pericardial disease. These subjects underwent 3D assessment of mitral and tricuspid valve. The right ventricular and left ventricular inflow were

interrogated for E, A, and deceleration time. All (14 of 14) mitral and tricuspid flow velocity data were successfully acquired and analyzed in a mean time of less than 15 minutes. The mean mitral valve E and A velocities were higher than those of the tricuspid valve: 71.2 ± 20.5 and 49.8 ± 22.1 cm/s versus 46.79 ± 13.45 and 32.2 ± 10.4 cm/s, respectively ($P = .0003$) (**Fig. 8**). However, there was no difference in E/A (P not significant). Of 14 subjects, 12 (86%; $P<.05$) had identical morphologic patterns for right and left ventricular diastolic function (seven impaired relaxation, one restrictive, four normal). The remaining two patients had discordant tricuspid and mitral flow (one ischemic cardiomyopathy patient had restrictive mitral flow pattern with a pseudonormal tricuspid flow; and the other patient referred for constriction had normal mitral and but restrictive tricuspid flow pattern). The deceleration time for the tricuspid valve was consistently higher when compared with that for the mitral valve (233 ± 65 versus 171 ± 35 ms; $P<.005$). This data demonstrate that right and left ventricular diastolic function can be readily, efficiently, and accurately assessed by CMR-PC. Clinically important, tricuspid flow data generally correspond morphologically with those of mitral flow patterns as expected, except in those cases where there is isolated ventricular pathology. The lower velocities, longer deceleration time, and shorter diastasis likely can be explained by lower atrioventricular pressure gradient compared with the left side. These findings represent important insights into right ventricular lusitropy.

It is now clear that assessment of the role of right ventricular diastolic function in determining the symptoms and prognosis of heart failure and

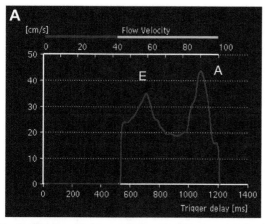
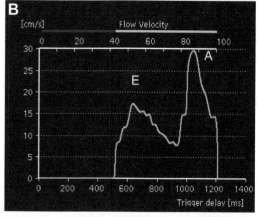

Fig. 8. Right and left ventricular diastolic function by CMR. Abnormal relaxation with prolonged deceleration time of mitral valve (*A*) and tricuspid valve (*B*) flow. Red bar indicates systole. Green bar indicates diastole. (*Data from* Rathi VK, Doyle M, Yamrozik J, et al. 3D diastolic function assessment of the right ventricle; interrogation by cardiovascular MRI [abstract]. J Cardiovasc Magn Reson 2005;7(1):abstract 505.)

pulmonary hypertension is warranted and elaborate studies on CMR-based tricuspid flow velocities, tricuspid annular velocities, and right ventricular strain or torsion should be performed to answer these key questions.

SUMMARY

The assessment of diastolic function has gained a firm foothold in the practice of cardiovascular disease. Even though problems related to diastolic function are increasingly recognized, their contribution to morbidity and mortality appear to continue unabated. Failure to address these problems stems in part from the complexities of treatment once the diagnosis is made. CMR has a demonstrated potential to define diastolic function and quantify its properties, in terms of active and passive stages, and its relaxation and compliance characteristics. CMR also gathers data related to inflow, myocardial, and untwisting properties of the chamber and myocardium, providing insights not fully available in the other invasive or noninvasive strategies. CMR, which offers the necessary capabilities to evaluate the complex structure of the right ventricle, can serve in the future as the standard for evaluating diastolic function as it currently does for systolic function.

REFERENCES

1. Apstein CS, Morgan JP. Cellular mechanisms underlying left ventricular diastolic dysfunction. In: Gaasch WH, LeWinter MM, editors. Left ventricular diastolic dysfunction and heart failure. Philadelphia: Lea & Febiger; 1994. p. 3–24.
2. Ingwall JS. Energetics of the normal and failing human heart: focus on the creatine kinase reaction. Adv Org Biol 1998;4:117–41.
3. Solaro RJ, Wolska BM, Westfall M. Regulatory proteins and diastolic relaxation. In: Lorell BH, Grossman W, editors. Diastolic relaxation of the heart. Boston: Kluwer Academic Publishers; 1987. p. 43–54.
4. Fishberg AM. Heart failure. Philadelphia: Lea & Febiger; 1937.
5. Rosamond W, Flegal K, Friday G, et al. American Heart Association Statistics Subcommittee. Circulation 2008;117(4):e25–146.
6. Grossman W. Diastolic dysfunction in congestive heart failure. N Engl J Med 1991;325:1557–64.
7. Zile MR, Baicu CF, Gaasch WH. Diastolic heart failure—abnormalities in active relaxation and passive stiffness of the left ventricle. N Engl J Med 2004;350(19):1953–9.
8. Zile MR, Brutsaert DL. New concepts in diastolic dysfunction and diastolic heart failure: part I: diagnosis, prognosis, and measurements of diastolic function. Circulation 2002;105(11):1387–93.
9. Zile MR, Brutsaert DL. New concepts in diastolic dysfunction and diastolic heart failure: part II: causal mechanisms and treatment. Circulation 2002; 105(12):1503–8.
10. Paulus WJ, Tschope C, Sanderson JE, et al. How to diagnose diastolic heart failure: a consensus statement on the diagnosis of heart failure with normal left ventricular ejection fraction by the Heart Failure and Echocardiography Associations of the European Society of Cardiology. Eur Heart J 2007; 28(20):2539–50.
11. Angeja BG, Grossman W. Evaluation and management of diastolic heart failure. Circulation 2003; 107(5):659–63.
12. Maurer MS, King DL, El-Khoury Rumbarger L, et al. Left heart failure with a normal ejection fraction: identification of different pathophysiologic mechanisms. J Card Fail 2005;11(3):177–87.
13. Maurer MS, El Khoury Rumbarger L, King DL. Ventricular volume and length in hypertensive diastolic heart failure. J Am Soc Echocardiogr 2005; 18(10):1051–7.
14. Kitzman DW, Little WC, Brubaker PH, et al. Pathophysiological characterization of isolated diastolic heart failure in comparison to systolic heart failure. JAMA 2002;288(17):2144–50.
15. Devereux RB, Roman MJ, Liu JE, et al. Congestive heart failure despite normal left ventricular systolic function in a population-based sample: the Strong Heart Study. Am J Cardiol 2000;86(10):1090–6.
16. Kass DA. Assessment of diastolic dysfunction. Invasive modalities. Cardiol Clin 2000;18(3):571–86.
17. Bonow RO, Bacharach SL, Green MV, et al. Impaired left ventricular diastolic filling in patients with coronary artery disease: assessment with radionuclide angiography. Circulation 1981;64:315–23.
18. Bacharach SL, Green MV, Borer JS, et al. Left ventricular peak ejection rate, filling rate, and ejection fraction: frame rate requirements at rest and exercise. J Nucl Med 1979;20:189.
19. van der Geest RJ, Reiber JH. Quantification in cardiac MRI. J Magn Reson Imaging 1999;10:602–8.
20. Fujita N, Hartiala J, O'Sullivan M, et al. Assessment of left ventricular diastolic function in dilated cardiomyopathy with cine magnetic resonance imaging: effect of an angiotensin converting enzyme inhibitor, benazepril. Am Heart J 1993;125:171–8.
21. Chatzimavroudis GP, Oshinski JN, Franch RH, et al. Evaluation of the precision of magnetic resonance phase velocity mapping for blood flow measurements. J Cardiovasc Magn Reson 2001;3(1):11–9.
22. Mohiaddin RH, Amanuma M, Kilner PJ, et al. MR phase-shift velocity mapping of mitral and pulmonary venous flow. J Comput Assist Tomogr 1991; 15(2):237–43.

23. Hartiala JJ, Mostbeck GH, Foster E, et al. Velocity-encoded cine CMR in the evaluation of left ventricular diastolic function: measurement of mitral valve and pulmonary vein flow velocities and flow volume across the mitral valve. Am Heart J 1993;125(4): 1054–66.

24. Karwatowski SP, Brecker SJ, Yang GZ, et al. Mitral valve flow measured with cine MR velocity mapping in patients with ischemic heart disease: comparison with Doppler echocardiography. J Magn Reson Imaging 1995;5(1):89–92.

25. Rathi VK, Doyle M, Yamrozik J, et al. Routine evaluation of left ventricular diasto-lic function by cardiovascular magnetic resonance: a practical approach. J Cardiovasc Magn Reson 2008;10(1):36.

26. Doyle M, Kortright E, Anayiotos AS, et al. Rapid velocity encoded cine imaging with Turbo-BRISK. J Cardiovasc Magn Reson 1999;1(3):223–32.

27. Kortright E, Doyle M, Anayiotos AS, et al. Validation of rapid velocity encoded cine imaging of a dynamically complex flow field using turbo block regional interpolation scheme for k space. Ann Biomed Eng 2001;29(2):128–34.

28. Karwatowski SP, Mohiaddin RH, Yang GZ, et al. Regional myocardial velocity imaged by magnetic resonance in patients with ischaemic heart disease. Br Heart J 1994;72(4):332–8.

29. Karwatowski SP, Brecker SJ, Yang GZ, et al. A comparison of left ventricular myocardial velocity in diastole measured by magnetic resonance and left ventricular filling measured by Doppler echocardiography. Eur Heart J 1996;17(5):795–802.

30. Paelinck BP, de Roos A, Bax JJ, et al. Feasibility of tissue magnetic resonance imaging: a pilot study in comparison with tissue Doppler imaging and invasive measurement. J Am Coll Cardiol 2005;45(7): 1109–16.

31. Zerhouni EA, Parish DM, Rogers WJ, et al. Human heart: tagging with MR imaging—a method for noninvasive assessment of myocardial motion. Radiology 1988;169(1):59–63.

32. Rademakers FE, Buchalter MB, Rogers WJ, et al. Dissociation between left ventricular untwisting and filling. Accentuation by catecholamines. Circulation 1992;85(4):1572–81, 1578.

33. Rogers WJ Jr, Shapiro EP, Weiss JL, et al. Quantification of and correction for left ventricular systolic long-axis shortening by magnetic resonance tissue tagging and slice isolation. Circulation 1991;84(2): 721–31.

34. Reichek N. CMR myocardial tagging. J Magn Reson Imaging 1999;10(5):609–16.

35. Beyar R, Yin F, Hausknecht M, et al. Dependence of left ventricular twist-radial shortening relations on cardiac cycle phase. Am J Physiol 1989;257: H1119–26.

36. Hansen DE, Daughters GT, Alderman EL, et al. Effect of acute human allograft rejection on left ventricular systolic torsion and diastolic recoil measured by intramyocardial markers. Circulation 1987;76:998–1008.

37. Bell SP, Nyland L, Tischler MD, et al. Alterations in the determinants of diastolic suction during pacing tachycardia. Circ Res 2000;87(3):235–40.

38. MacGowan GA, Shapiro EP, Azhari H, et al. Noninvasive measurement of shortening in the fiber and cross-fiber directions in the normal human left ventricle and in idiopathic dilated cardiomyopathy. Circulation 1997;96(2):535–41.

39. Rademakers FE, Bogaert J. Left ventricular myocardial tagging. Int J Cardiovasc Imaging 1997;13(3): 233–45.

40. Villari B, Vassalli G, Monrad ES, et al. Normalization of diastolic dysfunction in aortic stenosis late after valve replacement. Circulation 1995;91(9): 2353–8.

41. Beyar R, Dong SJ, Smith ER, et al. Ventricular interaction and septal deformation: a model compared with experimental data. Am J Physiol 1993;265: H2044–56.

42. Knudtson ML, Gaibraith PD, Hildebrand EL, et al. Dynamics of left ventricular apex rotation during angioplasty: a sensitive index of ischemic dysfunction. Circulation 1997;96:801–8.

43. Dong SJ, Hees PS, Siu CO, et al. CMR assessment of LV relaxation by untwisting rate: a new isovolumic phase measure of tau. Am J Physiol Heart Circ Physiol 2001;281(5):H2002–9.

44. Nagel E, Stuber M, Burkhard B, et al. Cardiac rotation and relaxation in patients with aortic valve stenosis. Eur Heart J 2000;21(7):582–9.

45. Stuber M, Scheidegger MB, Fischer SE, et al. Alterations in the local myocardial motion pattern in patients suffering from pressure overload due to aortic stenosis. Circulation 1999;100(4):361–8.

46. Biederman RW, Doyle M, Yamrozik J, et al. Physiologic compensation is supranormal in compensated aortic stenosis: Does it return to normal after aortic valve replacement or is it blunted by coexistent coronary artery disease? An intramyocardial magnetic resonance imaging study. Circulation 2005;112(9 Suppl):I429–36.

47. Moore CC, O'Dell WG, McVeigh ER, et al. Calculation of three-dimensional left ventricular strains from biplanar tagged MR images. J Magn Reson Imaging 1992;2(2):165–75.

48. Buchalter MB, Weiss JL, Rogers WJ, et al. Noninvasive quantification of left ventricular rotational

deformation in normal humans using magnetic resonance imaging myocardial tagging. Circulation 1990;81:1236–44.

49. Young AA, Axel L, Dougherty L, et al. Validation of tagging with MR imaging to estimate material deformation. Radiology 1993;188:101–8.

50. Osman NF, Kerwin WS, McVeigh ER, et al. Cardiac motion tracking using CINE harmonic phase (HARP) magnetic resonance imaging. Magn Reson Med 1999;42:1048–60.

51. Pye MP, Pringle SD, Cobbe SM. Reference values and reproducibility of Doppler echocardiography in the assessment of the tricuspid valve and right ventricular diastolic function in normal subjects. Am J Cardiol 1991;67:269–73.

52. Yu CM, Sanderson JE, Chan S, et al. Right ventricular diastolic dysfunction in heart failure. Circulation 1996;93(8):1509–14.

53. Gan CT, Holverda S, Marcus JT, et al. Right ventricular diastolic dysfunction and the acute effects of sildenafil in pulmonary hypertension patients. Chest 2007;132(1):11–7.

54. Rathi VK, Doyle M, Yamrozik J, et al. 3D Diastolic function assessment of the right ventricle; interrogation by cardiovascular MRI. J Cardiovasc Magn Reson 2005;7(1) [abstract 505].

Risk Stratification for Therapeutic Management and Prognosis

Otavio R. Coelho-Filho, MD, Leelakrishna Nallamshetty, MD,
Raymond Y. Kwong, MD, MPH, FACC*

KEYWORDS

- Heart failure • CMR imaging • Risk stratification
- Prognosis

Heart failure is a multifaceted clinical syndrome that has high hospitalization and mortality rates. The incidence of new heart failure diagnosis is high and is increasing, approaching 10 per 1000 in the elderly population.[1] Its main cause in developed countries is coronary artery disease (CAD). In patients who have CAD, the role of noninvasive imaging to assess myocardial viability has long been recognized to have great therapeutic and prognostic importance. The meta-analysis by Allman and colleagues[2] has helped establish the current understanding that mechanical coronary revascularization can improve clinical outcome only if substantial myocardial viability exists (**Fig. 1**). In addition, because the clinical success of improved medical therapies makes them an alternative to coronary revascularization[3] and because of the known morbidity from coronary revascularization, the risks and benefits of revascularization should be evaluated using noninvasive risk-stratification techniques that examine the physiology of CAD rather than coronary anatomy alone. In many reports cardiac magnetic resonance (CMR) has been shown to be highly accurate in its noninvasive detection of CAD. In CAD, CMR imaging offers the unique advantage of integrating several types of pulse-sequence examinations (eg, myocardial perfusion, cine wall motion, T2-weighted imaging for myocardial edema, late gadolinium enhancement, and CMR angiography) that can provide anatomic, functional, and physiologic information about the heart in a single imaging session. Because of this ability to interrogate myocardial physiology using different pulse sequence techniques within a single CMR session, this technique has been recognized increasingly in many centers as the test of choice for assessing patients who present with cardiomyopathy of undetermined cause. This article first reviews the current evidence supporting the prognosticating role of CMR in assessing CAD and then discusses CMR applications and prognostication in many non-coronary cardiac conditions.

CORONARY ARTERY DISEASE
Characterizing Myocardial Ischemia Using Stress Cardiac Magnetic Resonance Cine Imaging

CMR imaging is used increasingly to detect the presence of significant CAD and to assess the hemodynamic significance of coronary stenosis. The development of rapid magnetic resonance gradient systems and consequently high temporal resolution allows high-resolution cine cardiac imaging to be performed at rest and under stress at high heart rates. Cine steady-state free precession techniques provide imaging of cardiac structure and function with excellent definition of the endomyocardial border without the need for any contrast agent. Nagel and colleagues[4] performed dobutamine stress cine CMR and dobutamine

Brigham and Women's Hospital, Boston, MA, USA
* Corresponding author. Cardiovascular Division, Department of Medicine, Brigham and Women's Hospital, 75 Francis Street, Boston, MA 02115.
E-mail address: rykwong@partners.org (R.Y. Kwong).

Heart Failure Clin 5 (2009) 437–455
doi:10.1016/j.hfc.2009.02.010
1551-7136/09/$ – see front matter © 2009 Elsevier Inc. All rights reserved.

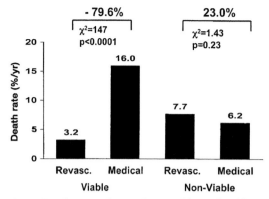

Fig. 1. Death rates for patients with and without myocardial viability treated by revascularization or medical therapy. There is a 79.6% reduction in mortality for patients who have viability treated by revascularization ($P < .0001$). In patients who do not have myocardial viability, there was no significant difference in mortality with revascularization or medical therapy. (*From* Allman KC, Shaw LJ, Hachamovitch R, et al. Myocardial viability testing and impact of revascularization on prognosis in patients who have coronary artery disease and left ventricular dysfunction: a meta-analysis. J Am Coll Cardiol 2002;39(7):1155; with permission.)

stress echocardiography in 208 patients who subsequently underwent clinically indicated coronary angiography. The authors reported high rates of sensitivity (86%) and specificity (86%), which compared favorably with echocardiography (sensitivity of 74% and specificity of 70%) in detecting angiographically significant coronary stenosis. In 153 patients who had a poor acoustic window for stress echocardiography, Hundley and colleagues[5] reported that dobutamine stress cine alone detected coronary lesions of more than 50% luminal stenosis with both a sensitivity and a specificity of 83%. These authors later reported the prognostic value of dobutamine stress cine CMR in a larger study of 279 patients.[6] The presence of a new abnormality in regional wall motion during dobutamine stress cine CMR that is consistent with inducible ischemia identifies patients at risk of myocardial infarction (MI) and cardiac death, independent of the presence of traditional risk factors for CAD or left ventricular ejection fraction (LVEF) (**Fig. 2**). A low cardiac event rate was demonstrated in cases with a negative dobutamine stress cine CMR (2% over 2 years for patients who had an LVEF > 40% and 0% over 2 years for patients who had an LVEF ≥ 60%). The same imaging techniques have been used to assess preoperative cardiac risk in patients undergoing non-cardiac surgery. A low cardiac event rate was demonstrated in cases of negative testing (2% over 2 years for patients who had an

LVEF > 40% and 0% over 2 years for patients who had ad LVEF ≥ 60%).[7]

Recently Jahnke and colleagues[8] sought to determine the prognostic value of magnetic resonance perfusion during adenosine stress and wall motion imaging during dobutamine stress in predicting cardiac death and nonfatal MI in a patient cohort that had known or suspected CAD. They enrolled 513 patients who had symptoms suggesting myocardial ischemia and followed them for a median of 2.3 years (range, 0.06–4.55 years). The 3-year event-free survival rates were 99.2% for patients who had normal adenosine myocardial perfusion and dobutamine stress cine function and 83.5% for those who had abnormal adenosine myocardial perfusion and dobutamine stress cine function. The presence of an abnormal result by adenosine myocardial perfusion or dobutamine stress cine function on CMR increased the likelihood of death or nonfatal MI over that obtained by the analysis of clinical risk factors (χ^2, 16.0–34.3 or 29.5, respectively; both $P < .001$). Although both CMR imaging techniques identified patients at high risk for future cardiac events (cardiac death or nonfatal MI), this study demonstrated that patients who had ischemia detected by either adenosine myocardial perfusion or dobutamine stress cine function had a 12- or 5-fold increased risk, respectively, for experiencing a subsequent cardiac event. Either adenosine myocardial perfusion or dobutamine stress cine function was effective in risk-stratifying patients who presented with chest pain syndromes suitable for noninvasive imaging. Because stepwise dobutamine infusion has well-known vasodilating effects during the intermediate dose, at Brigham and Women's Hospital myocardial perfusion usually is performed during the intermediate stage as well as the usual stages of cine stress wall motion imaging; the two techniques have been found to have complementary diagnostic roles (**Fig. 3**A, B; please also refer to the corresponding videos, which may be accessed in the online version of this article at http://www.heartfailure.theclinics.com/).

Dobutamine stress CMR also can be a helpful tool for predicting cardiac events in individuals who have reduced LVEF. Dall'Armellina and colleagues[9] assessed the prognostic implication of dobutamine stress CMR in 200 patients who had CAD and reduced left ventricular (LV) global function. The authors reported that in patients who had mild to moderate reductions (40%–50%) in LVEF, dobutamine-induced changes in regional wall motion quantified by a wall motion score index can forecast hard cardiac events (MI and cardiac death) incremental to the predictive value of resting

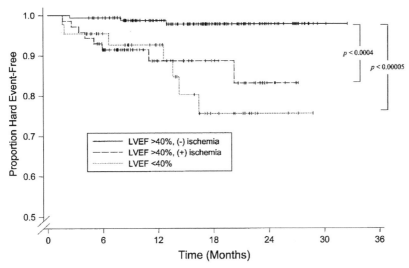

Fig. 2. Kaplan-Meier event-free survival curves in patients who have an LVEF of less than 40% or equal to or greater than 40%, with or without inducible ischemia. Compared with patients who have an LVEF of greater or equal than 40% and no evidence of inducible ischemia, event-free survival was significantly lower in patients who had inducible ischemia ($P < .0004$) or an LVEF of less than 40% ($P < .00005$). (*From* Hundley WG, Morgan TM, Neagle CM, et al. Magnetic resonance imaging determination of cardiac prognosis. Circulation 2002; 106(18):2331; with permission.)

LVEF alone. In patients who have moderate to severe LVEF (< 40%), however, the wall motion score index did not provide additional prognostic information beyond LVEF. It is conceivable that in patients who have moderate to severe LV dysfunction from CAD, the low resting LVEF and the dobutamine-induced global wall motion score index are highly correlated parameters describing the burden of myocardial ischemia; thus considering each parameter alone did not provide additional prognostic information adjusted to the effect of the other parameter. CMR has the unique advantage of allowing myocardial perfusion, late gadolinium enhancement (LGE) scar imaging, and stress cine to be performed in the same imaging session; thus imaging data from these other components may provide incremental prognostic information by describing other aspects of the altered myocardial physiology. Prospective clinical studies are necessary to assess the prognostic usefulness of combining these techniques within the same CMR examination.

Characterizing Myocardial Ischemia Using Cardiac Magnetic Resonance Myocardial Perfusion Imaging

First-pass CMR perfusion imaging collects a series of T1-weighted fast gradient-recalled echo images during a rapid injection of an intravenously administered contrast bolus that results in enhancement of perfused myocardium. On a technical level,

CMR perfusion offers in-plane spatial resolution of 2 mm, which is several folds higher than possible with nuclear imaging techniques such as single-proton emission computed tomography (SPECT) and positron emission tomography (PET), allows differentiation between subendocardial and subepicardial perfusion, and does not involve ionizing radiation. Like PET, CMR perfusion techniques can quantify myocardial perfusion in absolute terms at different hemodynamic states.[10–12] CMR myocardial perfusion data that cover multiple short- and long-axis locations can be acquired in less than 1 minute without the need for patient breathholding, at rest and during pharmacologic stress, respectively[13,14] With hardware improvements, the signal-to-noise ratio has improved, and the burden from artifacts has been reduced. On a clinical level, CMR myocardial perfusion imaging is becoming more widely accepted as a sensitive and reproducible diagnostic modality for detecting regional myocardial hypoperfusion during vasodilating stress caused by significant coronary stenosis. Numerous single-center[13,15–17] and multicenter[18,19] studies have demonstrated its excellent results in detecting CAD. CMR distinguishes subendocardial perfusion from epicardial perfusion and has been shown to provide corollary evidence about the cause of chest pain symptoms in women in the absence of epicardial coronary artery stenosis. Panting and colleagues[14] were able to show subjective evidence of subendocardial myocardial

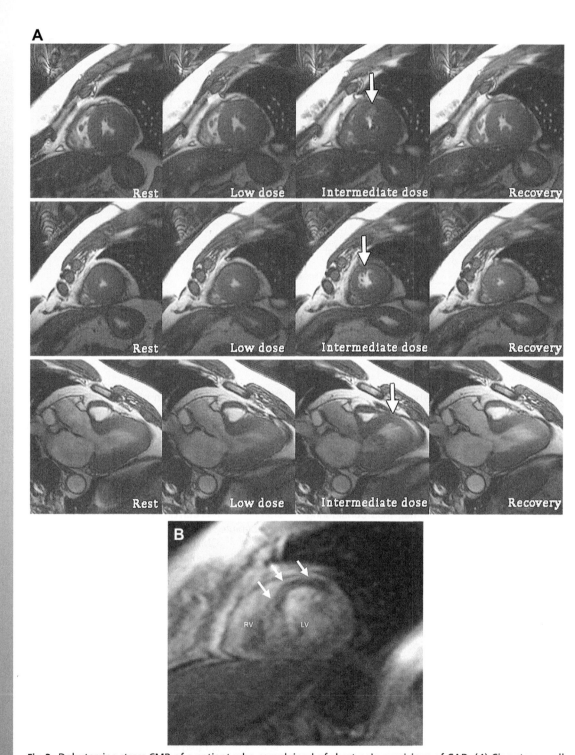

Fig. 3. Dobutamine stress CMR of a patient who complained of chest pain suspicious of CAD. (*A*) Cine stress wall motion imaging (short-axis and three-chamber views) demonstrated an inducible wall motion abnormality (*white arrows*) in the anterior wall at intermediate-dose stage (30 µg/kg/min). (*B*) Myocardial perfusion during intermediate dobutamine stage confirmed evidence of hypoperfusion secondary to a flow-limiting coronary stenosis by demonstrating a perfusion defect in the anterior wall (*white arrows*). This patient was found to have a severe proximal left anterior descending coronary artery. (Also refer to movie clips of **Fig. 3**A and 3B).

hypoperfusion with occurrence of chest pain during adenosine infusion in patients who had chest pain without epicardial coronary stenosis. Although the investigators could not establish a mechanism of subendomyocardial ischemia in these patients based on their semiquantitative measurement of myocardial perfusion reserve, this study provided evidence of abnormal coronary microcirculation in a disease entity that many long had considered to be psychological and non-cardiac.

Over the past years, as the technique has been increasingly used in patient care, prognostic values for perfusion imaging in more common clinical scenarios have been accumulating. Ingkanison and colleagues[20] demonstrated that an adenosine CMR perfusion can determine prognosis in patients presenting to an emergency department with chest pain, nondiagnostic EKG, and negative serial serum troponins for infarction. In that study a normal adenosine CMR perfusion had an excellent negative predictive value for a subsequent diagnosis of CAD or an adverse outcome. After a negative adenosine perfusion CMR, none of the subjects was diagnosed with an adverse event during 1-year follow-up (**Fig. 4**). In an earlier report, Kwong and colleagues[21] reported that a rest perfusion in conjunction with function and LGE imaging by CMR was effective in triaging patients who presented to the emergency room with chest pain. More recently, Schwitter and colleagues[22] published the first multicenter CMR perfusion study, which evaluated CMR perfusion employing multi-vendor scanners

and compared it with nuclear scintigraphy. The investigators first determined the accuracy of CMR diagnoses relative to quantitative coronary angiography by using five different doses of the CMR contrast medium. They reported that a 0.1-mmol/kg dose of gadolinium-based contrast yielded the highest accuracy in detecting coronary artery disease (> 50% stenosis in one or more vessels). Using this dose, Schwitter and colleagues[22] assessed the diagnostic usefulness of CMR myocardial perfusion imaging and SPECT performed at 18 experienced centers using imaging systems from different vendors. A core laboratory was established to interpret all data in a blinded fashion. The authors reported that, based on receiver operator analyses (ROC), the diagnostic performance of CMR perfusion was similar to that of all gated SPECT studies. In patients who had multivessel disease, however, or when compared with all SPECT studies (gated and ungated combined), CMR myocardial perfusion performed better than SPECT (**Fig. 5**). For future development, opinions from several experienced centers (including Brigham and Women's Hospital) indicate that CMR perfusion at 3 Tesla is highly promising. Several authors had reported significant improvement for CMR perfusion at 3 Tesla, compared with 1.5 Tesla, in both signal-to-noise ratio and contrast-to-noise ratio.[23,24] Most recently Cheng and colleagues[25] showed that CMR perfusion at 3 Tesla is superior to 1.5 Tesla for predicting significant single- and multivessel coronary disease (**Fig. 6**). The higher diagnostic accuracy of 3-Tesla perfusion found in that study was attributed to an increased signal-to-noise-ratio, allowing an accurate detection of reduced endocardial perfusion.

Sensitive Detection and Characterization of Myocardial Infarction

LGE after chelated gadolinium injection provides a highly reliable quantitation of the presence and the extent of infarcted myocardial tissue.[26] Kim and colleagues[27,28] showed that LGE delineates the transmural extent of infarction and distinguishes between reversible and irreversible myocardial injury regardless of the extent of wall motion at rest, the age of the infarct, or the reperfusion status. In a landmark study of patients who had CAD, the probability of improvement in regional contractility after successful coronary revascularization was inversely proportional to the transmural extent of LGE before revascularization (**Fig. 7**).[29] With four- to sixfold higher spatial resolution and a higher contrast-to-noise ratio than nuclear scintigraphy, LGE imaging has been

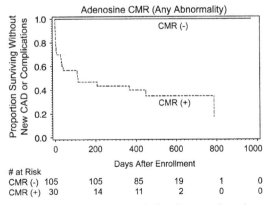

Fig. 4. Kaplan-Meier survival distributions based on the presence or absence of any abnormalities on CMR imaging. A normal adenosine perfusion has 100% event-free survival (100% negative predictive value). (*From* Ingkanisorn WP, Kwong RY, Bohme NS, et al. Prognosis of negative adenosine stress magnetic resonance in patients presenting to an emergency department with chest pain. J Am Coll Cardiol 2006;47(7):1430; with permission.)

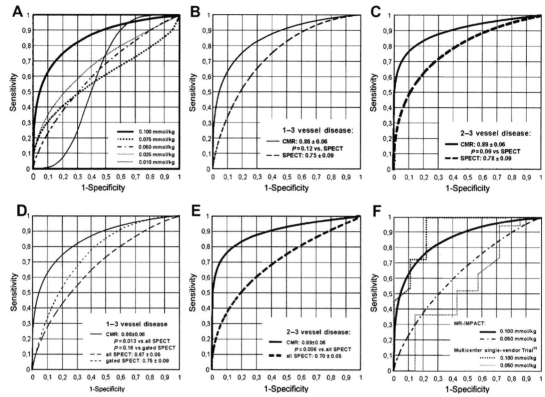

Fig. 5. (*A*) The diagnostic performance (ROCs) for different doses of contrast medium ranging from 0.01 to 0.10 mmol/kg Gd-DTPA-BMA. Best performance is achieved at the highest dose of 0.10 mmol/kg (*thick line*, dose 5). (*B*) In a head-to-head comparison, there is no significant difference in performance in the area under the receiver operating characteristic (AUROC) curve between the 0.10-mmol/kg dose (0.86 ± 0.06) and SPECT (0.75 ± 0.09, *P* = .12). (*C*) Similarly, in the patients who had two- or three-vessel disease, no significant difference was observed in the head-to-head comparison of the two techniques (*P* = .09). (*D*) When perfusion CMR performance is compared with SPECT in the entire population, the AUROC curve is larger for CMR than for SPECT (0.86 ± 0.06 versus 0.67 ± 0.5, *P* = .013). The difference between perfusion CMR and gated SPECT did not reach statistical significance. (*E*) For multivessel disease, the performance of perfusion CMR is superior to SPECT in the entire population (area under the receiver operating characteristic curve: 0.89 ± 0.06 versus. 0.70 ± 0.5, P = 0.006). The performance of perfusion CMR in this trial is consistent with findings in an earlier smaller multicenter single-vendor trial shown in (*F*) assessing doses of 0.10 and 0.05 mmol/kg. Numbers indicate mean ± SE of the area under the receiver operating characteristic curve. (*From* Schwitter J, Wacker CM, van Rossum AC, et al. MR-IMPACT: comparison of perfusion-cardiac magnetic resonance with single-photon emission computed tomography for the detection of coronary artery disease in a multicentre, multivendor, randomized trial. Eur Heart J 2008;29(4):485; with permission.)

shown to be consistently more sensitive and specific than nuclear techniques in detecting and sizing the spatial extent of MI[30,31] and should be the technique of choice for such indications in experienced centers. In addition, the transmural extent of LGE can predict accurately the response of LV function to beta-blocker therapy in patients who have heart failure.[32] In another study Orn and colleagues[33] found that scar size assessed by CMR was the strongest independent predictor of LVEF and LV volumes in patients who had acute MI and heart failure.

Because of its technical advantages, imaging unrecognized MI is one of the clinical situations

in which CMR has been shown to provide a strong prognostic value exceeding that of the available clinical tools. Population-based studies have shown that that one fourth of MI demonstrated by Q waves on the ECG are clinically unrecognized.[34] In fact, the true prevalence of unrecognized MI may be even higher, because of the insensitivity of Q waves.[35] A recent paper from Barbier and colleagues[36] examined the prevalence of this condition using CMR to detect clinically unrecognized MI noninvasively and found that 72 of 248 patients (29%) had abnormal LGE; in 49 of the patients who had abnormal LGE (20% of the cohort) an unrecognized MI was

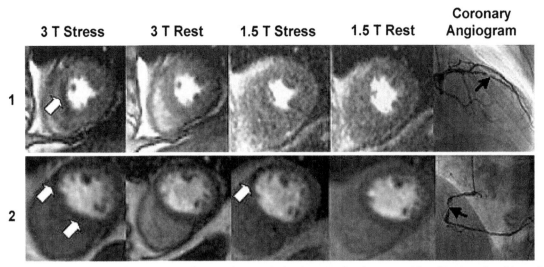

Fig. 6. ROC curves for visual assessment of 1.5- and 3-T perfusion imaging for the correct identification of multivessel disease. The diagnostic performance of 3-T perfusion imaging was significantly greater ($P = .05$). (*From* Cheng AS, Pegg TJ, Karamitsos TD, et al. Cardiovascular magnetic resonance perfusion imaging at 3-Tesla for the detection of coronary artery disease: a comparison with 1.5-Tesla. J Am Coll Cardiol 2007;49(25):2445; with permission.)

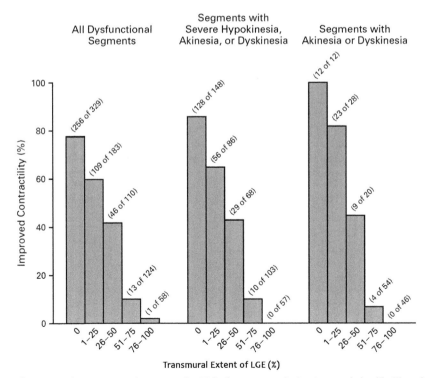

Fig. 7. Relation between the transmural extent of LGE before revascularization and the likelihood of increased contractility after revascularization. For all three analyses, there was an inverse relation between the transmural extent of LGE and the likelihood of improvement in contractility. (*From* Kim RJ, Wu E, Rafael A, et al. The use of contrast-enhanced magnetic resonance imaging to identify reversible myocardial dysfunction. N Engl J Med 2000;343(20):1450; with permission.)

confirmed on clinical grounds. In the same clinical cohort, the ECG detection rate of unrecognized MI by Q wave criteria was only 1%.

Unrecognized MI is a devastating condition; its 10-year mortality is estimated to be 45% to 55%, comparable to or higher than that in patients who have recognized MI.[37] In a study of 195 patients clinically referred for CMR who were suspected of having CAD but who did not have a history of MI, the authors' group at Brigham and Women's Hospital found that the presence of even a very small amount of myocardial scar portends a substantial risk for cardiac events, including death, when compared with outcomes in persons without scar (**Fig. 8**).[38] This prognostic association was strongly incremental to common risk markers such as LVEF, regional wall motion abnormality score, ECG markers of ischemia or infarction, and clinical risk factors. The authors found that the presence of a very small subendocardial scar, often missed by other imaging techniques, was associated with a high burden of coronary stenosis and thus supported the observed "threshold effect" for cardiac hard outcomes (**Fig. 9**).

Diabetics are a subgroup of patients who seem to be at particular risk of unrecognized MI, possibly because presenting symptoms of acute coronary syndromes may be atypical or absent. The authors' group recently investigated the prognostic association of LGE imaging in diabetic patients who had no history or ECG evidence of MI and compared their survival distribution with that of a control group of diabetic patients who had a known history of MI.[39] In this study the diabetic patients who were found to have unrecognized MI by LGE had poor survival outcomes, similar to those of diabetic patients who had experienced a clinical MI, and were nearly fourfold more

likely to suffer cardiac death during the study period than patients who did not have LGE (**Fig. 10**). More work is needed to assess whether CMR LGE can be used as a prospective screening or monitoring tool for high-risk diabetics.

Pilot evidence suggests that, in addition to detecting MI and scar, novel information with prognostic significance may be obtained by using the high contrast-to-noise ratio and spatial resolution of LGE and characterizing the components of infarction. Schmidt and colleagues[40] characterized the border zone of infarction using quantitative analysis of the LGE imaging signal intensity. They reported that the border zone of intermediate signal intensity was associated more strongly than LVEF with electrophysiologic substrates of ventricular arrhythmias (**Fig. 11**). In a pilot study, the authors' group found that, either in terms of absolute mass of myocardium involved or as a percent of the total infarct mass, this border zone was strongly associated with post-MI mortality in a small group of post-MI patients (**Fig. 12**).[41] In addition, the myocardial extent of no-reflow (microvascular obstruction) despite successful coronary revascularization after acute MI has an independent and significant prognostic significance. Wu and colleagues[42] reported significant associations of the extent of MI and microvascular obstruction seen by CMR with subsequent cardiac events, independent of infarct size. In a similar study, Hombach and colleagaues[43] described a similar pattern of increased cardiac mortality but also reported an association with adverse LV remodeling. Recently, T2-weighted fast spin-echo or gradient-echo techniques have been used to characterize the extent of myocardial edema as the "region at risk" because of ischemia.[44] Although the contrast-to-noise ratio of this technique is currently low in

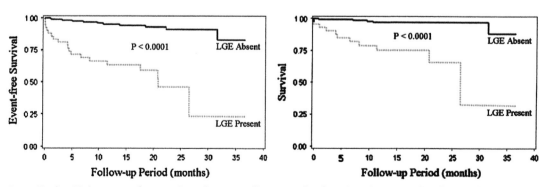

Fig. 8. Kaplan-Meier curves for a major adverse cardiac event (*top*) and cardiac mortality (*bottom*) stratified by LGE as an evidence of unrecognized MI. (*From* Kwong RY, Chan AK, Brown KA, et al. Impact of unrecognized myocardial scar detected by cardiac magnetic resonance imaging on event-free survival in patients presenting with signs or symptoms of coronary artery disease. Circulation 2006;113(23):2739; with permission.)

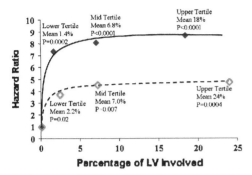

Fig. 9. Percent LGE (*closed blue diamonds curve*) and percent total wall motion score (*red diamond curve*) in tertiles and hazard ratio for a major adverse cardiac event. (*From* Kwong RY, Chan AK, Brown KA, et al. Impact of unrecognized myocardial scar detected by cardiac magnetic resonance imaging on event-free survival in patients presenting with signs or symptoms of coronary artery disease. Circulation 2006; 113(23):2740; with permission.)

the 1.5-T environment, early applications in the clinical setting where acute coronary syndrome is common have shown encouraging results. Cury and colleagues[45] assessed 62 patients who presented to the emergency room with chest pain and found that the addition of T2-weighted imaging for myocardial edema improved the differentiation of acute versus chronic CAD (**Fig. 13**). T2-weighted imaging enhanced the positive predictive value in detecting acute coronary syndrome from 55% to 85%. After an acute MI, infarct remodeling continues to take place over months governed by the status of coronary reflow,

ongoing ischemia, collateral formation, and infarct location. Thus it is expected that novel CMR techniques that can capture different aspects of myocardial physiology will continue to increase the prognostic value of CMR beyond that of total infarct size and LV function.

PROGNOSTIC VALUE OF CARDIAC MAGNETIC RESONANCE IN NON-ISCHEMIC CARDIOMYOPATHY

The prognosis of patients who have non-ischemic cardiomyopathy is poor with a 10-year survival rate of less than 60%.[46] A significant cause of mortality in these patients is sudden cardiac death. Primary prevention is performed with an implantable cardioverter-defibrillator (ICD) when LV systolic function is less than 35%.[47] Overall prognosis is not based on LV function alone, however. A combination of diagnostic features, including LV function, myocardial fibrosis, valvular dysfunction, and pericardial constriction, provides a more accurate prediction of outcomes in these patients.

Myocardial fibrosis leads to rigidity of the left ventricle resulting in both systolic and diastolic dysfunction. Myocardial fibrosis occurs in nonischemic cardiomyopathy as a result of a cascade of adrenergic activation, myocyte dysfunction, apoptosis, and fibroblast hyperplasia. This process is thought to be the cause of myocardial re-entry resulting in ventricular tachycardia.[48,49] Extensive data has been published regarding the ability of CMR to characterize and quantify myocardial fibrosis accurately using LGE imaging.

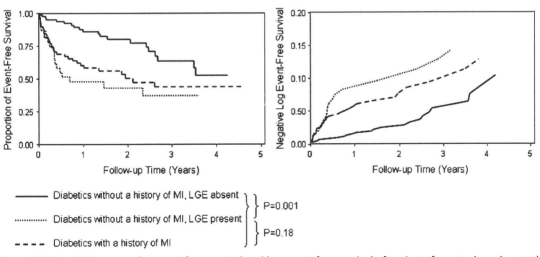

Fig. 10. Kaplan–Meier curves for event-free survival and log event-free survival of patients from study and control groups combined. (*From* Kwong RY, Sattar H, Wu H, et al. Incidence and prognostic implication of unrecognized myocardial scar characterized by cardiac magnetic resonance in diabetic patients who did not have clinical evidence of myocardial infarction</bibarticle>. Circulation 2008;118(10):1018; with permission.)

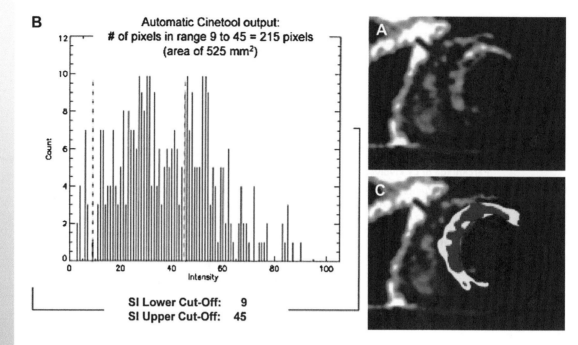

Gray zone = Area with SI between 9 and 45
Core = Area with SI > 45
Gray + core = Area with SI > 9 (gray+core)

Fig. 11. Gray zone measurement. (*A*) Late gadolinium-enhanced short-axis MRI of a patient who has an anterior infarct. In this example the peak signal intensity (SI) within the remote, non-infarcted region was 9. Abnormal enhancement is defined as SI greater than 9. (*B*) The histogram of SI within the hyperenhanced region. In this example, the peak SI within the high SI region is 90. The upper threshold for gray zone extent is 50% of the peak SI (in this example, 90 × 0.50 = 45). (*C*) The gray zone (*yellow area*) is the region with SI between 9 and 45. The core region (*red area*) is the region with SI greater than 45. (*From* Schmidt A, Azevedo CF, Cheng A, et al. Infarct tissue heterogeneity by magnetic resonance imaging identifies enhanced cardiac arrhythmia susceptibility in patients who have LV dysfunction. Circulation 2007;115(15):2008; with permission.)

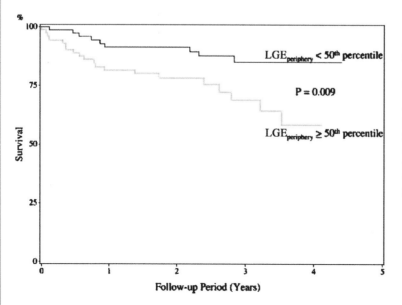

Fig. 12. Kaplan-Meier survival curves for all-cause mortality, stratified by the median percentage of LGE_Periphery. (*From* Yan AT, Shayne AJ, Brown KA, et al. Characterization of the peri-infarct zone by contrast-enhanced cardiac magnetic resonance imaging is a powerful predictor of post-myocardial infarction mortality. Circulation 2006;114(1):36; with permission.)

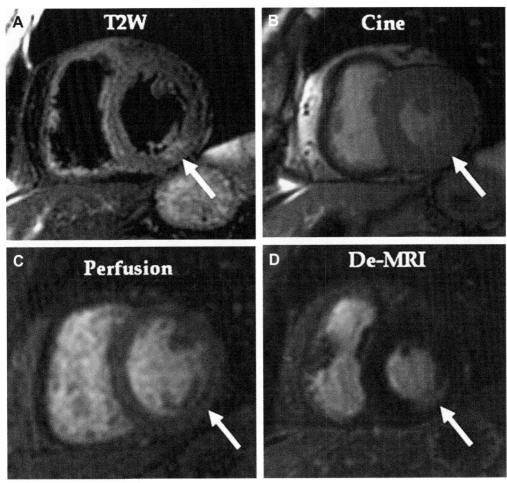

Fig.13. A patient who has non-ST elevation MI. CMR was performed in a 63-year-old man 1 hour after his arrival at the emergency department with initial normal cardiac enzymes. It revealed (*A*) a small area of T2 hyperintensity in the inferolateral wall (myocardial edema) with (*B*) associated subtle hypokinesis, (*C*) a resting perfusion defect, and (*D*) late gadolinium enhancement (myocardial necrosis) in the same area (*arrows*). (*From* Cury RC, Shash K, Nagurney JT, et al. Cardiac magnetic resonance with T2-weighted imaging improves detection of patients who have acute coronary syndrome in the emergency department. Circulation 2008;118(8):841; with permission.)

Gadolinium-based contrast agents become trapped in areas of fibrosis and demonstrate delayed washout characteristics compared with normal myocardium.

Increasing evidence has been reported that the extent of myocardial fibrosis as determined by LGE on CMR is inversely proportional to both LV function and clinical symptoms in patients who have heart failure. This correlation holds true for all patients, despite their therapeutic profile, be it medical, surgical, device, or revascularization therapy. The overall incidence of LGE in patients who have nonischemic cardiomyopathy has been reported to be approximately 35%.[50] Assomull and colleagues[50] evaluated outcomes in patients who had nonischemic cardiomyopathy based on the presence of LGE of the LV myocardium. They demonstrated that the presence of any LGE is associated with increased all-cause mortality and hospitalizations and has an increased hazard ratio of 3.1. These findings were confirmed in a recent study by Wu and colleagues.[51] During a 17-month follow-up, patients who had LGE had an eightfold higher risk of hospitalizations for heart failure, appropriate ICD firing, and sudden cardiac death than patients who did not demonstrate any LGE.

Idiopathic Dilated Cardiomyopathy

The typical LGE pattern in idiopathic cardiomyopathy is mid-wall, most predominantly affecting the basal and mid septum (**Fig. 14**). In these patients a transmural extent of LGE greater than 25% indicates increased risk of inducible ventricular

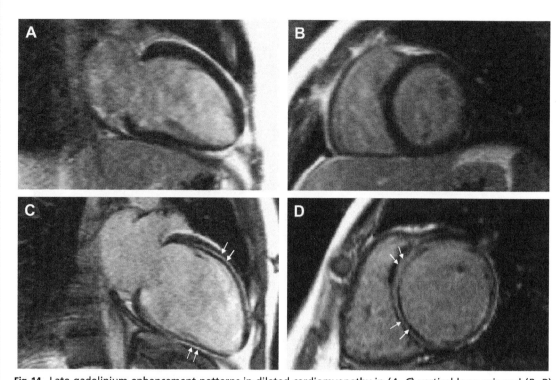

Fig. 14. Late gadolinium enhancement patterns in dilated cardiomyopathy in (*A, C*) vertical long axis and (*B, D*) short axis. *A* and *B* show a patient without late enhancement. *C* and *D* show a patient with marked mid-wall enhancement. The enhancement pattern (*arrows*) is distinct from that associated with coronary artery disease because of endocardial sparing and non-coronary territory distribution. (*From* Assomull RG, Prasad SK, Lyne J, et al. Cardiovascular magnetic resonance, fibrosis, and prognosis in dilated cardiomyopathy. J Am Coll Cardiol 2006;48(10):1979; with permission.)

arrhythmias on electrophysiology studies.[52] Inducible sustained ventricular tachycardia is associated with poor prognosis. Patients who have LGE have poorer recovery following aggressive medical management than patients who do not demonstrate any scarring. Assomull and colleagues[50] demonstrated that approximately 35% of patients who have idiopathic cardiomyopathy have LGE, and that the presence of LGE predicts the occurrence of both primary all-cause mortality of death and sudden cardiac death or ventricular tachycardia with a hazard ratio of 5.2 (*P* = .3) (**Fig. 15**). Statistical analyses demonstrate that LGE is more predictive for these primary and secondary end points than ejection fraction, which currently is used more widely to determine the need for ICD placement.

Hypertrophic Cardiomyopathy

Cine CMR has become a very useful tool in the quantification of hypertrophy in patients who have hypertrophic cardiomyopathy (HCM). Several studies have demonstrated that, especially in apical HCM, hypertrophied segments

may be missed or underestimated with standard echocardiography.[53,54] More severe LV hypertrophy increases the risk of sudden cardiac death and arrhythmias.[55] Therefore, accurate measurements of LV wall thickness and mass are crucial for optimizing management of these patients.

In addition to LV mass quantification using cine CMR imaging, LGE is seen within hypertrophic segments. The typical enhancement pattern in HCM is patchy areas of mid-wall enhancement most characteristically at the right ventricular (RV) insertion sites. Moon and colleagues[56] have shown that the amount of myocardial scarring, as indicated by LGE, is increased in patients who have HCM and two or more risk factors for sudden cardiac death (**Fig. 16**). Also, the extent of enhancement is inversely related to the LVEF.

Finally phase-contrast imaging can be used to evaluate the obstructive physiology through the LV outflow tract resulting in systolic anterior motion. Because CMR can assess accurately assess LV mass, areas of fibrosis with LGE, and valvular pathology, it plays an important role in the initial diagnosis of HCM. In addition, CMR can be used to follow the response to therapeutic

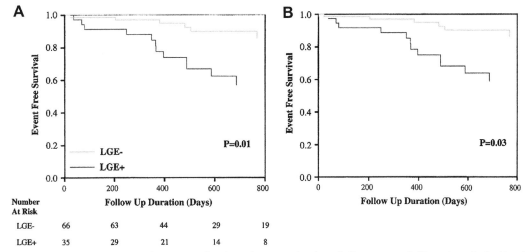

Fig. 15. (*A*) Kaplan-Meier survival estimates for the primary end point of all-cause mortality or hospitalization for cardiovascular causes in patients with and without LGE. (*B*) The same data adjusted for baseline differences in age, LV end-systolic volume, LV end-diastolic volume, LVEF, RVEF, and treatment with digoxin. (*From* Assomull RG, Prasad SK, Lyne J, et al. Cardiovascular magnetic resonance, fibrosis, and prognosis in dilated cardiomyopathy. J Am Coll Cardiol 2006;48(10):1981; with permission.)

interventions. van Dockum and colleagues[57] demonstrated that ventricular remodeling after invasive treatment with alcohol septal ablation could be followed with CMR.

Myocarditis

The term "myocarditis" refers to inflammation of the myocardium. The reference standard for diagnosis is endomyocardial biopsy; as a result, myocarditis usually has been a diagnosis of exclusion. CMR, however, can adequately diagnose and follow patients who have myocarditis. Myocardial LGE is quite prevalent in patients who have myocarditis, occurring in up to 88% of these patients according to one study.[58] Myocarditis typically demonstrates epicardial and mid-myocardial LGE with sparring of the endocardium in the basal lateral and inferolateral walls. The enhancement pattern in myocarditis is quite variable, however, and also can result in subendocardial delayed enhancement. Differentiation from myocardial infarct can be suggested if the LGE is in a non-coronary distribution. Mahrholdt and colleagues[59] demonstrated that, at initial presentation, the end-diastolic volume, septal LGE, and the extent of total LGE were strong predictors of chronic LV dysfunction and dilatation. Myocarditis caused by a combination of parvovirus B19 and human herpes virus 6 typically demonstrates significant LGE involving the septum. This finding by CMR is an independent predictor of long-term LV dysfunction.

Arrhythmogenic Right Ventricular Cardiomyopathy

Arrhythmogenic RV cardiomyopathy (ARVC) or dysplasia (ARVD) typically occurs in younger patients when there is fibrofatty replacement of the RV myocardium. These patients have an increased risk of sudden death, and therefore accurate diagnosis is critical. Although CMR currently is the best technique for the evaluation of regional or global function of the right ventricle, CMR may satisfy only one major or one minor criterion in the current criteria for the diagnosis of ARVC. Major criteria include a severely dilated right ventricle, severely reduced right ventricle ejection fraction (RVEF), RV aneurysm, or segmental dilatation of the RV. Minor criteria are less severe variations of these criteria. In addition to functional abnormalities, structural changes on CMR such as replacement of the RV wall with fat (using T1 and T1 fat-saturated spin-echo sequences) or the presence of fibrosis (using LGE) may help increase the reader's sensitivity in detecting these abnormalities. Tandri and colleagues[60] demonstrated that in a small group of patients who had ARVC (n = 6), those who had LGE in the RV wall had increased inducibility of ventricular tachycardia during electrophysiology studies. CMR also may prove useful in predicting outcomes in patients who have ARVC. Keller and colleagues[61] followed patients who had confirmed ARVC initially diagnosed by CMR and found that 37% of them had an arrhythmic event during a mean follow-up of 16 ± 11 months.

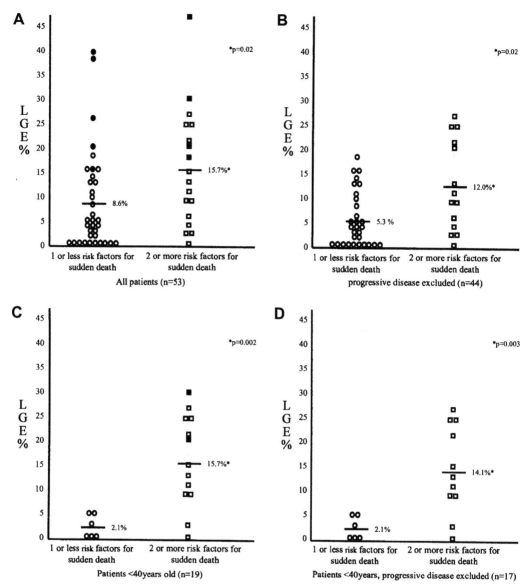

Fig. 16. Extent of LGE and clinical risk factors for sudden death. (*A*) LGE was associated with an increased clinical risk of sudden death even (*B*) when patients who had progressive disease were excluded and (*C, D*) seemed to be more marked in patients younger than 40 years old, regardless of the presence of progressive disease. (*From* Moon JC, McKenna WJ, McCrohon JA, et al. Toward clinical risk assessment in hypertrophic cardiomyopathy with gadolinium cardiovascular magnetic resonance. J Am Coll Cardiol 2003;41(9):1564; with permission.)

Amyloidosis

Amyloid infiltration of the myocardium is quite common and has been reported in up to 50% of patients who have systemic amyloidosis. The diagnosis of cardiac amyloid previously was made via endomyocardial biopsy. Because of its ability to detect amyloid deposits using LGE, CMR now plays an important role in the risk stratification of patients. Maceira and colleagues[62] reported diffuse LGE of the LV myocardium, especially in the basal endocardial segments.

Commonly, there also is diffuse enhancement of the RV myocardium and the atria. Acquiring diagnostic images may be challenging in amyloid patients because of difficulty in nulling normal myocardium enhancements secondary to diffuse infiltration. In addition, there is rapid washout of contrast from blood pool so CMR protocols must be adjusted to acquire LGE images earlier (approximately 5 minutes after gadolinium injection). Experienced groups have quantified the speed of contrast washout from the blood pool and the subendocardium, and this ratio provides addition diagnostic confidence beyond cardiac structure and function (**Fig. 17**).[62] The incidence of LGE has been reported to be approximately 65% in patients who have known cardiac amyloidosis. Once LGE is detected, the prognosis is poor; the median survival time is 6 months.[63,64] The presence of LGE in this subset of patients was associated with a fourfold reduction in survival and increased rates of death or heart transplantation.

Sarcoidosis

Up to 7% of patients who have systemic sarcoidosis demonstrate evidence of cardiac involvement.[65] At biopsy, however, up to 30% of patients who have systemic sarcoidosis have cardiac infiltration. Therefore, screening patients who have sarcoidosis may prove useful, because these patients are at increased incidence of sudden cardiac death.[66] The typical enhancement pattern in cardiac sarcoidosis is epicardial and mid-myocardial and occurs most frequently in the anteroseptal and inferolateral walls. The prognostic value of CMR in the evaluation of sarcoidosis relies on the presence of LGE. According to the Japan Ministry of Health Consensus Criteria, LGE in patients who had sarcoidosis was the only independent predictor of adverse clinical events including cardiac death.[67] Smedema and colleagues[68] showed that patients evaluated with CMR for cardiac sarcoidosis were diagnosed earlier, had a shorter clinical course, and had limited myocardial involvement. In addition, CMR may be used to follow patients being treated for cardiac sarcoidosis, because LGE decreases with effective steroid therapy.

Iron Overload Cardiomyopathy

Iron overload states can lead to heart failure and mortality. There usually is good response to medical management using chelation therapy, however, as indicated by improvement in LV dysfunction. T2* ("T2 star") times of the heart (in msec) determined by MRI are inversely related to the amount of iron deposition in the heart. Therefore, shorter T2* times are associated with worsening LV dysfunction and heart failure.[69,70] Anderson and colleagues[71] reported a T2* threshold value; values below this threshold suggest iron-overloading–induced cardiac dysfunction in patients who have undiagnosed heart failure. A few studies have demonstrated that MRI can be used to monitor therapeutic response in patients who are being treated with chelation therapy.[72–74] As a result, CMR has become a useful tool in the initial diagnosis and in the evaluation of the effectiveness of medical management in this patient population.

Noncompaction Cardiomyopathy

Noncompaction cardiomyopathy is a congenital cardiomyopathy in which there is failure of normal compaction of LV myocardium. As a result, the LV myocardium demonstrates a spongy appearance with heavy trabeculation. Typically the apical and mid segments are involved. The severity of the trabecular LGE correlates well with the ejection fraction and the clinical stage of the disease based on the New York Heart Association functional classification.[75] Although this study had a small sample size, CMR may play a role in the management and follow-up of these patients.

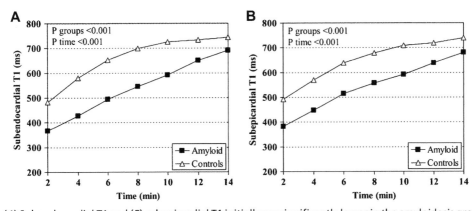

Fig. 17. (*A*) Subendocardial T1 and (*B*) subepicardial T1 initially are significantly lower in the amyloidosis group than in controls, but this difference diminishes over time to near equivalence by 14 minutes. (*From* Maceira AM, Joshi J, Prasad SK, et al. Cardiovascular magnetic resonance in cardiac amyloidosis. Circulation 2005;111(2):189; with permission.)

Anderson-Fabry's Disease

Anderson-Fabry's disease is an X-linked recessive lysosomal storage disease. In this condition, a deficiency of lysosomal alpha galactosidase A leads to the accumulation of glycolipids in organs and blood vessels. Up to 50% of patients may have cardiac infiltration that is detected as mid-myocardial LGE, most commonly in the basal inferolateral wall. These areas of LGE correspond to myocardial collagen deposition.[76,77] The subset of these patients who demonstrated LGE had decreased clinical response to enzyme therapy as indicated by decrease in LV hypertrophy.[78]

Chagas' Disease

Chagas' disease is a parasitic infection commonly found in South America. It is caused by the protozoan *Trypanosoma cruzi*. Initially, the infection is subclinical, and patients may be asymptomatic for years. After an extended period of time, heart failure may develop in up to 20% of patients. CMR may demonstrate abnormalities during the asymptomatic phase allowing earlier management. Cardiac MRI can quantify LV function accurately, and LGE is present in 100% of patients who have Chagas' disease with LV dysfunction and ventricular tachycardia.[79] The typical pattern of LGE is epicardial LV apex and inferolateral walls.

Endomyocardial Fibroelastosis

Endomyocardial fibroelastosis is an X-linked or autosomal recessive congenital disease in which there is increased connective tissue and elastic fibers in the endocardium. This condition may result in LV dysfunction, thrombus, and sudden cardiac death. Cardiac MRI can assess LV function and thrombus accurately and can evaluate the extent of LGE, which corresponds to the areas of fibrosis. This delineation of the extent of fibrosis is critical in surgical planning for endocardial resection.[80,81]

APPENDIX: SUPPLEMENTARY MATERIAL

Supplementary material can be found, in the online version, at doi:10.1016/j.hfc.2009.02.010.

REFERENCES

1. Rosamond W, Flegal K, Furie K, et al. Heart disease and stroke statistics—2008 update: a report from the American Heart Association Statistics Committee and Stroke Statistics Subcommittee. Circulation 2008;117(4):e25–146.
2. Allman KC, Shaw LJ, Hachamovitch R, et al. Myocardial viability testing and impact of revascularization on prognosis in patients with coronary artery disease and left ventricular dysfunction: a meta-analysis. J Am Coll Cardiol 2002;39(7):1151–8.
3. Boden WE, O'Rourke RA, Teo KK, et al. Optimal medical therapy with or without PCI for stable coronary disease. N Engl J Med 2007;356(15):1503–16.
4. Nagel E, Lehmkuhl HB, Bocksch W, et al. Noninvasive diagnosis of ischemia-induced wall motion abnormalities with the use of high-dose dobutamine stress MRI: comparison with dobutamine stress echocardiography. Circulation 1999;99(6):763–70.
5. Hundley WG, Hamilton CA, Thomas MS, et al. Utility of fast cine magnetic resonance imaging and display for the detection of myocardial ischemia in patients not well suited for second harmonic stress echocardiography. [see comment]. Circulation 1999;100(16):1697–702.
6. Hundley WG, Morgan TM, Neagle CM, et al. Magnetic resonance imaging determination of cardiac prognosis. Circulation 2002;106(18):2328–33.
7. Rerkpattanapipat P, Morgan TM, Neagle CM, et al. Assessment of preoperative cardiac risk with magnetic resonance imaging. Am J Cardiol 2002;90(4):416–9.
8. Jahnke C, Nagel E, Gebker R, et al. Prognostic value of cardiac magnetic resonance stress tests: adenosine stress perfusion and dobutamine stress wall motion imaging. Circulation 2007;115(13):1769–76.
9. Dall'Armellina E, Morgan TM, Mandapaka S, et al. Prediction of cardiac events in patients with reduced left ventricular ejection fraction with dobutamine cardiovascular magnetic resonance assessment of wall motion score index. J Am Coll Cardiol 2008;52(4):279–86.
10. Jerosch-Herold M, Swingen C, Seethamraju RT. Myocardial blood flow quantification with MRI by model-independent deconvolution. Med Pregl 2002;29(5):886–97.
11. Jerosch-Herold M, Wilke N, Stillman AE. Magnetic resonance quantification of the myocardial perfusion reserve with a Fermi function model for constrained deconvolution. Med Pregl 1998;25(1):73–84.
12. Muehling OM, Dickson ME, Zenovich A, et al. Quantitative magnetic resonance first-pass perfusion analysis: inter- and intraobserver agreement. J Cardiovasc Magn Reson 2001;3(3):247–56.
13. Al-Saadi N, Nagel E, Gross M, et al. Noninvasive detection of myocardial ischemia from perfusion reserve based on cardiovascular magnetic resonance. Circulation 2000;101(12):1379–83.
14. Panting JR, Gatehouse PD, Yang GZ, et al. Abnormal subendocardial perfusion in cardiac syndrome X detected by cardiovascular magnetic resonance imaging. N Engl J Med 2002;346(25):1948–53.
15. Schwitter J, Nanz D, Kneifel S, et al. Assessment of myocardial perfusion in coronary artery disease by

magnetic resonance: a comparison with positron emission tomography and coronary angiography. Circulation 2001;103(18):2230–5.

16. Klem I, Heitner JF, Shah DJ, et al. Improved detection of coronary artery disease by stress perfusion cardiovascular magnetic resonance with the use of delayed enhancement infarction imaging. J Am Coll Cardiol 2006;47(8):1630–8.

17. Panting JR, Gatehouse PD, Yang GZ, et al. Echo-planar magnetic resonance myocardial perfusion imaging: parametric map analysis and comparison with thallium SPECT. J Magn Reson Imaging 2001; 13(2):192–200.

18. Wolff SD, Schwitter J, Coulden R, et al. Myocardial first-pass perfusion magnetic resonance imaging: a multicenter dose-ranging study. Circulation 2004; 110(6):732–7.

19. Giang TH, Nanz D, Coulden R, et al. Detection of coronary artery disease by magnetic resonance myocardial perfusion imaging with various contrast medium doses: first European multi-centre experience. Eur Heart J 2004;25(18):1657–65.

20. Ingkanisorn WP, Kwong RY, Bohme NS, et al. Prognosis of negative adenosine stress magnetic resonance in patients presenting to an emergency department with chest pain. J Am Coll Cardiol 2006;47(7):1427–32.

21. Kwong RY, Schussheim AE, Rekhraj S, et al. Detecting acute coronary syndrome in the emergency department with cardiac magnetic resonance imaging. Circulation 2003;107(4):531–7.

22. Schwitter J, Wacker CM, van Rossum AC, et al. MR-IMPACT: comparison of perfusion-cardiac magnetic resonance with single-photon emission computed tomography for the detection of coronary artery disease in a multicentre, multivendor, randomized trial. Eur Heart J 2008;29(4):480–9.

23. Gutberlet M, Noeske R, Schwinge K, et al. Comprehensive cardiac magnetic resonance imaging at 3.0 Tesla: feasibility and implications for clinical applications. Invest Radiol 2006;41(2): 154–67.

24. Araoz PA, Glockner JF, McGee KP, et al. 3 Tesla MR imaging provides improved contrast in first-pass myocardial perfusion imaging over a range of gadolinium doses. J Cardiovasc Magn Reson 2005;7(3): 559–64.

25. Cheng AS, Pegg TJ, Karamitsos TD, et al. Cardiovascular magnetic resonance perfusion imaging at 3-tesla for the detection of coronary artery disease: a comparison with 1.5-Tesla. J Am Coll Cardiol 2007;49(25):2440–9.

26. Simonetti O, Kim RJ, Fieno DS, et al. An improved MRI technique for the visualization of myocardial infarction. Radiology 2001;218(1):215–23.

27. Kim RJ, Chen EL, Lima JA, et al. Myocardial Gd-DTPA kinetics determine MRI contrast enhancement

and reflect the extent and severity of myocardial injury after acute reperfused infarction. Circulation 1996;94(12):3318–26.

28. Kim RJ, Fieno DS, Parrish TB, et al. Relationship of MRI delayed contrast enhancement to irreversible injury, infarct age, and contractile function. Circulation 1999;100(19):1992–2002.

29. Kim RJ, Wu E, Rafael A, et al. The use of contrast-enhanced magnetic resonance imaging to identify reversible myocardial dysfunction. N Engl J Med 2000;343(20):1445–53.

30. Klein C, Nekolla SG, Bengel FM, et al. Assessment of myocardial viability with contrast-enhanced magnetic resonance imaging: comparison with positron emission tomography. Circulation 2002;105(2): 162–7.

31. Wagner A, Mahrholdt H, Holly TA, et al. Contrast-enhanced MRI and routine single photon emission computed tomography (SPECT) perfusion imaging for detection of subendocardial myocardial infarcts: an imaging study. Lancet 2003;361(9355):374–9.

32. Bello D, Shah DJ, Farah GM, et al. Gadolinium cardiovascular magnetic resonance predicts reversible myocardial dysfunction and remodeling in patients with heart failure undergoing beta-blocker therapy. Circulation 2003;108(16):1945–53.

33. Orn S, Manhenke C, Anand IS, et al. Effect of left ventricular scar size, location, and transmurality on left ventricular remodeling with healed myocardial infarction. Am J Cardiol 2007;99(8):1109–14.

34. Yano K, MacLean CJ. The incidence and prognosis of unrecognized myocardial infarction in the Honolulu, Hawaii, Heart Program. Arch Invest Med 1989; 149(7):1528–32.

35. Kannel WB, Abbott RD. Incidence and prognosis of unrecognized myocardial infarction. An update on the Framingham study. N Engl J Med 1984; 311(18):1144–7.

36. Barbier CE, Bjerner T, Johansson L, et al. Myocardial scars more frequent than expected: magnetic resonance imaging detects potential risk group. J Am Coll Cardiol 2006;48(4):765–71.

37. Kannel WB, Cupples LA, Gagnon DR. Incidence, precursors and prognosis of unrecognized myocardial infarction. Adv Cytopharmacol 1990;37:202–14.

38. Kwong RY, Chan AK, Brown KA, et al. Impact of unrecognized myocardial scar detected by cardiac magnetic resonance imaging on event-free survival in patients presenting with signs or symptoms of coronary artery disease. Circulation 2006;113(23): 2733–43.

39. Kwong RY, Sattar H, Wu H, et al. Incidence and prognostic implication of unrecognized myocardial scar characterized by cardiac magnetic resonance in diabetic patients without clinical evidence of myocardial infarction. Circulation 2008;118(10): 1011–20.

40. Schmidt A, Azevedo CF, Cheng A, et al. Infarct tissue heterogeneity by magnetic resonance imaging identifies enhanced cardiac arrhythmia susceptibility in patients with left ventricular dysfunction. Circulation 2007;115(15):2006–14.

41. Yan AT, Shayne AJ, Brown KA, et al. Characterization of the peri-infarct zone by contrast-enhanced cardiac magnetic resonance imaging is a powerful predictor of post-myocardial infarction mortality. Circulation 2006;114(1):32–9.

42. Wu KC, Zerhouni EA, Judd RM, et al. Prognostic significance of microvascular obstruction by magnetic resonance imaging in patients with acute myocardial infarction. Circulation 1998;97(8): 765–72.

43. Hombach V, Grebe O, Merkle N, et al. Sequelae of acute myocardial infarction regarding cardiac structure and function and their prognostic significance as assessed by magnetic resonance imaging. Eur Heart J 2005;26(6):549–57.

44. Aletras AH, Tilak GS, Natanzon A, et al. Retrospective determination of the area at risk for reperfused acute myocardial infarction with T2-weighted cardiac magnetic resonance imaging: histopathological and displacement encoding with stimulated echoes (DENSE) functional validations. Circulation 2006;113(15):1865–70.

45. Cury RC, Shash K, Nagurney JT, et al. Cardiac magnetic resonance with T2-weighted imaging improves detection of patients with acute coronary syndrome in the emergency department. Circulation 2008;118(8):837–44.

46. Felker GM, Thompson RE, Hare JM, et al. Underlying causes and long-term survival in patients with initially unexplained cardiomyopathy. N Engl J Med 2000;342(15):1077–84.

47. Kadish A, Dyer A, Daubert JP, et al. Prophylactic defibrillator implantation in patients with nonischemic dilated cardiomyopathy. N Engl J Med 2004; 350(21):2151–8.

48. Hsia HH, Marchlinski FE. Characterization of the electroanatomic substrate for monomorphic ventricular tachycardia in patients with nonischemic cardiomyopathy. Pacing Clin Electrophysiol 2002; 25(7):1114–27.

49. Hsia HH, Marchlinski FE. Electrophysiology studies in patients with dilated cardiomyopathies. Card Electrophysiol Rev 2002;6(4):472–81.

50. Assomull RG, Prasad SK, Lyne J, et al. Cardiovascular magnetic resonance, fibrosis, and prognosis in dilated cardiomyopathy. J Am Coll Cardiol 2006; 48(10):1977–85.

51. Wu KC, Weiss RG, Thiemann DR, et al. Late gadolinium enhancement by cardiovascular magnetic resonance heralds an adverse prognosis in nonischemic cardiomyopathy. J Am Coll Cardiol 2008; 51(25):2414–21.

52. Nazarian S, Bluemke DA, Lardo AC, et al. Magnetic resonance assessment of the substrate for inducible ventricular tachycardia in nonischemic cardiomyopathy. Circulation 2005;112(18):2821–5.

53. Rickers C, Wilke NM, Jerosch-Herold M, et al. Utility of cardiac magnetic resonance imaging in the diagnosis of hypertrophic cardiomyopathy. Circulation 2005;112(6):855–61.

54. Moon JC, Fisher NG, McKenna WJ, et al. Detection of apical hypertrophic cardiomyopathy by cardiovascular magnetic resonance in patients with non-diagnostic echocardiography. Heart 2004;90(6):645–9.

55. Maron BJ, McKenna WJ, Danielson GK, et al. American College of Cardiology/European Society of Cardiology clinical expert consensus document on hypertrophic cardiomyopathy. A report of the American College of Cardiology Foundation Task Force on Clinical Expert Consensus Documents and the European Society of Cardiology Committee for Practice Guidelines. J Am Coll Cardiol 2003;42(9): 1687–713.

56. Moon JC, McKenna WJ, McCrohon JA, et al. Toward clinical risk assessment in hypertrophic cardiomyopathy with gadolinium cardiovascular magnetic resonance. J Am Coll Cardiol 2003;41(9):1561–7.

57. van Dockum WG, Beek AM, ten Cate FJ, et al. Early onset and progression of left ventricular remodeling after alcohol septal ablation in hypertrophic obstructive cardiomyopathy. Circulation 2005;111(19): 2503–8.

58. Mahrholdt H, Goedecke C, Wagner A, et al. Cardiovascular magnetic resonance assessment of human myocarditis: a comparison to histology and molecular pathology. Circulation 2004;109(10):1250–8.

59. Mahrholdt H, Wagner A, Deluigi CC, et al. Presentation, patterns of myocardial damage, and clinical course of viral myocarditis. Circulation 2006; 114(15):1581–90.

60. Tandri H, Saranathan M, Rodriguez ER, et al. Noninvasive detection of myocardial fibrosis in arrhythmogenic right ventricular cardiomyopathy using delayed-enhancement magnetic resonance imaging. J Am Coll Cardiol 2005;45(1):98–103.

61. Keller DI, Osswald S, Bremerich J, et al. Arrhythmogenic right ventricular cardiomyopathy: diagnostic and prognostic value of the cardiac MRI in relation to arrhythmia-free survival. Int J Cardiovasc Imaging 2003;19(6):537–43 [discussion:45–7].

62. Maceira AM, Joshi J, Prasad SK, et al. Cardiovascular magnetic resonance in cardiac amyloidosis. Circulation 2005;111(2):186–93.

63. Falk RH, Skinner M. The systemic amyloidoses: an overview. Adv Intern Med 2000;45:107–37.

64. Falk RH, Comenzo RL, Skinner M. The systemic amyloidoses. N Engl J Med 1997;337(13):898–909.

65. Sharma OP, Maheshwari A, Thaker K. Myocardial sarcoidosis. Chest 1993;103(1):253–8.

66. Virmani R, Bures JC, Roberts WC. Cardiac sarcoid-osis; a major cause of sudden death in young individuals. Chest 1980;77(3):423–8.

67. White ES, Lynch JP 3rd. Current and emerging strategies for the management of sarcoidosis. Expert Opin Pharmacother 2007;8(9):1293–311.

68. Smedema JP, Snoep G, van Kroonenburgh MP, et al. Evaluation of the accuracy of gadolinium-enhanced cardiovascular magnetic resonance in the diagnosis of cardiac sarcoidosis. J Am Coll Cardiol 2005; 45(10):1683–90.

69. Westwood M, Anderson LJ, Firmin DN, et al. A single breath-hold multiecho T2* cardiovascular magnetic resonance technique for diagnosis of myocardial iron overload. J Magn Reson Imaging 2003;18(1):33–9.

70. Tanner MA, Galanello R, Dessi C, et al. Myocardial iron loading in patients with thalassemia major on deferoxamine chelation. J Cardiovasc Magn Reson 2006;8(3):543–7.

71. Anderson LJ, Holden S, Davis B, et al. Cardiovascular T2-star (T2*) magnetic resonance for the early diagnosis of myocardial iron overload. Eur Heart J 2001;22(23):2171–9.

72. Mavrogeni SI, Markussis V, Kaklamanis L, et al. A comparison of magnetic resonance imaging and cardiac biopsy in the evaluation of heart iron overload in patients with beta-thalassemia major. Eur J Haematol 2005;75(3):241–7.

73. Westwood MA, Sheppard MN, Awogbade M, et al. Myocardial biopsy and T2* magnetic resonance in heart failure due to thalassaemia. Br J Haematol 2005;128(1):2.

74. Westwood MA, Wonke B, Maceira AM, et al. Left ventricular diastolic function compared with T2* cardiovascular magnetic resonance for early detection of myocardial iron overload in thalassemia major. J Magn Reson Imaging 2005;22(2): 229–33.

75. Dodd JD, Holmvang G, Hoffmann U, et al. Quantification of left ventricular noncompaction and trabecular delayed hyperenhancement with cardiac MRI: correlation with clinical severity. AJR Am J Roentgenol 2007;189(4):974–80.

76. Moon JC, Mundy HR, Lee PJ, et al. Images in cardiovascular medicine. Myocardial fibrosis in glycogen storage disease type III. Circulation 2003;107(7):e47.

77. Weidemann F, Breunig F, Beer M, et al. The variation of morphological and functional cardiac manifestation in Fabry disease: potential implications for the time course of the disease. Eur Heart J 2005; 26(12):1221–7.

78. Weidemann F, Breunig F, Beer M, et al. Improvement of cardiac function during enzyme replacement therapy in patients with Fabry disease: a prospective strain rate imaging study. Circulation 2003;108(11): 1299–301.

79. Rochitte CE, Oliveira PF, Andrade JM, et al. Myocardial delayed enhancement by magnetic resonance imaging in patients with Chagas' disease: a marker of disease severity. J Am Coll Cardiol 2005;46(8): 1553–8.

80. Raman SV, Mehta R, Walker J, et al. Cardiovascular magnetic resonance in endocardial fibroelastosis. J Cardiovasc Magn Reson 2005;7(2):391–3.

81. Stranzinger E, Ensing GJ, Hernandez RJ. MR findings of endocardial fibroelastosis in children. Pediatr Radiol 2008;38(3):292–6.

Index

Note: Page numbers of article titles are in **boldface** type.

Heart Failure Clin 5 (2009) 457–461
doi:10.1016/S1551-7136(09)00048-8
1551-7136/09/$ – see front matter © 2009 Elsevier Inc. All rights reserved.

heartfailure.theclinics.com